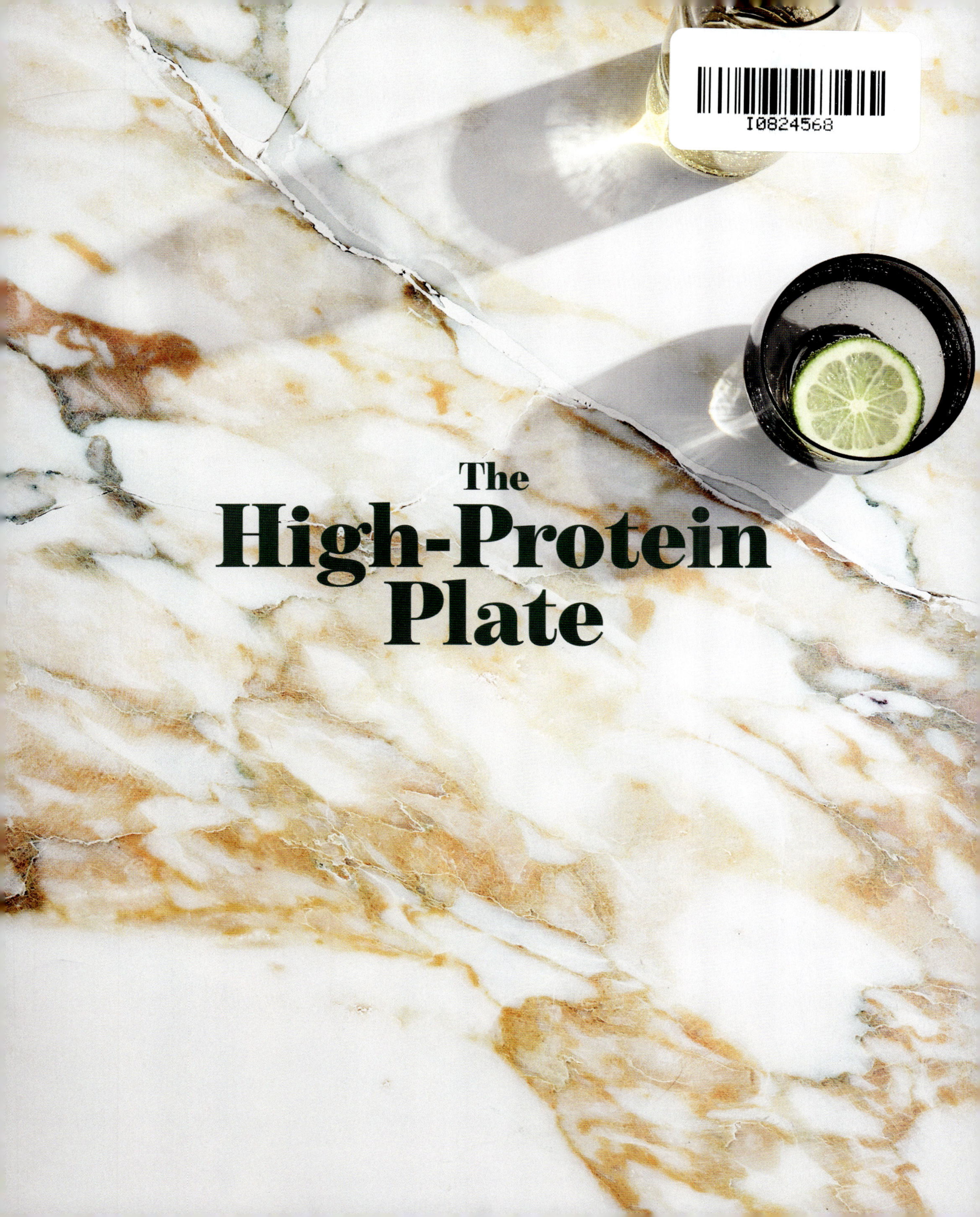

# The High-Protein Plate

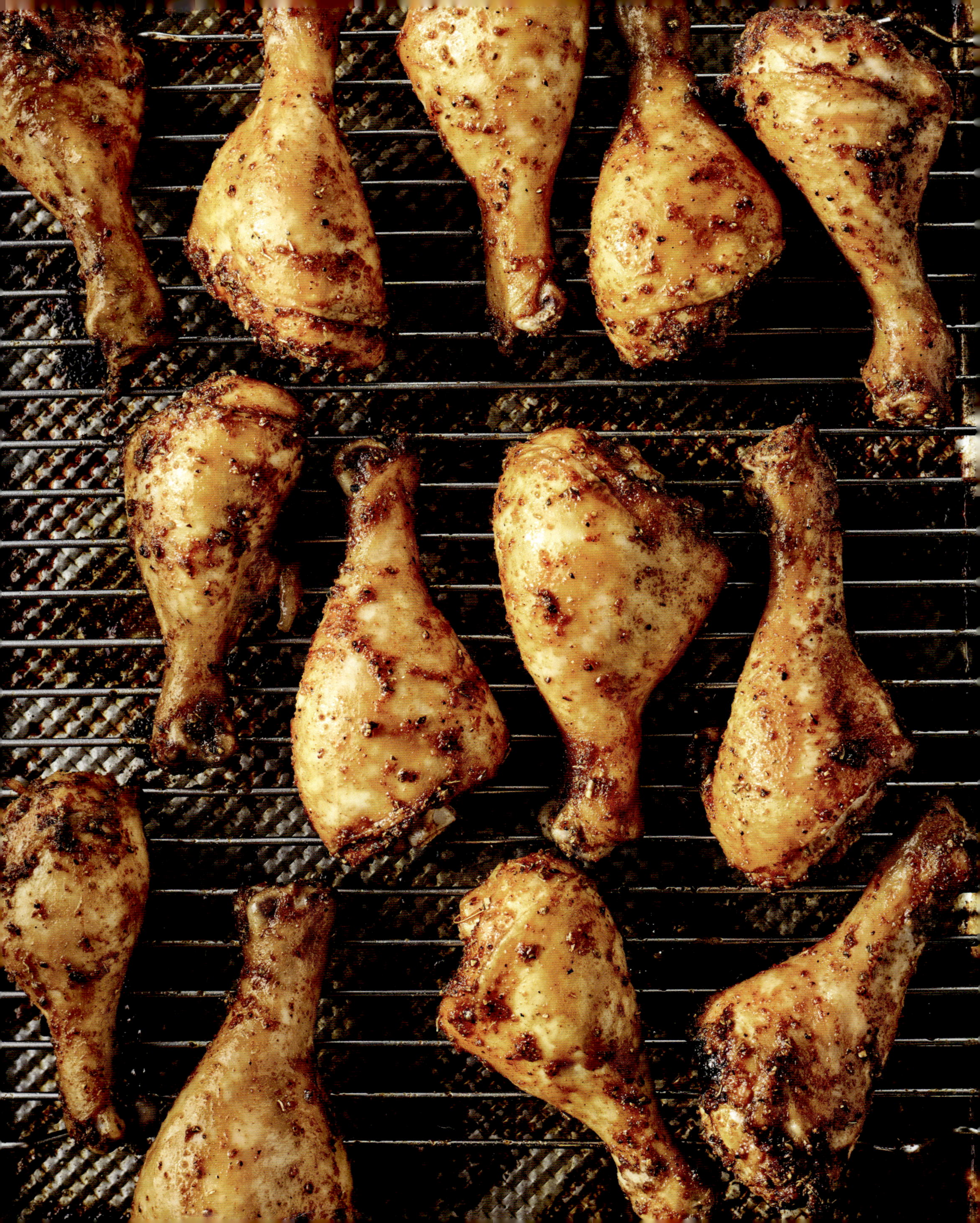

100 SATISFYING EVERYDAY RECIPES

# The High-Protein Plate


Rachael DeVaux, RD

Photography by Eva Kolenko



SIMON ELEMENT

NEW YORK AMSTERDAM/ANTWERP LONDON
TORONTO SYDNEY/MELBOURNE NEW DELHI

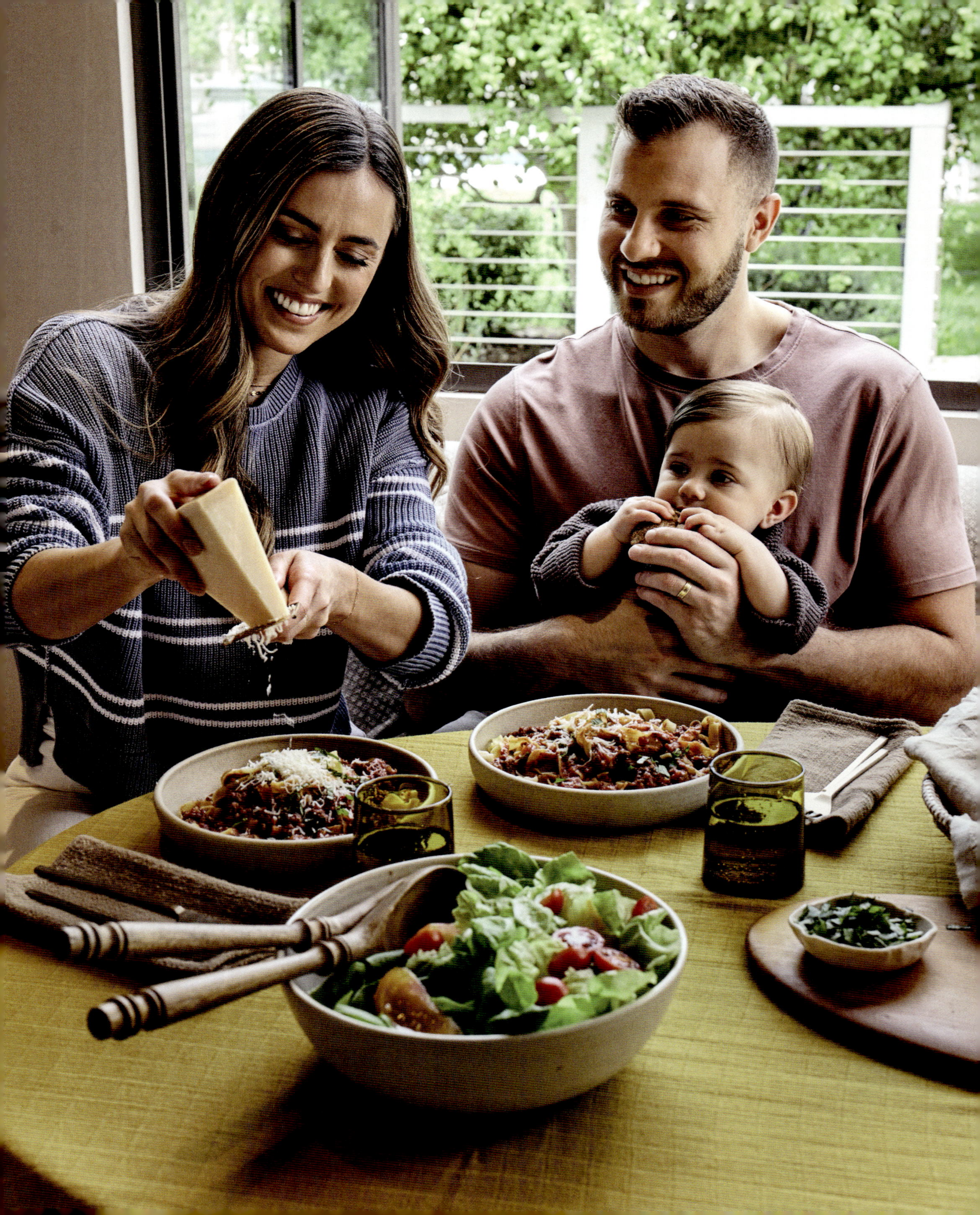

# *Praise for* The High-Protein Plate

"Rachael delivers what we're all looking for in eating well: approachability, variety, and meals that truly satisfy. This book is packed with flavor and protein-forward recipes that keep you nourished, energized, and excited to make them again and again."

**—ARASH HASHEMI, *New York Times* bestselling author of *Shred Happens: So Easy, So Good***

"Rachael's high-protein cookbook proves that nutritious can still mean seriously flavorful. . . . *The High-Protein Plate* is a must-have for anyone looking to fuel their body and enjoy every bite."

**—KYLIE SAKAIDA, MS, RD, *New York Times* bestselling author of *So Easy So Good***

"Rachael's ability to effortlessly add high-protein recipes into everyday life makes her a go-to resource for anyone looking to feel stronger, more satisfied, and confident in the kitchen. *The High-Protein Plate* is more than a collection of nutrient-packed meals—it's your guide to making every meal count, from breakfast to dessert!"

**—CARISSA STANTON, *New York Times* bestselling author of *Seriously, So Good***

"Long before Rachael was my peer (and now friend), she was instrumental in shaping my own healthy cooking journey. Her unwavering commitment to helping people live better through mindful food choices is captured beautifully in this cookbook—a must-have for deeply nourishing, easy-to-make, impactful recipes you'll want on repeat!"

**—OLIVIA ADRIANCE, creator of @olivia.adriance**

"This is the book you'll actually cook from. Rachael's high-protein meals are flavorful, practical, and made for busy lives, not perfect ones. Her approach connects because it's honest, approachable, and helps you feel your best with what you've got, what you can afford, and the time you have."

**—KEVIN CURRY, author of *Fit Men Cook***

"As someone who prioritizes nutritious, protein-packed meals, I know *The High-Protein Plate* will be a staple for me. From Everything Bagel Egg Wraps to Philly Cheesesteak–Stuffed Poblanos to Chipotle Chicken and Avocado Bowls, these recipes make it easy to get dinner on the table whether it's a thirty-minute meal, a one-pan wonder, or a make-ahead dish for a healthy week. This book is perfect for anyone looking to bring more high-protein meals into everyday life!"

**—ALEX SNODGRASS, *New York Times* bestselling author of *The Defined Dish*, *Dinner Tonight*, and *The Comfortable Kitchen***

"Rachael's recipes are as nourishing as they are crave-worthy, and this cookbook quickly became a go-to for me, my boys, and my clients! Every recipe serves up the amino acids you need to satisfy cravings, build better body composition, and easily avoid snacking, all without feeling restrictive. This is a must-have for anyone who wants to support their body with every bite!"

**—KELLY LeVEQUE, author of *Body Love***

"Gone are the days of bland chicken-and-rice, gym-bro meals. Rachael delivers refreshing, approachable, and delicious takes on protein-packed recipes fit for any occasion. This book will have you eating well, feeling great, and looking your best."

**—RONNY JOSEPH LVOVSKI, author of *The Primal Gourmet Cookbook***

**To Bridger and Hayes—**
*who make my life feel full in every way.*

# Contents


9 **Introduction**

## Breakfast

**FIRST THINGS FIRST**

46 Savory Herb and Turkey-Bacon Quiche
49 Cinnamon-Apple Protein Pancakes
50 Honey-Blackberry Overnight Oats
53 Roasty Breakfast Potato Hash
54 Everything Bagel Egg Wraps
57 Maple-Chicken Breakfast Patties
58 Chorizo-Style Breakfast Tacos
61 Berry Crumble Yogurt Bowls
62 Ready-When-You-Are Breakfast Sandwiches
65 Make-Ahead Coconut-Mango Chia Pudding
66 Cheesy Bacon and Chive Egg Muffins
69 Better-than-a-Bagel-Run Bagels

**SMOOTHIES**

72 Pick-Me-Up Mocha Smoothie
75 Strawberry Shortcake Smoothie
76 Salted Peanut Butter Cup Smoothie
79 Passionberry Smoothie
80 Pumpkin Pie Smoothie

## Everyday Mains

**DINNERS WORTH REPEATING**

86 Korean Beef with Glass Noodles
88 Chili-Lime Grilled Steak with Zesty Avocado Salsa
91 Seasoned Crispy Drumsticks
92 Greek-Style Smash Burgers
95 Chicken Milanese with Homemade Alfredo
99 Steak and Chimichurri Baguette Sandwiches
100 Blackened Shrimp Tacos with Pineapple-Avocado Salsa
103 Philly Cheesesteak–Stuffed Poblanos
104 Rosemary-Garlic Lamb Chops with Veggies

**DINNERS WORTH REPEATING (cont.)**

107 Szechuan Chicken Lettuce Wraps
108 Beef Bolognese
110 Tomato-Basil Chicken with Spaghetti Squash
112 Seared Halloumi and Chickpea Bowls with Herby Tahini

**30-MINUTES OR LESS MAINS**

117 Honey-Harissa Salmon with Asparagus
118 Super Crispy Chicken Tenders with Homemade BBQ Sauce
121 Chipotle Chicken and Avocado Bowls
122 Saucy Coconut-Curry Turkey Meatballs
125 Air-Fryer Garlic-Butter Salmon Bites
126 Oven-Baked Beefy Burritos
129 Chili Crisp Tofu and Quinoa Power Bowls
130 Chicken and Peanut Pad Thai Bowls
133 20-Minute Shredded Chicken Verde
134 Grilled Mahi Mahi with Mango Salsa
137 Mexican Meatballs in Creamy Enchilada Sauce
138 Shredded Chicken Quesadillas
141 Loaded Chicken Pesto Panini
142 My Weeknight Hero: Ginger-Garlic Turkey Skillet

**SLOW COOKER MAINS**

146 Tangy Pulled Pork Sandwiches
148 Buffalo Chicken Baked Tacos
151 Sesame-Ginger Pot Roast
152 Short Ribs with Bone Broth Polenta
155 Slow Cooker Picadillo
156 Brothy Beans with Zesty Chimichurri

**ONE-PAN MEALS**

160 Marry Me Chicken
163 Beef Fried Rice
164 Sheet-Pan Brats and Potatoes

**ONE-PAN MEALS (cont.)**
167 Crispy Lemon-Garlic Chicken Thighs
168 Pesto-Crusted Baked Cod
171 Egg Roll in a Bowl
172 One-Pan Beef and Broccoli
175 Salsa Verde Shrimp and Rice
176 Sloppy Joe Bowls
179 Double Double-Cheeseburger Bowls
180 Sheet-Pan Turmeric Chicken with Romesco

**Simple One-Pan Sides**
182 Sautéed Greens with Lemon and Olive Oil
182 Farro
183 Roasted Japanese Sweet Potatoes
183 Garlicky Roasted Broccolini

## Soups, Salads, and Satisfying Snacks

**SIDES AND SALADS**
188 Southwest Steak Salad Bowls
190 Italian-Style Chop Salad
193 Next-Level Mac and Cheese
194 Harvest Cobb Salad with Maple-Dijon Dressing
197 5-Minute Pesto Chicken Salad
198 Bone Broth Jasmine Rice Three Ways
201 Grilled Summer Pasta Salad
202 Roasted Sweet Potatoes with Spiced Chickpeas and Tahini Drizzle
205 Zucchini Fritters with Lemon-Dill Sauce
206 The Rachael Salad
209 Moroccan-Spiced Carrots with Hummus
210 Cheesy Bone Broth Mashed Potatoes
212 Sheet-Pan Greek Chicken and Chickpea Salad
215 Spicy Tuna Spring Rolls

**SOUPS**
218 Slow Cooker Beef Stew
221 Creamy Tuscan Chicken Soup
222 Sausage, White Bean, and Kale Soup
225 Hearty Protein-Packed Chili
226 Golden Chicken Bone Broth
228 Roasted Butternut Squash Soup with Coconut-Lime Crema

**SATISFYING SNACKS**
232 Lemon-Pepper Wings with Dilly Ranch
234 Birthday Cake Bliss Balls
237 Game-Day Buffalo Chicken Dip
238 Savory Beefy Queso Dip
241 Crispy Ranch Air-Fryer Chickpeas
242 Savory Cottage Cheese Bowls
245 Avocado Whipped Feta
246 Banana Bread Protein Muffins
248 Magic Shell Yogurt Bowl

## Yes, There's Protein in Dessert

**DESSERTS**
254 Ninja Creami Ice Cream Two Ways
257 Chocolate-Coconut Caramel Tart
258 Fudge Brownies
261 Raspberry-Vanilla Protein Mug Cake
262 Sweet and Salty Candy Bark
265 Mini Apple Tarts
266 Peppermint Patties
269 Protein Muddy Buddies
270 Brown Butter–Chocolate Chip Cookies
273 Strawberry Cheesecake Pudding

275 **Acknowledgments**
278 **Index**

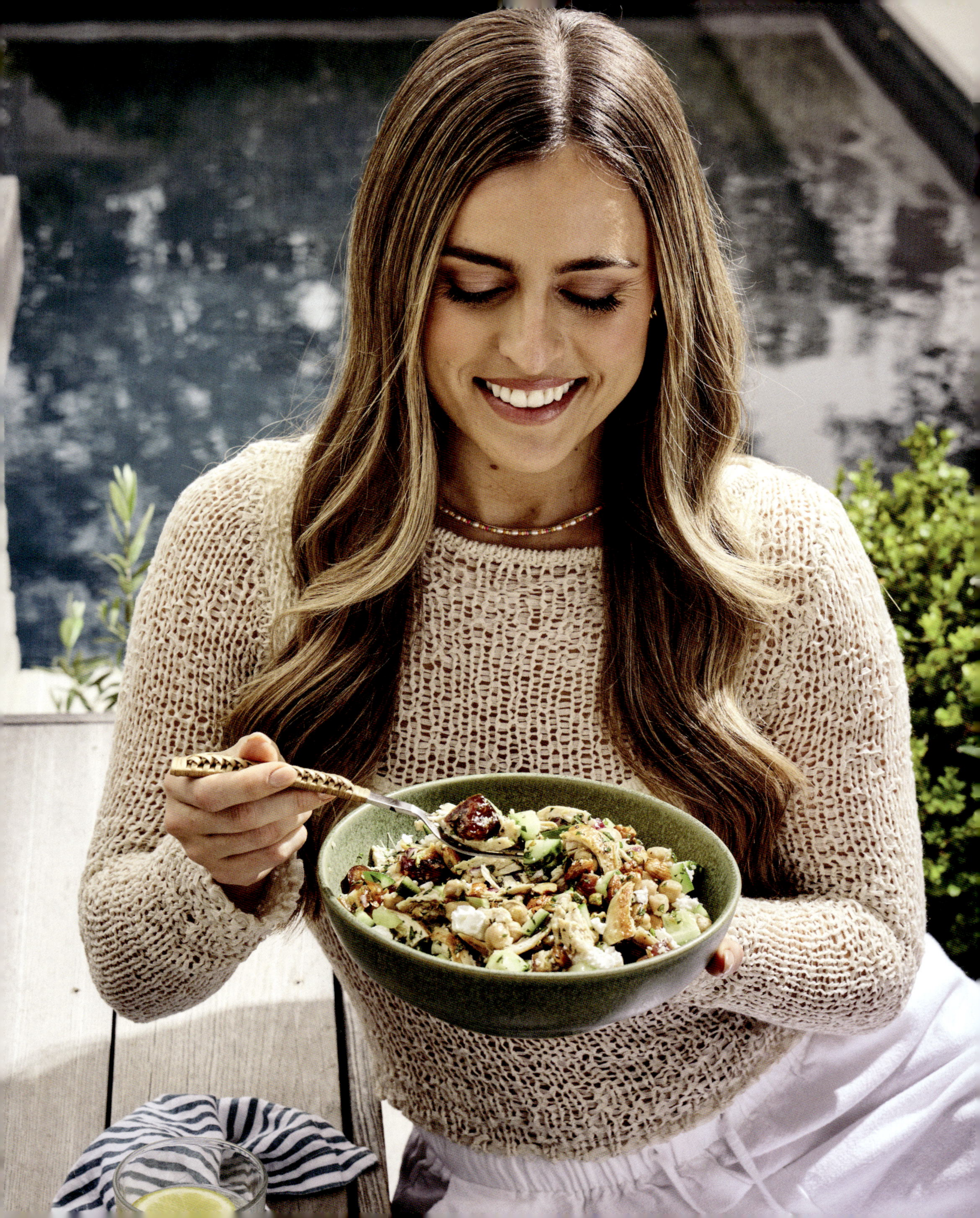

# Introduction

For as long as I can remember, food has been at the center of my life. Not just as fuel, but as a way to bring comfort, connect with friends and family, and celebrate the little (and big!) moments. I grew up believing that cooking and eating well should actually feel good. It should be something you look forward to, not a chore or something dragged down by restriction. That philosophy has guided not just how I cook and share recipes, but the entire foundation of my career as a dietitian. To me, food should nourish your body. And it should also bring you joy.

Over the years, I've worked with everyone—teens, new moms, busy professionals, older adults—and the same struggle pops up over and over: food burnout. Some people can't seem to get enough protein, while others think eating healthy means sacrificing flavor and fun. Too often we're led to believe nutritious food has to be boring, or all about chasing numbers—weight loss, better labs, more muscle—or just . . . blah. And honestly, the hardest part is often just finding the time and energy to make it all happen in real life.

That's why people come to me: they want recipes that solve what I call the *triple challenge* of eating well—easy to make, actually taste amazing, *and* help you feel like your best self. I get it—I've been there. Between work, family, and all the chaos in between, I've had seasons where I needed meals that didn't exhaust all my free time and still made me excited to sit down and eat. If I'm not genuinely looking forward to a meal, I'm grabbing whatever's convenient—and let's be real, it's usually not all that great.

You and your family deserve recipes that make healthy eating simple and satisfying, without screaming "health food."

The past few years especially, protein has taken center stage for good reason—it's the MVP for feeling full, strong, and energized. But one of the top questions I get is: *How do I actually eat more protein without the same three meals on repeat?* That's the challenge, right? You want variety. You want flavor. You want options that fit a busy life (aka always). That's exactly why I wrote this book.

It's filled with meals that actually work in day-to-day—full of flavor, never boring, with a major emphasis on protein. I've packed it with nutrient-dense recipes for every single meal of the day (yes, even dessert). Basically, if you cook from this book, you won't need anything else.

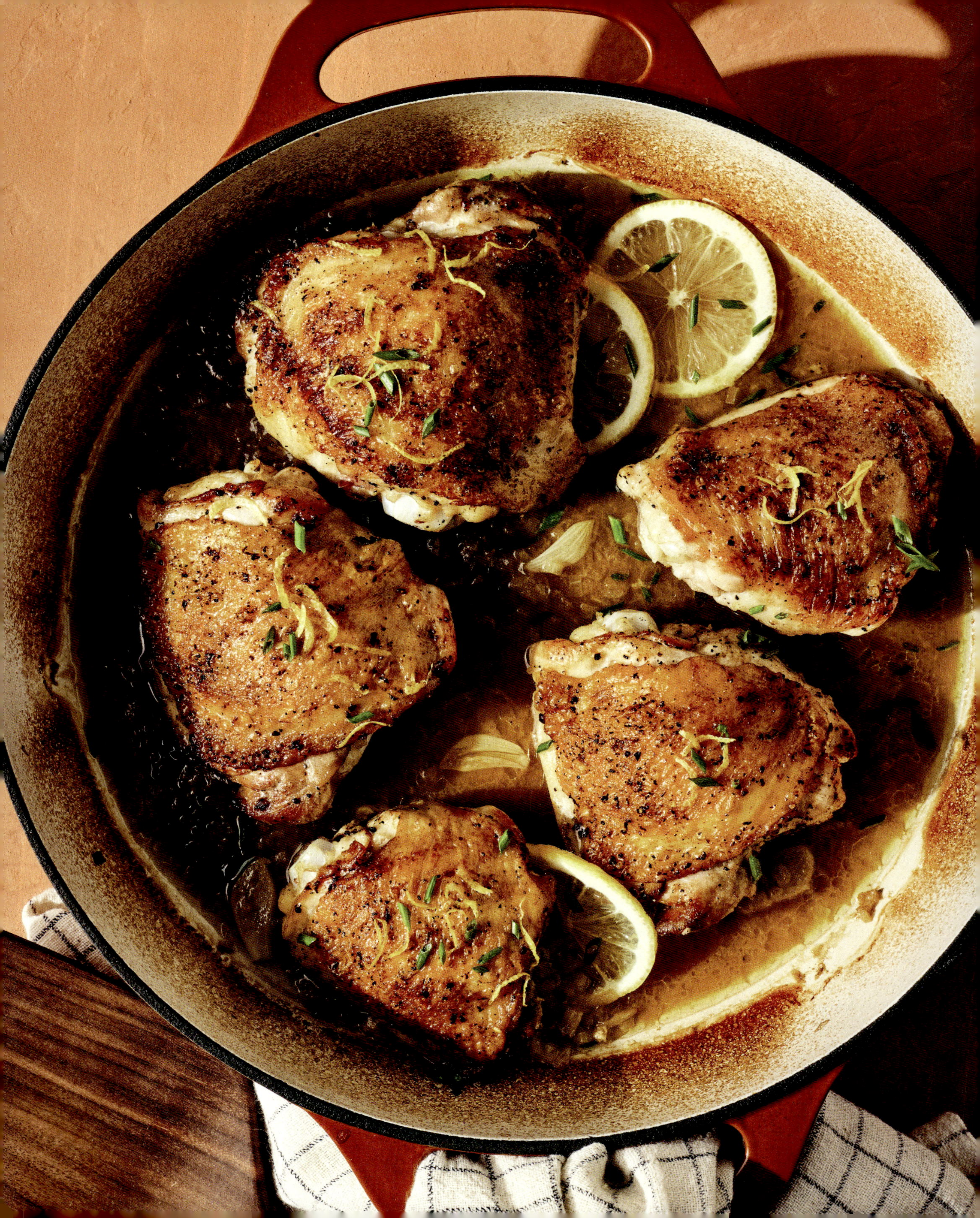

# The Power of Protein

Here's something I've seen time and time again: When people start eating more protein, everything changes. They have more energy. Fewer cravings. Better workouts. Their meals satisfy them and they don't feel hungry a few hours later.

I used to be the person constantly grabbing a granola bar or a handful of crackers an hour after lunch, and I could never figure out why I was still hungry. Turns out, I wasn't eating enough protein in the first place. Once I started building my meals around protein, everything shifted—it was like flipping a switch, and I've never looked back.

Protein isn't just for building muscle—it's key for a healthy metabolism, balanced hormones, and steady blood sugar. All of which keeps you from getting hangry, helps you recover faster (whether from a workout or just a really active day), and makes your body run the way it's supposed to: energized, strong, and steady.

This book is all about making protein a no-brainer. I want you to flip through these pages, see a recipe, and think, *yep, I want that.* You'll look forward to making these recipes because they are so easy and deliver on taste—and they just happen to be doing your body a whole lot of good too.

If there were two things I'd recommend to just about anyone wanting to feel better and live healthier, it'd be these: Eat more protein and scale back on added sugar. These two shifts, which are really not complicated, make a big difference—and that's why every recipe in this book reflects that approach. You'll see clear labels on each one—dairy-free, gluten-free, grain-free, no added sugar, Paleo—so you know exactly what you're getting. I want this to be a book you trust and turn to for food that fuels you and fits your life.

When I set out to write a high-protein cookbook, I thought about the different people I've worked with and the many life stages—and life goals—where nutrition plays a key role: Adolescence, when kids need nutrients to fuel growth and stay strong for their active lives. Adulthood, when men and women decide *this* is the year they'll finally focus on building lean muscle and gaining lasting mass—whether for general strength or more noticeable results at the gym. Pregnancy (been there, done that!), when nourishment matters not just for the baby (of course), but also for mom—something too many women downplay. And then there's the hormonal roller coaster that starts around age forty, when the ups and downs can really affect how we feel.

The common need here? *A lot of protein*.

Regardless of age or life stage, protein is an essential building block—yet most of us don't get enough of it. This book will give you the tools and recipes to incorporate protein into your meals in a way that is both doable and also exciting. Because once you see how good you feel, you won't want to stop.

As a registered dietitian, I've heard all the nutrition noise—the one-size-fits-all plans, the protein panic, the overhyped superfoods or supplements. Let's cut through it. I'll simplify the science so you can focus on eating foods that you love—and that support your goals—and that also help you build strength and provide the energy for everything your life demands.

The best part? Eating more protein doesn't mean giving up your favorite meals or forcing yourself to eat plain chicken breast at every meal. Flavor is king, right? I have you covered for breakfast, lunch, dinner, and in between with food that you'll actually crave. I promise, eating a high-protein plate will never feel like a trade-off.

## *Why Protein Matters*

Protein is so much more than just a muscle-building nutrient; it's the unsung hero behind the scenes, quietly working to support nearly every function in your body. It plays a crucial role in keeping your immune system strong by contributing to the creation of antibodies that fight off infections and illnesses. Without enough protein, your body's defenses take a hit, making you more prone to getting sick.

Protein is also a key player when it comes to hormone regulation. Essential hormones like insulin (controls blood sugar), leptin (regulates hunger), and growth hormone (supports tissue repair and muscle growth) all rely on protein.

And let's not forget about muscle recovery—protein is the ultimate repair crew. Most strength and higher-intensity workouts create tiny micro-tears in your muscles, and protein steps in to rebuild and restore them—making you stronger, less sore, and ready for what's next.

Plus, when you eat more protein, you naturally stabilize blood sugar, control hunger, and reduce cravings. Even better, you can hit your protein goals without overcomplicating your meals or spending hours in the kitchen. This book is packed with flavorful, creative, protein-rich recipes that make eating well easy and enjoyable.

## *What Does Eating "High-Protein" Mean, and Are You Eating Enough?*

Here's the thing: Eating high-protein isn't about following some restrictive diet or counting macros until your brain hurts. High-protein eating simply means putting nutrient-dense foods front and center on your plate—foods that support muscle recovery, promote steady energy (rather than the spike and crash of refined carbs and sugar), and improve hunger control. When protein meets big flavor and easy ingredients, eating well stops feeling like a diet and starts becoming something you crave.

One of the biggest mistakes I see among my nutrition clients is that they underestimate how much protein they really need—not just to maintain muscle, but also to feel their best. While everyone's needs are different, a solid starting point is aiming for around 100 grams of protein per day. That might look like 30 to 40 grams for each main meal, with additional protein coming from snacks.

If you want to get more specific, aim for 0.8 to 1 gram of protein per pound of your goal body weight. For example, if your goal weight is 150 pounds, that's 120 to 150 grams protein a day. Divide that total across your meals—if you eat five meals, that's about 30 grams per meal. Prefer fewer meals? Go for 40 to 50 grams protein per main meal.

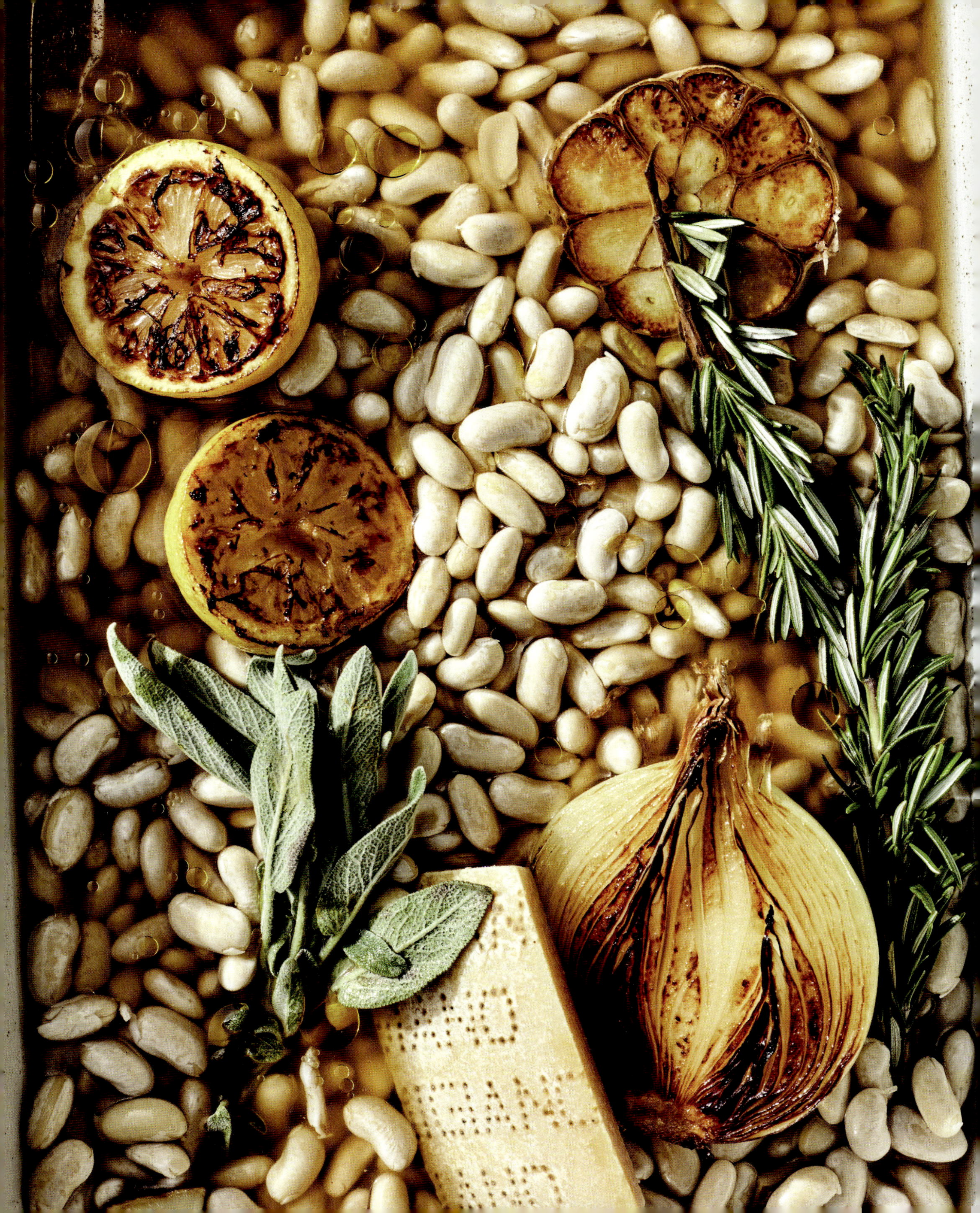

I know calorie and macro tracking works really well for some people—but personally, it's not my thing, and I don't usually recommend it for most. In my experience, it can add pressure and take away the flexibility that makes eating enjoyable. That said, I *do* think it's worth tracking your protein for a day or two. Most people are surprised to see they're not getting nearly enough—and once you see the numbers, it's so much easier to make small, intentional changes that actually stick.

### *Your Body Runs on Protein—Here's How to Get It Right*

Because most of us don't have the time or inclination to dive into textbook-level nutrition science, let me lay it out real quick: Protein is made up of building blocks called amino acids. Some of them, known as *essential* amino acids, can come only from the food you eat. That's why high-quality protein matters—it gives your body what it needs for energy, strength, recovery, hormone balance, and appetite regulation, without you needing to micromanage your meals.

Animal proteins like eggs, fish, beef, and chicken provide all nine essential amino acids in the most bioavailable form, meaning your body can absorb and use them efficiently. They're effective because they closely match the amino acid profile we need, which makes digestion, muscle repair, and the body's ability to use them overall pretty seamless.

Beyond being an efficient source of protein, animal proteins also deliver essential nutrients that support muscle function, energy, metabolism, and general health. Nutrients like heme iron, zinc, B vitamins (especially B12), and omega-3s are naturally abundant in animal-based foods, making them some of the most efficient, nutrient-rich options available.

Plant-based proteins can absolutely meet your needs, too, but they often require strategic pairings to provide all essential amino acids—for example, combining black beans and rice, hummus and whole grain pita, or lentils and quinoa. Plant proteins also tend to be higher in fiber and contain compounds called antinutrients (like phytates and oxalates), which can slightly reduce the absorption of certain minerals. That's why, throughout this book, I focused on high-quality animal protein sources, while including a handful of plant-based options to keep meals balanced and versatile—and I make sure there's plenty of fiber as well. Even in the meat-based dishes, you'll find plenty of veggies woven in to support a nutrient-dense, well-rounded plate.

Most of the recipes in this book are naturally gluten-free, many are dairy-free, and all are refined sugar-free—because eating this way helps amplify the benefits of a high-protein diet. When your meals are built around quality protein and supported by real, whole ingredients, it becomes a lot easier to stay energized, satisfied, and feeling your best.

### *Why Muscle Matters (and How to Keep It After Thirty)*

After age thirty, we naturally start losing muscle, about 3 to 8 percent per decade. Yikes, right? And if we don't take steps to maintain our strength, this decline *will* speed up after sixty. By the time we reach our seventies or eighties, we could lose up to 50 percent of our muscle mass. Why? Because our bodies become less efficient at building and preserving muscle as we age, especially if we're not consistently challenging those muscles through movement and nutrition. The more muscle mass you build and maintain *early* in life, the more "reserve" you have to draw from later—so the decline is slower and less impactful. The

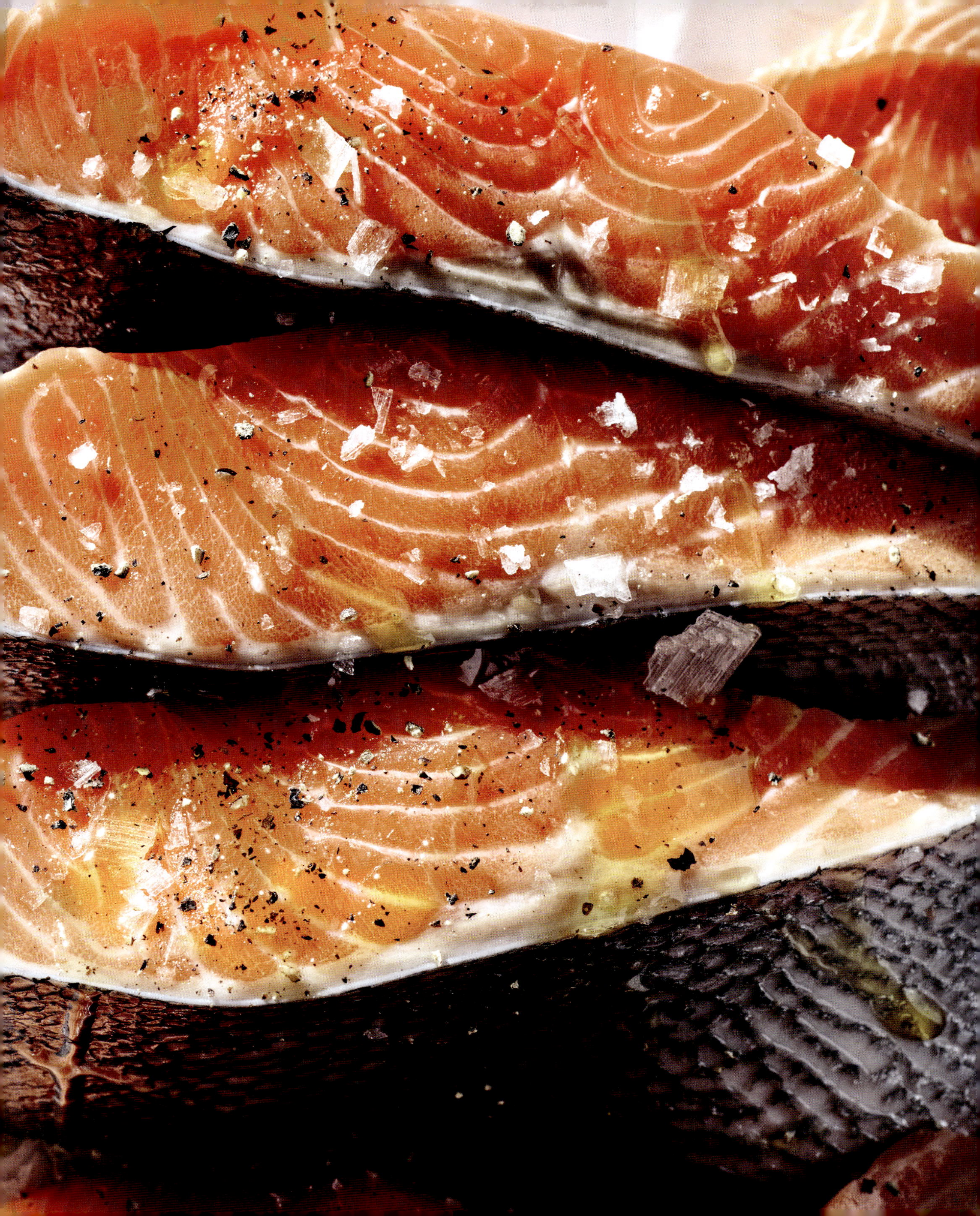

good news is you can slow (and even reverse) age-related muscle loss with the right nutrition and strength training.

Here's the truth: Muscle isn't just about aesthetics—it plays a major role in how your body functions, both now and decades from now. It revs your metabolism, helps regulate blood sugar, protects your bones and joints, and supports everything from daily movement to long-term health. It even helps you burn more calories at rest. And let's be honest—having more muscle just makes life easier, whether you're carrying groceries, chasing your littles, or going for a long walk. Build it now, and future-you will be so glad you did.

## *Putting the High-Protein Plate into Action*

This book isn't just a collection of recipes—it's a reflection of how I've learned to cook and fuel my body through different seasons of life. There were days when I had the time to cook elaborate meals for myself and my husband, Bridger, and others when I was playing hostess for family and friends, preparing dishes that brought everyone together. Then came pregnancy and postpartum, when quick, protein-forward meals became my literal lifeline. From slow cooker meals I could set and forget, to breakfasts that kept me full while juggling all the things, I leaned hard on simple, nutrient-dense recipes.

Because I know firsthand how unpredictable life can be, I've filled this book with recipes that make healthy eating feel second nature. Chapters covering one-pan meals (page 159), slow cooker recipes (page 145), and 30-minutes or less dishes (page 115) are designed for when you're short on time and energy, or just need something easy that still tastes amazing and keeps you full. I'm not kidding when I say I rely on these recipes constantly—they make eating well realistic and enjoyable, even when life gets messy.

I have tested (and tested, and retested) every recipe so that you can confidently rely on how they come out, and know they're built for real life. They're here for you when you need to meal prep for the week, are searching for a one-pot slow cooker number, or have only a few minutes to whip up a quick dinner.

I hope this book empowers you to eat with confidence and, most of all, gets you excited to cook—whether for yourself or your people. These recipes make it so that nourishing your body doesn't have to be complicated, restrictive, or boring.

## *Front-Load Protein*

One of the best strategies for hitting your protein goals without feeling overwhelmed is to front-load your protein earlier in the day. Starting strong with a protein-rich breakfast and lunch ensures you're not relying on dinner to make up for any shortfalls. Options like Cinnamon-Apple Protein Pancakes (page 49), Ready-When-You-Are Breakfast Sandwiches (page 62), or a Berry Crumble Yogurt Bowl (page 61) kick off your day with flavor and fuel, setting you up for success. And because these recipes are also low in sugar, they help regulate steady energy throughout the day. One of the easiest and quickest ways to get a heaping serving of protein early in the day is with smoothies—you've got five delicious ones waiting for you on pages 72–80.

Boosting your protein in a pinch can be simpler than you think—especially with a few smart staples on hand. A quality protein powder can be your best friend as it's easy to blend into smoothies, stir into oatmeal, or mix into baked goods to boost your intake without much effort. Keep high-protein snacks handy, such as grass-fed meat sticks, hard-boiled eggs, and cottage cheese, along with lean proteins like cooked ground turkey and salmon. These are lifesavers when you're hungry and need a quick fix.

Prepping two proteins and one side at the start of the week makes all the difference. It's a simple system that gives me tons of mix-and-match options. On the weekend, I'll make something like 20-Minute Shredded Chicken Verde (page 133), Slow Cooker Beef Stew (page 218), and a batch of Bone Broth Jasmine Rice (page 198), then build meals from there. Chicken and rice with sautéed greens. Stew over rice with avocado on the side. You get the idea. Having these basics ready to go means you can throw together a high-protein meal in minutes—even when your day gets a little wild.

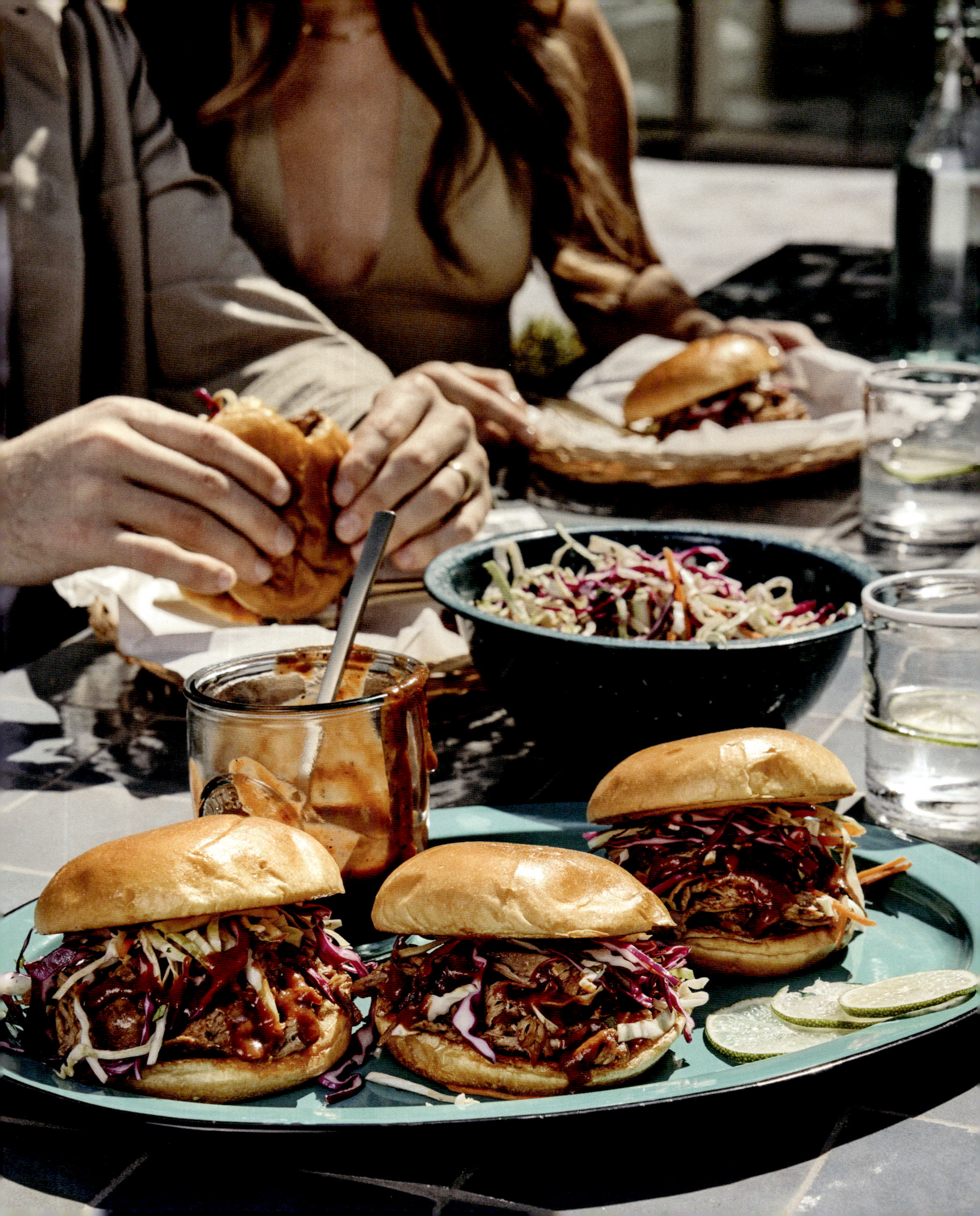

# Choosing the Best Protein Sources

When it comes to protein, quality matters just as much as quantity. You can hit your daily protein goals with just about any source, but if you want to fuel your body in the best way possible, go for the good stuff—ingredients that are organic, grass-fed, grass-finished, pasture-raised, wild-caught, and/or full-fat. Not only do they provide the protein your body needs, they also deliver added health benefits—higher levels of omega-3s, more antioxidants and vitamins (like A and E), and fewer inflammatory additives than conventional proteins.

Grass-fed and grass-finished organic beef is considered the gold standard when it comes to red meat. "Grass-fed" alone can mean the cattle started on grass but were later finished on grain. In contrast, "grass-finished" ensures the animal eats grass for its entire life. This results in better-quality fats—including more omega-3s, more CLA (conjugated linoleic acid), and a better balance of nutrients to support hormone production, brain function, heart health, and inflammation control. Plus, grass-finished beef is leaner overall while still delivering plenty of protein.

The same logic applies to organic, pasture-raised poultry and eggs. Chickens raised on pasture get to roam freely and eat a natural diet, which boosts the vitamin D, choline, and antioxidant content in their eggs—key nutrients for brain health, energy, and cellular repair. Choline, in particular, is a big deal for nervous system health, memory, and cellular repair.

And if you're a seafood lover, wild-caught fish like salmon, cod, tuna, and mahi mahi are naturally higher in omega-3s, iodine, and essential trace minerals than farmed options. They also tend to be lower in contaminants, which makes them a cleaner choice for your high-protein meals.

That said, meals don't have to be perfect 100 percent of the time. Not every dish has to be organic or wild-caught. Just aim to do your best with what's available. Even conventional proteins can absolutely help you build strong, balanced meals.

### *Why Full-Fat Dairy Is the Best Choice*

When choosing dairy, full-fat wins. For years, we were told low-fat was better—but the research now says otherwise. Full-fat dairy keeps you fuller, helps regulate hormones, and improves your body's ability to absorb fat-soluble vitamins like A, D, E, and K.

The fat in dairy slows digestion and buffers blood sugar, keeping your energy steady and reducing the crash-and-snack cycle. Plus, full-fat options like Greek yogurt, cottage cheese, and raw cheese offer healthy fats like CLA, which may support metabolism and reduce inflammation.

If you tolerate dairy well, go for the highest-quality options you can find: grass-fed, full-fat, and ideally organic. You'll get more omega-3s, vitamin K2, and gut-friendly probiotics from these versions. But don't stress if you can't find grass-fed every time—even a basic full-fat dairy option is still a smart choice.

### *Making the Best Choices for You*

The bottom line: you don't need to overhaul your grocery list to eat well. Start where you are and aim to level up when you can. Choosing grass-fed or pasture-raised proteins when possible is a simple way to make your meals more nutrient-dense and supportive of long-term health.

Whether that means stocking up on grass-fed beef when it's on sale, choosing wild-caught salmon when it's available, or grabbing the best full-fat yogurt your store carries, each small upgrade helps you squeeze more nutrition out of every bite and gives your meals added value beyond solely hitting your protein target.

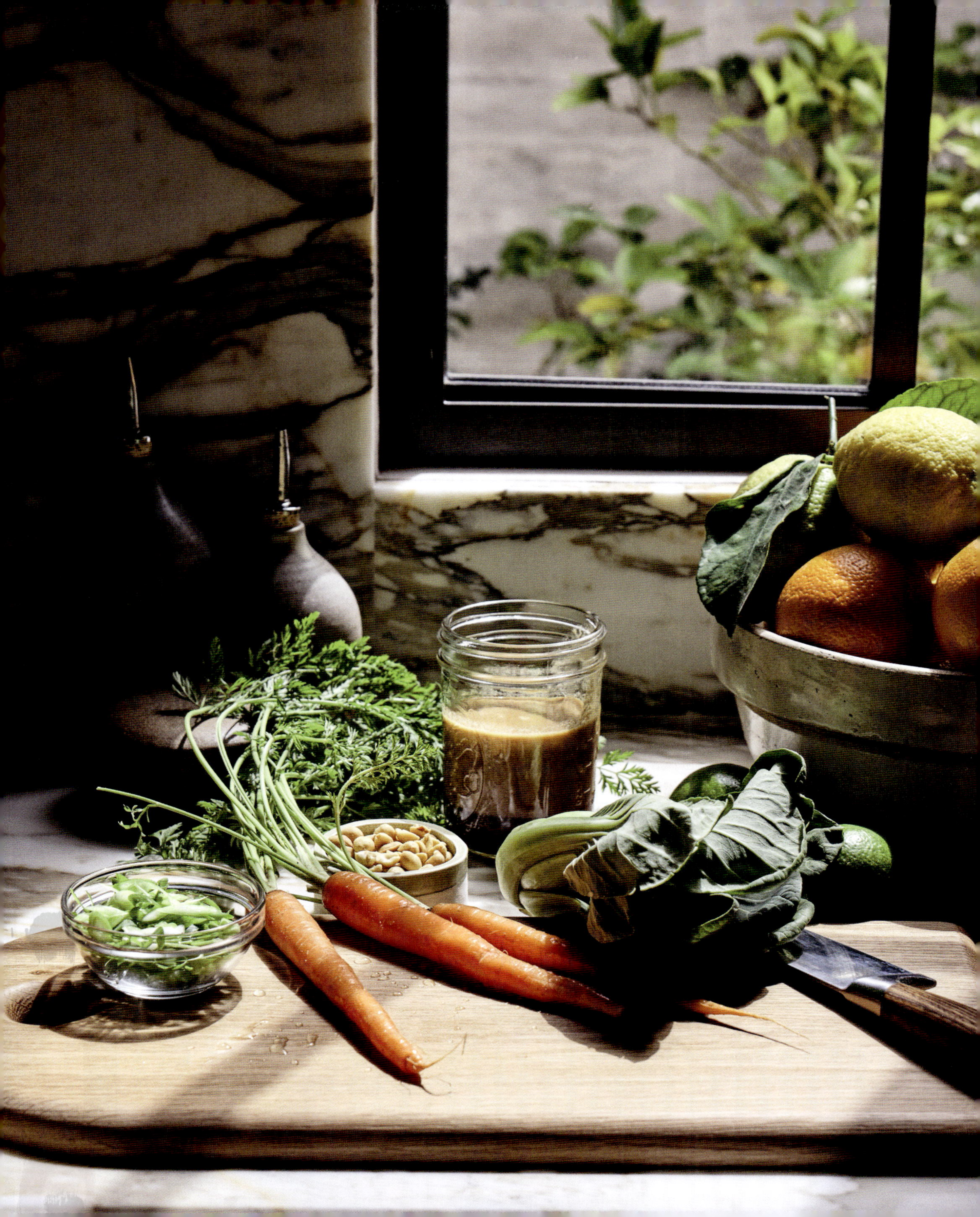

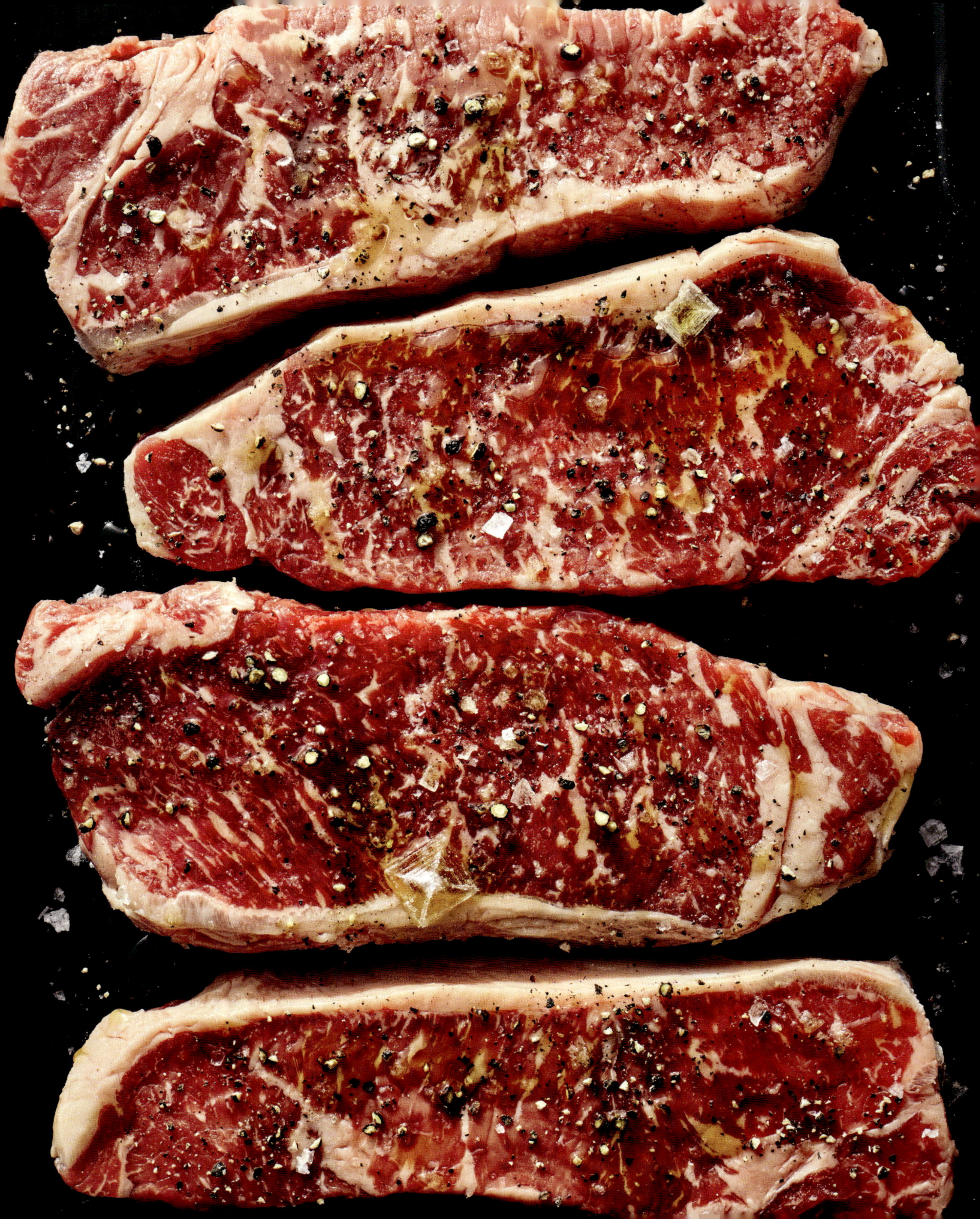

# Let's Break It Down

I put together this quick protein guide so you can easily see how much protein is in common everyday foods—whether you're planning meals, meal-prepping, or trying to hit your daily goal.

| NUTS & SEEDS | SERVING SIZE | AMOUNT OF PROTEIN |
|---|---|---|
| **Almonds** | ¼ cup | 7g protein |
| **Brazil nuts** | ¼ cup | 5g protein |
| **Cashews** | ¼ cup | 5g protein |
| **Chia seeds** | ¼ cup | 12g protein |
| **Flaxseed** | ¼ cup | 8g protein |
| **Hazelnuts** | ¼ cup | 5g protein |
| **Hemp seeds** | ¼ cup | 13g protein |
| **Peanut butter** | 2 tbsps | 7g protein |
| **Peanuts** | ¼ cup | 9g protein |
| **Pistachios** | ¼ cup | 6g protein |
| **Pumpkin seed butter** | 2 tbsps | 8g protein |
| **Pumpkin seeds** | ¼ cup | 9g protein |
| **Sesame seeds** | ¼ cup | 7g protein |
| **Sunflower seeds** | ¼ cup | 7g protein |
| **Walnuts** | ¼ cup | 5g protein |

| ANIMAL PROTEINS | SERVING SIZE | AMOUNT OF PROTEIN |
|---|---|---|
| **Chicken, organic (canned in water)** | 6 oz | 40g protein |
| **Chicken breast, organic (cooked)** | 6 oz | 40g protein |
| **Chicken sausage ,organic (cooked)** | 6 oz | 28g protein |
| **Chuck roast, grass-fed (cooked)** | 6 oz | 46g protein |
| **Ground beef, grass-fed, 80% lean (cooked)** | 6 oz | 44g protein |
| **Ground beef, grass-fed, 90% lean (cooked)** | 6 oz | 44g protein |
| **Ground chicken, organic (cooked)** | 6 oz | 42g protein |
| **Ground turkey, organic (cooked)** | 6 oz | 46g protein |
| **New York strip steak, grass-fed (cooked)** | 6 oz | 45g protein |
| **Pork chop, pasture-raised (cooked)** | 6 oz | 45g protein |
| **Pork sausage, pasture-raised (cooked)** | 6 oz | 28g protein |
| **Turkey sausage, organic (cooked)** | 6 oz | 26g protein |
| **Wild cod (cooked)** | 6 oz | 40g protein |
| **Wild salmon (cooked)** | 6 oz | 44g protein |
| **Wild tuna (canned in water)** | 6 oz | 40g protein |
| **Wild tuna (cooked)** | 6 oz | 40g protein |

| VEGETABLES | SERVING SIZE | AMOUNT OF PROTEIN |
|---|---|---|
| **Artichoke hearts (cooked)** | 1 cup | 5g protein |
| **Asparagus (cooked)** | 1 cup | 3g protein |
| **Avocado** | ⅓ medium | 1g protein |
| **Bell peppers** | 1 cup | 1g protein |
| **Broccoli (cooked)** | 1 cup | 4.5g protein |
| **Brussels sprouts (cooked)** | 1 cup | 4g protein |
| **Cauliflower (cooked)** | 1 cup | 2g protein |
| **Collard greens (cooked)** | 1 cup | 5g protein |
| **Edamame (cooked)** | 1 cup | 17g protein |
| **Green beans (cooked)** | 1 cup | 2g protein |
| **Kale (cooked)** | 1 cup | 3g protein |
| **Mushrooms, white (cooked)** | 1 cup | 3g protein |
| **Spinach (cooked)** | 1 cup | 5g protein |
| **Spinach (raw)** | 1 cup | 1g protein |
| **Sweet potato (baked)** | 1 cup | 4g protein |
| **Zucchini (cooked)** | 1 cup | 2g protein |

| LEGUMES & GRAINS | SERVING SIZE | AMOUNT OF PROTEIN |
|---|---|---|
| **Black beans (cooked)** | 1 cup | 15g protein |
| **Fava beans (cooked)** | 1 cup | 9g protein |
| **Garbanzo beans (chickpeas), cooked** | 1 cup | 15g protein |
| **Lentils (cooked)** | 1 cup | 18g protein |
| **Lentil or chickpea pasta (cooked)** | 1 cup | 13g protein |
| **Oats (organic, dry)** | ½ cup | 5g protein |
| **Peas (cooked)** | 1 cup | 8g protein |
| **Quinoa (cooked)** | 1 cup | 8g protein |
| **Rice, brown (cooked)** | 1 cup | 5g protein |
| **Rice, white (cooked)** | 1 cup | 4g protein |
| **Sprouted bread (like Ezekiel)** | 1 slice | 5g protein |
| **White beans (cannellini, navy, great northern), cooked** | 1 cup | 17g protein |

| EGGS & EGG WHITES | SERVING SIZE | AMOUNT OF PROTEIN |
|---|---|---|
| **Egg, whole** | 1 large | 6g protein |
| **Egg whites** | from 3 large eggs | 10g protein |

| DAIRY (organic and full-fat, when possible) | SERVING SIZE | AMOUNT OF PROTEIN |
|---|---|---|
| **Cottage cheese** | 1 cup | 28g protein |
| **Cow's milk** | 1 cup | 8g protein |
| **Goat cheese** | 1 oz | 5g protein |
| **Greek yogurt (unsweetened, plain)** | 1 cup | 20g protein |
| **Kefir (unsweetened)** | 1 cup | 9g protein |
| **Sharp cheddar cheese** | 1 oz | 7g protein |
| **Skyr (unsweetened)** | 1 cup | 20g protein |

| BAKING INGREDIENTS | SERVING SIZE | AMOUNT OF PROTEIN |
|---|---|---|
| **All-purpose baking flour** | ¼ cup | 3–4g protein |
| **Almond flour** | ¼ cup | 6g protein |
| **Cassava flour** | ¼ cup | 1g protein |
| **Coconut flour** | ¼ cup | 6g protein |
| **Gluten-free baking flour** | ¼ cup | 3–4g protein |

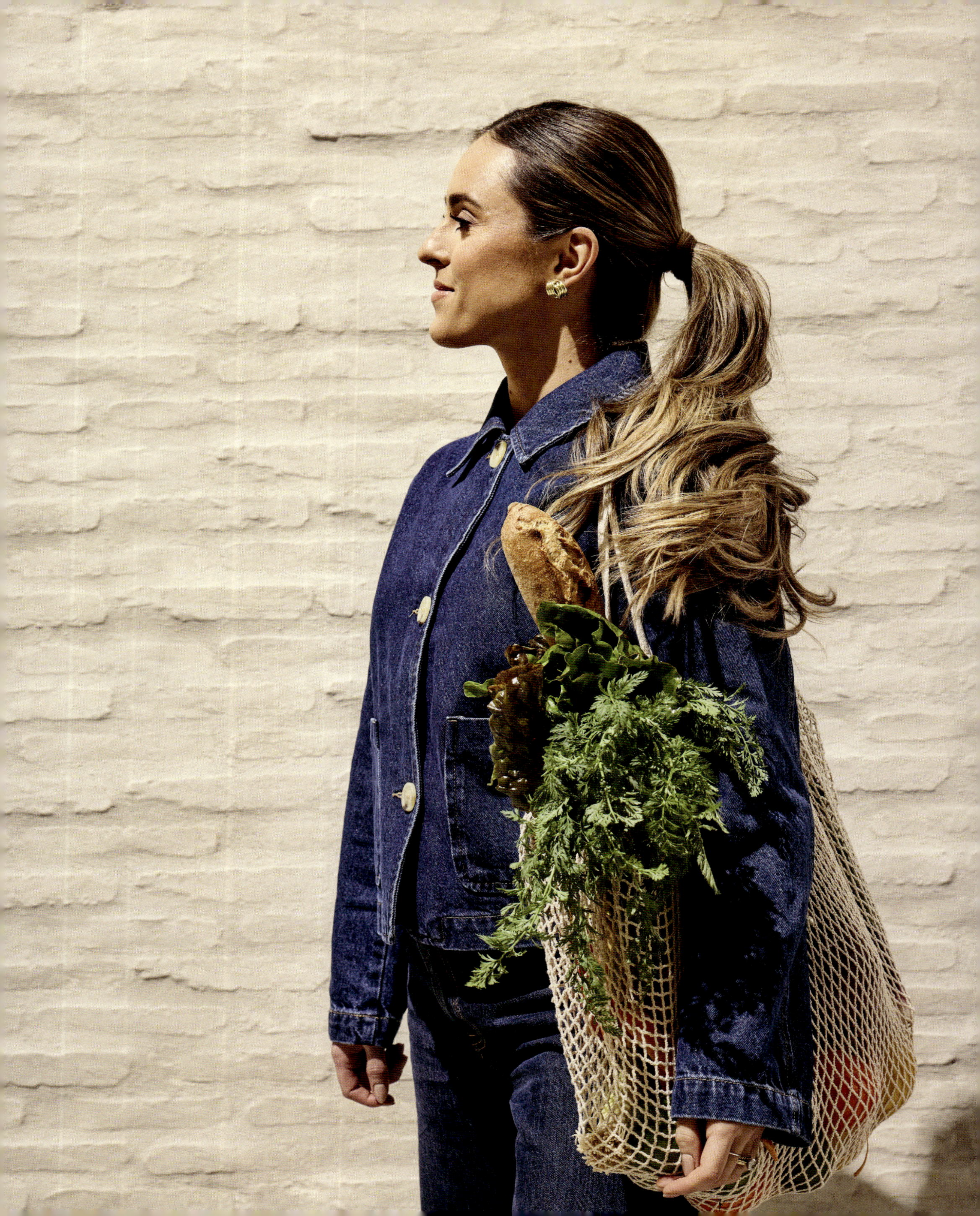

# The Power Pantry

If there's one thing I've learned, it's that eating well starts with a power pantry. A few smart staples and suddenly dinner is less "What the heck do I make?" and more "Wow, that was easy." Stocking the right ingredients means fewer last-minute grocery runs (okay, those still happen!) and way less mealtime stress.

These are the things that make high-protein cooking second nature—the pantry, fridge, and freezer favorites I reach for every single week to whip up meals that are both bold and fuss-free.

## *Baking Flours*

### ALMOND FLOUR

My go-to for grain-free baking. Perfect for cookies, muffins, and pancakes thanks to its subtly sweet nutty flavor and soft, tender texture. I use almond flour in savory dishes, too, when I want to give fish or chicken a crisp, golden crust. Almond flour is rich in protein, vitamin E, and healthy fats—one of the most nutrient-dense flours out there. **Pro tip:** Do not use almond flour in sauces or gravies—it can turn gritty. Arrowroot powder (right) is a better thickener.

### COCONUT FLOUR

Light, slightly sweet, and ultra-absorbent. A little goes a long way—just ¼ cup coconut flour replaces 1 cup regular flour. It's rich in fiber and helps support steady blood sugar. Since it soaks up a lot of liquid, always add extra moisture and eggs when baking with it—typically, 1 egg for every ¼ cup of coconut flour, plus additional liquid as needed.

### CASSAVA FLOUR

The closest grain-free alternative to all-purpose flour. It's mild, light, and nut-free, making it great for allergy-friendly recipes. Use it as a 1:1 replacement for all-purpose flour in savory dishes. But for baking, be mindful that it absorbs more liquid. Follow recipes closely, and if needed, add a splash of water to loosen batters.

### GLUTEN-FREE ALL-PURPOSE FLOUR

The flour I reach for when I need structure and reliability in gluten-free baking. I love Bob's Red Mill Gluten-Free All-Purpose Baking Flour—it's sturdy, versatile, and creates a great texture in everything from muffins to pancakes.

### ARROWROOT POWDER

Also called arrowroot starch and arrowroot flour. A fine, neutral thickener great for soups, sauces, and crispy coatings. It works similarly to cornstarch but without the GMO concerns.

### *Cooking Oils and Fats*

**EXTRA-VIRGIN OLIVE OIL**

The gold standard. Look for cold-pressed, organic EVOO in a dark glass bottle to preserve its nutrients. Best for drizzling, dressing, and finishing.

**AVOCADO OIL**

One of my top picks for high-heat cooking. It has a neutral flavor, a high smoke point, and is full of monounsaturated fats that support heart health.

**COCONUT OIL**

Great for baking, stir-frying, and even in coffee. It's rich in MCTs (medium-chain triglycerides), which offer quick energy and support metabolism.

**GHEE**

Ghee is clarified butter—meaning the milk solids (lactose and casein) have been removed, making it a great option for those who are lactose intolerant. (I'm sensitive to lactose, and ghee never gives me any issues.) It has a rich, nutty flavor and a high smoke point, which makes it perfect for high-heat cooking like roasting, sautéing, and searing. I love stirring it into warm dishes like Bone Broth Jasmine Rice (page 198) for a layer of buttery richness. Plus, it's full of fat-soluble vitamins like A, D, E, and K, which support brain function, skin health, and hormone balance. Trust me—it's a total game-changer in the kitchen. My favorite brand is 4th & Heart.

**GRASS-FED BUTTER**

Worth keeping around if you tolerate dairy. Grass-fed butter has a rich flavor and is a good source of fat-soluble vitamins—especially K2, which supports bone and heart health. I personally stick to ghee since I'm sensitive to lactose, but for anyone who isn't, this is a great go-to for lower-temp cooking or adding richness to foods like mashed potatoes or toast.

### *Pantry MVPs*

**BONE BROTH**

Liquid gold. Rich in collagen, amino acids, and minerals that support gut, skin, and joint health. Sip it, cook with it, or use it as a base for soups, stews, and grains. I love the Kettle & Fire and Bonafide Provisions brands when I'm not making my own (see page 226).

**CANNED COCONUT MILK**

A must-have for creamy sauces, curries, soups—and even desserts. Always go for full-fat, unsweetened for the best texture and flavor. You'll find it in recipes like my Saucy Coconut-Curry Turkey Meatballs (page 122), Roasted Butternut Squash Soup with Coconut-Lime Crema (page 228), and Make-Ahead Coconut-Mango Chia Pudding (page 65).

**COCONUT AMINOS**

A gluten-free, slightly sweet alternative to soy sauce. Lower in sodium and perfect for stir-fries, sauces, and marinades. Just know it's not a 1:1 sub for soy sauce—if you're swapping, you'll need to dilute the soy sauce. A good rule of thumb? If a recipe calls for 2 tablespoons coconut aminos, try using 1 tablespoon soy sauce mixed with 1 tablespoon water to balance the saltiness.

**DIJON AND STONE-GROUND MUSTARDS**

A little goes a long way. Mustards add tang and richness to dressings, marinades, and sauces. I keep a jar in my fridge or pantry.

**GLUTEN-FREE ORGANIC PROTEIN OATS**

I always have a bag of Bob's Red Mill Protein Oats in my pantry. They're hearty, gluten-free, and perfect for my Honey-Blackberry Overnight Oats (page 50).

**JARRED ROASTED RED PEPPERS**

Shortcut ingredient that adds smoky sweetness and depth. Great in dips and sauces (hello, Romesco, page 180).

### NUT BUTTERS

Look for brands with just nuts and sea salt—no added sugars or oils. Almond, peanut, and cashew butters are great for boosting protein in smoothies, oats, and energy bites.

### SEEDS

Tiny but mighty: chia, flax, and hemp add protein, fiber, and omega-3s to smoothies, oatmeal, baked goods, and even sprinkled over salads.

### PROTEIN POWDER

An easy way to hit your protein goals fast—whether you're tossing it in a smoothie, stirring it into oats, or baking it into a snack. Look for short ingredient lists, no artificial sweeteners, and third-party tested sourcing. I share my go-to brands on my website.

### UNFLAVORED COLLAGEN PEPTIDES

One of my frequent protein-boosting add-ins, collagen peptides are flavorless and dissolve effortlessly into both hot and cold foods. I mix them into soups, sauces, and even desserts for a little extra protein without changing the texture or taste. You'll see them show up in quite a few recipes throughout this book. Plus, collagen is great for skin, hair, nails, and joint support—so it's a win-win all around.

### QUICK SNACKS

Sometimes you just need something simple and protein-forward to hold you over. These are the ones I reach for most:

**Grass-fed meat sticks:** Quick 10+ grams of protein with clean ingredients. Chomps, Archer, Lineage Provisions, and Paleovalley brands are in heavy rotation at our house.

**Single-pack pitted olives:** Great source of healthy fats with zero prep.

**Dry-roasted nuts and seeds:** Almonds, cashews, pistachios, Brazil nuts, macadamia nuts, and pumpkin seeds are always stocked in my pantry. (Be sure to look for options without added oils, since they tend to be the inflammatory class of vegetable oils.)

**Nut butter packets:** Great to have on hand for a quick protein boost, whether drizzled over fruit or eaten straight from the packet.

### Protein Powders

Whole, nutrient-dense foods should always be the foundation of your diet, but protein powders are convenient, especially on busy days or when you need a quick way to meet your protein goals. I recommend choosing a high-quality protein powder with simple ingredients and no unnecessary additives. When reading the label, here's what I recommend looking for:

- A short, recognizable ingredient list
- No artificial sweeteners like sucralose, aspartame, or acesulfame potassium
- No artificial colors or flavors
- No fillers or gums like carrageenan, or excessive guar or xanthan gum (which can cause digestive issues for some)
- Transparent sourcing (like grass-fed whey or organic pea protein)
- Third-party testing to ensure quality and purity (look for it on the brand's website or packaging—it's not always listed front and center)

I use protein powder in smoothies and baked goods, and I even stir it into oatmeal. If you're looking for more tips on picking the best protein powder, check out my site, Rachael's Good Eats.

**STORE-BOUGHT SALSA**

Easy for quick, flavorful meals. Once you try my 20-Minute Shredded Chicken Verde (page 133), I know you'll understand.

**SUN-DRIED TOMATOES**

Loaded with umami, these can be tossed into salads, blended into sauces, or stirred into pastas and grain bowls. The ones stored in extra-virgin olive oil are my pick for big flavor.

**TAHINI**

A nutty, creamy staple made from sesame seeds. Tahini is perfect for dressings, sauces, and even desserts. It adds richness and depth to both sweet and savory dishes, like the creamy dressing in the Chili Crisp Tofu and Quinoa Power Bowls (page 129), or in the Chocolate Tahini Chunk Cookies from my first cookbook.

**TINNED FISH (SALMON, SARDINES, TUNA, MACKEREL) AND CHICKEN**

These protein powerhouses deliver omega-3s and essential nutrients, making them ideal for quick lunches, salads, or mashing into an easy spread with lemon and mustard. I always keep a few cans of the chicken on hand for my 5-Minute Pesto Chicken Salad (page 197).

**WHITE WINE VINEGAR**

Bright and tangy, white wine vinegar adds acidity to dressings, marinades, and even cooked dishes. It's great for balancing flavors and adding a little zest—and as a fermented food, it can also support gut health in small amounts.

## *Sweeteners*

**RAW HONEY**

My sweetener of choice! Raw honey delivers natural enzymes, antioxidants, and trace minerals that support immunity and digestion—but those benefits can diminish when heated above 104°F. I still use it in baked goods for flavor and texture, but if you want the full nutritional perks, drizzle it on after cooking or stir into something cool.

**MAPLE SYRUP**

This unrefined sweetener adds layers of flavor to everything from pancakes to marinades. Look for 100 percent pure maple syrup to get the most benefits.

**PITTED MEDJOOL DATES**

Nature's candy! Dates are naturally sweet and full of fiber, making them a great alternative to processed sugar. Blend into smoothies, chop into energy bites, or use to sweeten desserts, like my Chocolate-Coconut Caramel Tart (page 257).

**COCONUT SUGAR**

A lower-glycemic alternative to refined sugar, coconut sugar adds a mild caramel-like sweetness to treats. It works well as a 1:1 replacement for white sugar in most recipes and is less processed and less likely to cause the energy spike and crash that often comes with conventional sugar.

## *Fridge Staples*

I don't always have every single one of these in my fridge at once, but I like to rotate through them so I have fresh options to pull for meals throughout the week.

**DELI MEATS (ORGANIC TURKEY AND CHICKEN)**

Perfect for quick, high-protein snacks or adding to wraps and sandwiches. But not all deli meats are created equal so I stick with organic, high-quality options that have minimal ingredients, no added sugars, and no artificial preservatives. When you choose well, deli meats can absolutely be part of a balanced, protein-forward plate.

**FRESH PRODUCE**

I love rotating seasonal produce, but there are a few produce picks I almost always have on hand:

**Avocados** are a must for healthy fats and creamy texture, whether mashed into guac, sliced over bowls, or blended into smoothies.

**Bell peppers**, especially red peppers since they're rich in vitamin C, add the perfect crunch to salads, wraps, and quick sautés. You'll notice they make a lot of cameos in this book—what can I say, they never let me down! Feel free to swap in whatever peppers you love or already have on hand.

Crunchy **Persian cucumbers** are an excellent grab for snacking and dipping, while **zucchini** is incredibly versatile for stir-fries, baking, and spiralizing as a pasta swap.

I also keep a steady rotation of **dark leafy greens** like spinach, kale, and arugula for scrambles, sautés, salads, and smoothies,

**Fresh herbs** like cilantro, parsley, basil, dill, and mint brighten up any meal.

### FULL-FAT GREEK YOGURT AND COTTAGE CHEESE

The forgotten protein powerhouses that make meals filling and satisfying. Greek yogurt and cottage cheese are also rich in probiotics, which support gut health. I recommend the full-fat versions—they taste better, keep you fuller longer, and help your body absorb fat-soluble vitamins like A, D, E, and K, which, again, support everything from immune function to bone health.

### GRASS-FED CHEESE (SHARP CHEDDAR, GOAT CHEESE, PARMESAN, FETA)

Full of protein and healthy fats to add depth and richness to dishes. Goat milk products don't upset my stomach the way cow's milk does—likely because goat milk has less lactose and smaller fat globules, which can make it easier to digest. Aged cheeses like Parmesan and sharp cheddar are also lower in lactose, which makes them good options for those who are sensitive. I add feta to salads, goat cheese to bowls or wraps, and sharp cheddar to eggs, roasted veggies, or anything that needs an extra punch of flavor.

### HUMMUS

A great source of fiber and plant-based protein. Hummus pairs well with veggies, wraps, or as a topping for bowls. Look for brands made with extra-virgin olive oil instead of seed oils.

### ORGANIC GRASS-FED MEATS (CHICKEN, BEEF, TURKEY, LAMB, PORK, SAUSAGE)

I usually keep a handful of various proteins that I plan to cook within the next few days in the fridge. This could be pasture-raised chicken, grass-fed beef (always in the mix), or wild-caught salmon—whatever I have planned for dinners that week.

### ORGANIC PASTURE-RAISED EGGS

One of the highest-quality protein sources, full of choline, B vitamins, and essential amino acids. I eat eggs daily, whether plain, or in scrambles, frittatas, or baked goods.

### WILD-CAUGHT FISH (SALMON, MAHI MAHI, COD, TUNA, SHRIMP)

Loaded with omega-3s, protein, and essential minerals to support muscle recovery and brain health. Frozen shrimp and salmon fillets are always in my freezer for quick meals.

## *Freezer Staples*

This is where I keep my go-to protein sources so they are always available for quick meals.

### DARK CHOCOLATE AND DESSERT BITES

Of course I aim to get most of my protein from meals and snacks throughout the day, but I'm never mad about having a freezer stash of treats that sneak in a little protein too. Peppermint Patties (page 266) and Sweet and Salty Candy

Bark (page 262) love to make their way into rotation.

### FROZEN BONE BROTH

During the weeks when I'm on top of my game, I make a big batch of homemade bone broth (page 226) and freeze it in portions to use for soups, stews, and sauces. It adds rich flavor and an extra hit of protein to recipes like my Slow Cooker Beef Stew (page 218) and Bone Broth Jasmine Rice (page 198).

### FROZEN BERRIES AND BANANAS

Essential for smoothies, baking, and throwing into yogurt bowls. I always have frozen berries and halved bananas in reusable silicone ziplock bags. You'll find them in several of my most-loved smoothies (pages 72–80).

### FROZEN VEGGIES

A lifesaver when I don't have time to prep fresh veggies. I will toss frozen peas, corn, and spinach into stir-fries.

### FROZEN GLUTEN-FREE BREAD OR TORTILLAS

I usually keep a pack of grain-free tortillas (like Siete) or a loaf of gluten-free sourdough in the freezer to pull out as needed. I'm obsessed with tacos—for breakfast, lunch, and dinner—so tortillas are a non-negotiable in my freezer. You'll see them in recipes like my Chorizo-Style Breakfast Tacos (page 58).

### FROZEN GRASS-FED, PASTURE-RAISED MEATS (BEEF, CHICKEN, TURKEY, LAMB)

I love keeping extra proteins in the freezer so I can easily defrost what I need for dinner without running to the store. Ground meats, chicken thighs, and steak are always stocked.

### FROZEN PITTED DATES

Soft Medjool dates live in my freezer at all times. Just one or two add natural sweetness to smoothies, and that yummy caramel flavor makes everything taste a little more indulgent.

### FROZEN WILD-CAUGHT FISH (SALMON, COD, TUNA, MAHI MAHI)

Wild-caught fish is rich in omega-3s, quick to cook, and freezes—and defrosts—well, making it an endlessly convenient choice when I need to throw together a quick, feel-good lunch or dinner.

**TIP:** *Whenever possible, double-batch soups, stews, and chilis and freeze half for an easy, no-effort meal later. To do this, let the extra portion cool completely, then transfer to a freezer-safe container or lay it flat in a freezer bag (This saves space!). Label with the name and date, and when you're ready to eat, just reheat it on the stove with a splash of water or broth to bring it back to life—or microwave it in a covered, microwave-safe dish in sixty- to ninety-second intervals, stirring in between, until warmed through.*

# A Few Tips Before You Get Cooking

Season to your taste: I give measurements for seasonings, but don't be afraid to adjust based on what you like. Love heat? Add more chili flakes. Need a little more salt? Go for it. Cooking should be flexible!

**Ingredient swaps are welcome:** If you need to swap ingredients, don't stress. I include plenty of suggestions, and I always encourage making a recipe work for you. Just keep in mind that changing ingredients—especially protein sources—will affect the protein amount listed. If hitting a certain protein goal is important for you, consider using a food-tracking app to get an accurate breakdown based on your changes.

**TIP:** *If you want a great starting point, Cronometer is my recommendation for quick, easy nutrition tracking.*

**Read through the entire recipe before you start:** Sounds obvious, but trust me: I know that people don't do this! It makes cooking so much easier when you know what's coming next. Also, it *truly, truly* helps to do all your chopping and prepping before you start cooking—rather than winging it while your protein is already in the pan and on the verge of overcooking. Get everything out and measured, and cooking will be much less of a hassle.

**Meal prep = your best friend:** Many of these recipes are great for prepping ahead. If you're short on time during the week, making a batch of shredded chicken, roasted veggies, or a higher-protein sauce (like Romesco, page 180, or Southwest Sauce, page 188) can be a game-changer for quick meals.

**Use the right pan for the job:** A crowded pan leads to steaming, not searing. That means no golden edges and more bland, soggy results. So if a recipe calls for a large skillet or baking sheet, it's not just being fancy. Give your ingredients some breathing room—you'll get better texture and flavor every time.

**Protein is key, but so is balance:** If I could give two simple recommendations for feeling your best, they'd be this: prioritize protein (this book has you covered there!) and be mindful of added sugar. It's hidden in store-bought ingredients and is one of the biggest culprits behind energy crashes, cravings, and metabolic issues. If you want to take it a step further, check out my e-book *7-Day Added Sugar Detox* at shopgoodeats.com.

**Store it right:** Most proteins and roasted or raw veggies will keep well in the fridge for up to 5 days, and all the sauces in this book will last about a week. Store everything in airtight containers and make weekday meals effortless.

# The Plug-and-Play Meal Prep Guide

Prep a few staples from this guide at the start of the week, and you'll be set up for fast, feel-good, protein-rich meals every day. The chart makes it easy: you can either follow each row straight across for the full meal I've mapped out, or mix and match your favorite protein, base, sauce, and veggies from the full list to build your own combos.

| PROTEIN | SAUCE | GRAIN / BASE | VEGETABLE |
|---|---|---|---|
| **Maple-Chicken Breakfast Patties (page 57)** | Smoky chipotle yogurt sauce (mix ½ cup plain Greek yogurt, 1½ tbsps lime juice, ½ tsp chipotle powder, 1 small garlic clove, ¼ tsp sea salt) | Bone Broth Jasmine Rice (page 198) | Garlic-roasted zucchini (toss sliced zucchini with olive oil, garlic powder, and sea salt; roast at 425°F for 20–25 minutes) |
| **Hard-boiled eggs (boil 8–10 minutes, add to ice bath, peel)** | Pesto (page 141) or chimichurri (page 156) | Roasty Breakfast Potato Hash (page 53) | Sautéed Greens with Lemon and Olive Oil (page 182) |
| **Shredded rotisserie chicken** | Southwest Sauce (page 188) | Cauliflower rice | Chopped onion, celery, and carrots |
| **Canned wild tuna or salmon (drain and mash with lemon and Dijon)** | Dijon and olive oil vinaigrette | Mexican Rice (page 198) | Arugula and cherry tomatoes |
| **Chili Crisp Tofu (page 129)** | Peanut Pad Thai Sauce (page 130) | Rice noodles | Shredded cabbage and bell peppers |

| PROTEIN | SAUCE | GRAIN / BASE | VEGETABLE |
|---|---|---|---|
| **Ground beef or turkey sautéed with onion, garlic, and smoked paprika** | Coconut aminos and garlic (sauté together until fragrant for a quick, savory sauce) | Roasted Japanese Sweet Potatoes (page 183) | Steamed green beans |
| **Grilled chicken thighs (season with salt, pepper, and paprika)** | Herby Tahini Sauce (page 112) | Quinoa | Garlicky Roasted Broccolini (page 183) |
| **Chili-Lime Grilled Steak (page 88)** | Hummus and chili crisp (mix with olive oil to thin out and use as a dressing or sauce) | Farro (page 182) | Grilled onions and peppers |
| **20-Minute Shredded Chicken Verde (page 133)** | Avocado crema (blend 1 ripe avocado with 2 tbsps lime juice, 2 tbsps water, a small garlic clove, and a pinch of salt until smooth) | Cilantro-Lime Rice (page 198) | Fajita-style bell peppers |

# 28-Day Protein Reset

I don't just want to give you recipes—I also want to make it easy—and delicious—for you to increase the amount of protein you eat. I know that sometimes just *deciding* what to make can be an obstacle. The 28-Day Protein Reset takes out all the guesswork, using meals straight from this book to help you build better plates without overthinking it. Make it your own and swap things in, skip around, or follow it to a T if you're ready to go all in.

This is your game plan for building stronger, more satisfying meals without the tracking, counting, and getting caught up in every bite. Just follow the recipes, and you'll naturally start eating more whole foods, feeling fewer cravings, snacking less, staying fuller between meals, and noticing better energy throughout the day. OK, sue me—I'm in too. Let's do this!

**QUICK TIP:** *Leftovers are totally fair game! If you made a bigger batch, feel free to roll it into lunch or dinner the next day.*

| DAY | BREAKFAST / SMOOTHIE | LUNCH | SNACK | DINNER (MAIN + SIDE IF NEEDED) | DESSERT |
|---|---|---|---|---|---|
| **Day 1** | Berry Crumble Yogurt Bowls (page 61) | 5-Minute Pesto Chicken Salad (page 197) | Birthday Cake Bliss Balls (page 234) | Chili-Lime Grilled Steak (page 88) + Roasted Sweet Potatoes with Spiced Chickpeas and Tahini Drizzle (page 202) | Brown Butter–Chocolate Chip Cookies (page 270) |
| **Day 2** | Make-Ahead Coconut-Mango Chia Pudding (page 65) | Italian-Style Chop Salad (page 190) | Savory Cottage Cheese Bowls (page 242) | Buffalo Chicken Baked Tacos (page 148) | Brown Butter–Chocolate Chip Cookies (leftover) |
| **Day 3** | Cinnamon-Apple Protein Pancakes (page 49) | Game-Day Buffalo Chicken Dip (page 237) + veggies (using taco leftovers) | Magic Shell Yogurt Bowl (page 248) | Marry Me Chicken (page 160) + Garlicky Roasted Broccolini (page 183) | Birthday Cake Bliss Balls (leftover) |
| **Day 4** | Make-Ahead Coconut-Mango Chia Pudding (leftover) | Southwest Steak Salad Bowls (page 188) | Birthday Cake Bliss Balls (leftover) | Beef Fried Rice (page 163) | |
| **Day 5** | Honey-Blackberry Overnight Oats (page 50) | Beef Fried Rice (leftover) | Strawberry Shortcake Smoothie (page 75) | Korean Beef with Glass Noodles (page 86) | Fudge Brownies (page 258) |
| **Day 6** | Ready-When-You-Are Breakfast Sandwiches (page 62) | Shredded Chicken Quesadillas (page 138) | Honey-Blackberry Overnight Oats (leftover) | Steak and Chimichurri Baguette Sandwiches (page 99) + Moroccan-Spiced Carrots with Hummus (page 209) | Fudge Brownies (leftover) |
| **Day 7** | Honey-Blackberry Overnight Oats (leftover) | The Rachael Salad (page 206) | Avocado Whipped Feta (page 245) + veggies | Slow Cooker Beef Stew (page 218) | Fudge Brownies (leftover) |

| DAY | BREAKFAST / SMOOTHIE | LUNCH | SNACK | DINNER (MAIN + SIDE IF NEEDED) | DESSERT |
|---|---|---|---|---|---|
| **Day 8** | Ready-When-You-Are Breakfast Sandwiches (page 62) | Slow Cooker Beef Stew (leftover) and/or The Rachael Salad (leftover) | Crispy Ranch Air-Fryer Chickpeas (page 241) | My Weeknight Hero: Ginger-Garlic Turkey Skillet (page 142) + Bone Broth Jasmine Rice (page 198) | Strawberry Cheesecake Pudding (page 273) |
| **Day 9** | Pick-Me-Up Mocha Smoothie (page 72) | Ginger-Garlic Turkey Skillet (leftover) over greens or rice | Raspberry-Vanilla Protein Mug Cake (page 261) | Blackened Shrimp Tacos with Pineapple-Avocado Salsa (page 100) | |
| **Day 10** | Passionberry Smoothie (page 79) | Grilled Summer Pasta Salad (page 201) | Banana Bread Protein Muffins (page 246) | Seasoned Crispy Drumsticks (page 91) + Cheesy Bone Broth Mashed Potatoes (page 210) + Sautéed Greens with Lemon and Olive Oil (page 182) | Sweet and Salty Candy Bark (page 262) |
| **Day 11** | Ready-When-You-Are Breakfast Sandwiches (leftover, or new if needed) | Grilled Summer Pasta Salad (leftover) | Magic Shell Yogurt Bowl (page 248) | Szechuan Chicken Lettuce Wraps (page 107) | Banana Bread Protein Muffins (leftover) |
| **Day 12** | Savory Herb and Turkey-Bacon Quiche (page 46) | Sheet-Pan Greek Chicken and Chickpea Salad (page 212) | Raspberry-Vanilla Protein Mug Cake (page 261) | Honey-Harissa Salmon with Asparagus (page 117) | |
| **Day 13** | Savory Herb and Turkey-Bacon Quiche (leftover) | Sheet-Pan Greek Chicken and Chickpea Salad (leftover) | Super Crispy Chicken Tenders with Homemade BBQ Sauce (page 118) | Philly Cheesesteak-Stuffed Poblanos (page 103) | Sweet and Salty Candy Bark (leftover) |
| **Day 14** | Roasty Breakfast Potato Hash (page 53) | 5-Minute Pesto Chicken Salad (page 197) | Super Crispy Chicken Tenders with Homemade BBQ Sauce (leftover) | Mexican Meatballs in Creamy Enchilada Sauce (page 137) | |

| DAY | BREAKFAST / SMOOTHIE | LUNCH | SNACK | DINNER (MAIN + SIDE IF NEEDED) | DESSERT |
|---|---|---|---|---|---|
| **Day 15** | Everything Bagel Egg Wraps (page 54) | Mexican Meatballs in Creamy Enchilada Sauce (leftover) | Make-Ahead Coconut-Mango Chia Pudding (page 65) | Oven-Baked Beefy Burritos (page 126) | |
| **Day 16** | Make-Ahead Coconut-Mango Chia Pudding (leftover) | Oven-Baked Beefy Burritos (leftover) | Crispy Ranch Air-Fryer Chickpeas (page 241) | Saucy Coconut-Curry Turkey Meatballs (page 122) + Bone Broth Jasmine Rice (page 198) | Sweet and Salty Candy Bark (leftover) |
| **Day 17** | Chorizo-Style Breakfast Tacos (page 58) | Tomato-Basil Chicken with Spaghetti Squash (page 110) | Avocado Whipped Feta (page 245) + veggies | Salsa Verde Shrimp and Rice (page 175) | Sweet and Salty Candy Bark (leftover) |
| **Day 18** | Better-than-a-Bagel-Run Bagels (page 69) | Tomato-Basil Chicken with Spaghetti Squash (leftover) | Magic Shell Yogurt Bowl (page 248) | Double Double-Cheeseburger Bowls (page 179) | |
| **Day 19** | Berry Crumble Yogurt Bowls (page 61) | Tomato-Basil Chicken with Spaghetti Squash (leftover) | Savory Cottage Cheese Bowls (page 242) | Egg Roll in a Bowl (page 171) | Chocolate-Coconut Caramel Tart (page 257) |
| **Day 20** | Passionberry Smoothie (page 79) | Egg Roll in a Bowl (leftover) | Banana Bread Protein Muffins (page 246) | Sloppy Joe Bowls (page 176) | Chocolate-Coconut Caramel Tart (leftover) |
| **Day 21** | Roasty Breakfast Potato Hash (page 53) | 5-Minute Pesto Chicken Salad (page 197) | Birthday Cake Bliss Balls (page 234) | Air-Fryer Garlic-Butter Salmon Bites (page 125) + Sautéed Greens with Lemon and Olive Oil (page 182) | Chocolate-Coconut Caramel Tart (leftover) |
| **Day 22** | Everything Bagel Egg Wraps (page 54) | Sausage, White Bean, and Kale Soup (page 222) | Raspberry-Vanilla Protein Mug Cake (page 261) | Greek-Style Smash Burgers (page 92) | |

| DAY | BREAKFAST / SMOOTHIE | LUNCH | SNACK | DINNER (MAIN + SIDE IF NEEDED) | DESSERT |
|---|---|---|---|---|---|
| **Day 23** | Maple-Chicken Breakfast Patties (page 57) | Sausage, White Bean, and Kale Soup (leftover) | Golden Chicken Bone Broth (page 226) + Crispy Ranch Air-Fryer Chickpeas (page 241) | 20-Minute Shredded Chicken Verde (page 133) | Peppermint Patties (page 266) |
| **Day 24** | Strawberry Shortcake Smoothie (page 75) | 20-Minute Shredded Chicken Verde (leftover) | Savory Cottage Cheese Bowls (page 242) | Sheet-Pan Brats and Potatoes (page 164) | Peppermint Patties (leftover) |
| **Day 25** | Maple-Chicken Breakfast Patties (leftover) | The Rachael Salad (page 206) | Birthday Cake Bliss Balls (page 234) | Chicken and Peanut Pad Thai Bowls (page 130) | Ninja Creami Ice Cream Two Ways (page 234) |
| **Day 26** | Pumpkin Pie Smoothie (page 80) | The Rachael Salad (leftover) | Zucchini Fritters with Lemon-Dill Sauce (page 205) | Slow Cooker Picadillo (page 155) | Ninja Creami Ice Cream Two Ways (page 234) |
| **Day 27** | Roasty Breakfast Potato Hash (page 53) | Slow Cooker Picadillo (leftover) | Golden Chicken Bone Broth (page 226) | Sheet-Pan Turmeric Chicken with Romesco (page 180) + Bone Broth Jasmine Rice (page 198) | Mini Apple Tarts (page 265) |
| **Day 28** | Berry Crumble Yogurt Bowls (page 61) | 5-Minute Pesto Chicken Salad (page 197) | Salted Peanut Butter Cup Smoothie (page 76) | Crispy Lemon-Garlic Chicken Thighs (page 167) + Next-Level Mac and Cheese (page 193) | Mini Apple Tarts (leftover) |

## *How to Use the Recipes*

Each recipe includes a macro breakdown of protein, carbs, and fat per serving. These numbers reflect only the core ingredients—optional toppings, swaps, or sides aren't included to keep things consistent.

You can mix and match recipes based on your needs. If you're tracking closely, plug your full plate into an app like Cronometer or MacrosFirst for detailed breakdowns.

Dietary labels like gluten-free, dairy-free, grain-free, no added sugar, and Paleo are listed at the top of each recipe. These apply to the ingredients as written, so if you make substitutions, just note how they may affect those labels.

Now, let's get cookin'!

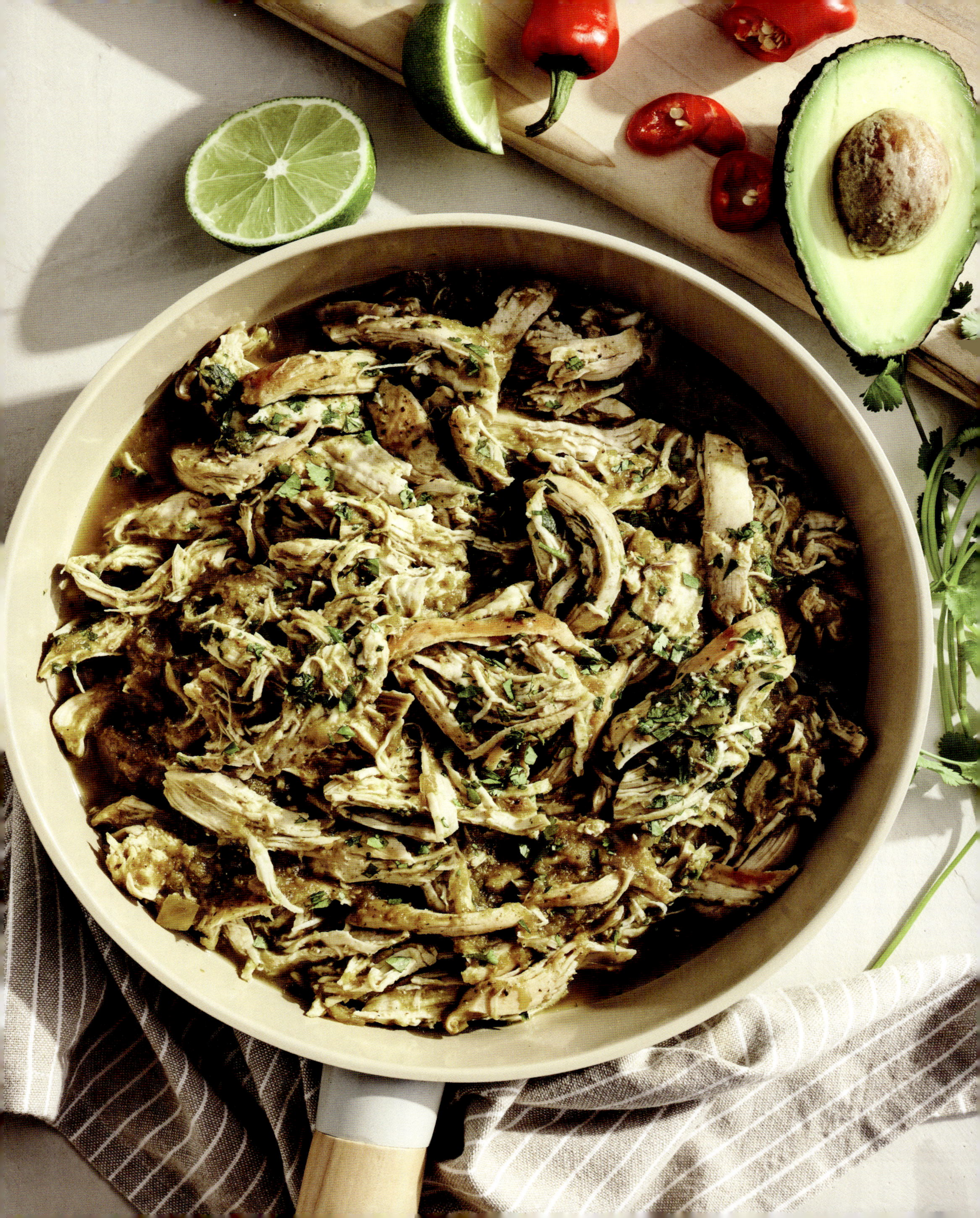

# Breakfast

FIRST THINGS FIRST 45

SMOOTHIES 71

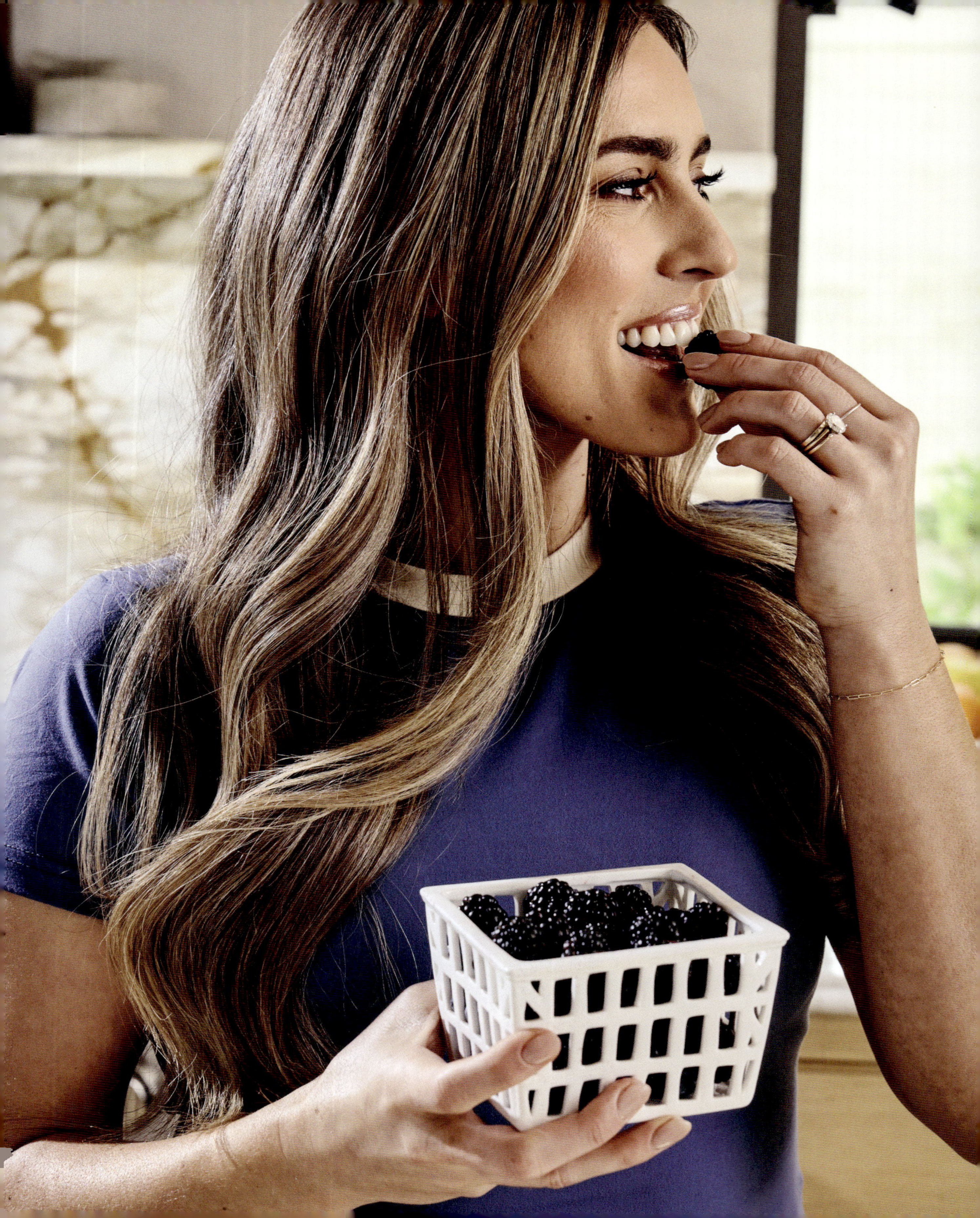

46 Savory Herb and Turkey-Bacon Quiche
49 Cinnamon-Apple Protein Pancakes
50 Honey-Blackberry Overnight Oats
53 Roasty Breakfast Potato Hash
54 Everything Bagel Egg Wraps
57 Maple-Chicken Breakfast Patties
58 Chorizo-Style Breakfast Tacos
61 Berry Crumble Yogurt Bowls
62 Ready-When-You-Are Breakfast Sandwiches
65 Make-Ahead Coconut-Mango Chia Pudding
66 Cheesy Bacon and Chive Egg Muffins
69 Better-than-a-Bagel-Run Bagels

# First Things First

Dairy-Free
Gluten-Free
No Added Sugar

# Savory Herb and Turkey-Bacon Quiche

**SERVES 6 • PREP TIME: 35 MINUTES • COOK TIME: 45 TO 50 MINUTES • TOTAL TIME: 1 HOUR 15 MINUTES**

If you're looking for a show-stopping brunch dish or an easy meal-prep breakfast that actually gets better as the week goes on, this quiche is it. The rosemary-infused crust provides the perfect savory herb touch, and the turkey bacon and cheddar cheese combo is unreal. Use a store-bought crust if you're short on time, swap in Italian sausage for the bacon (if that's what you have on hand or prefer), or load it up with extra veggies—this recipe makes good use of leftovers.

**FOR THE CRUST**

½ cup ghee
3 tablespoons almond milk
1¾ cups gluten-free flour
½ teaspoon sea salt
½ teaspoon baking powder
1 tablespoon fresh rosemary, minced
1 large egg, beaten

**FOR THE FILLING**

6 large eggs
½ cup unsweetened almond milk
1 teaspoon sea salt
½ teaspoon freshly ground black pepper
1 tablespoon avocado oil
6 slices turkey bacon
½ onion, diced
1 red or yellow bell pepper, seeded and diced (about 1 cup; or swap in sliced mushrooms or zucchini)
2 cups packed baby spinach
4 green onions, white and green parts, chopped
1 cup shredded cheddar (or preferred cheese)

1. Preheat the oven to 375°F. Grease a 9-inch pie pan.
2. **Make the crust:** In a small bowl, microwave the ghee for 30 to 60 seconds, until melted. Add the almond milk and set aside.
3. In a medium bowl, whisk together the flour, salt, baking powder, and rosemary. Add the ghee mixture and egg, mixing until the dough holds together when pressed with your fingers.
4. Transfer the dough to the pan and use your fingers to evenly press it onto the bottom and up the sides, ensuring a uniform thickness. Trim any excess dough from the edges.
5. **Make the filling:** Whisk together the eggs, almond milk, salt, and pepper in a medium bowl. Set aside.
6. In a medium skillet, heat the oil over medium heat. Add the bacon and cook for 3 to 4 minutes per side, until crisp. Transfer to a paper towel–lined plate and set aside until cool. Crumble or chop into small pieces.
7. In the same pan, sauté the onion and bell pepper for 4 to 5 minutes, until softened. Add the spinach and green onions and cook for 2 to 3 minutes, until wilted.
8. **Assemble the quiche:** In the pie shell, layer in the veggies, then the bacon, followed by the cheese. Pour the egg mixture over everything and gently smooth out to evenly distribute. Place the pie pan on a baking sheet. Bake for 45 to 50 minutes, until the filling is set. Let cool for 15 minutes before slicing and serving.

---

**PER SERVING**
Protein: 16g
Carbohydrates: 20g
Fat: 23g

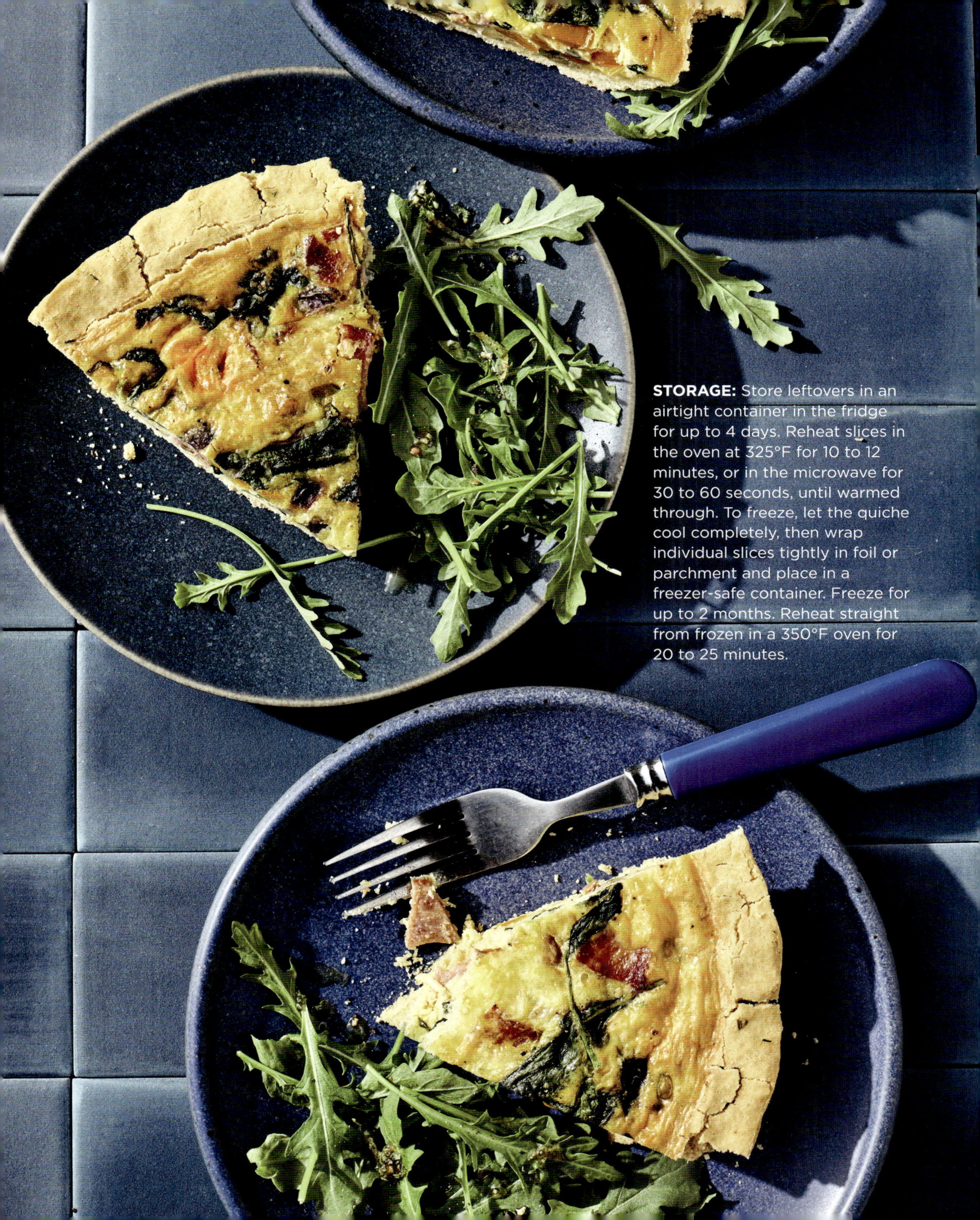

**STORAGE:** Store leftovers in an airtight container in the fridge for up to 4 days. Reheat slices in the oven at 325°F for 10 to 12 minutes, or in the microwave for 30 to 60 seconds, until warmed through. To freeze, let the quiche cool completely, then wrap individual slices tightly in foil or parchment and place in a freezer-safe container. Freeze for up to 2 months. Reheat straight from frozen in a 350°F oven for 20 to 25 minutes.

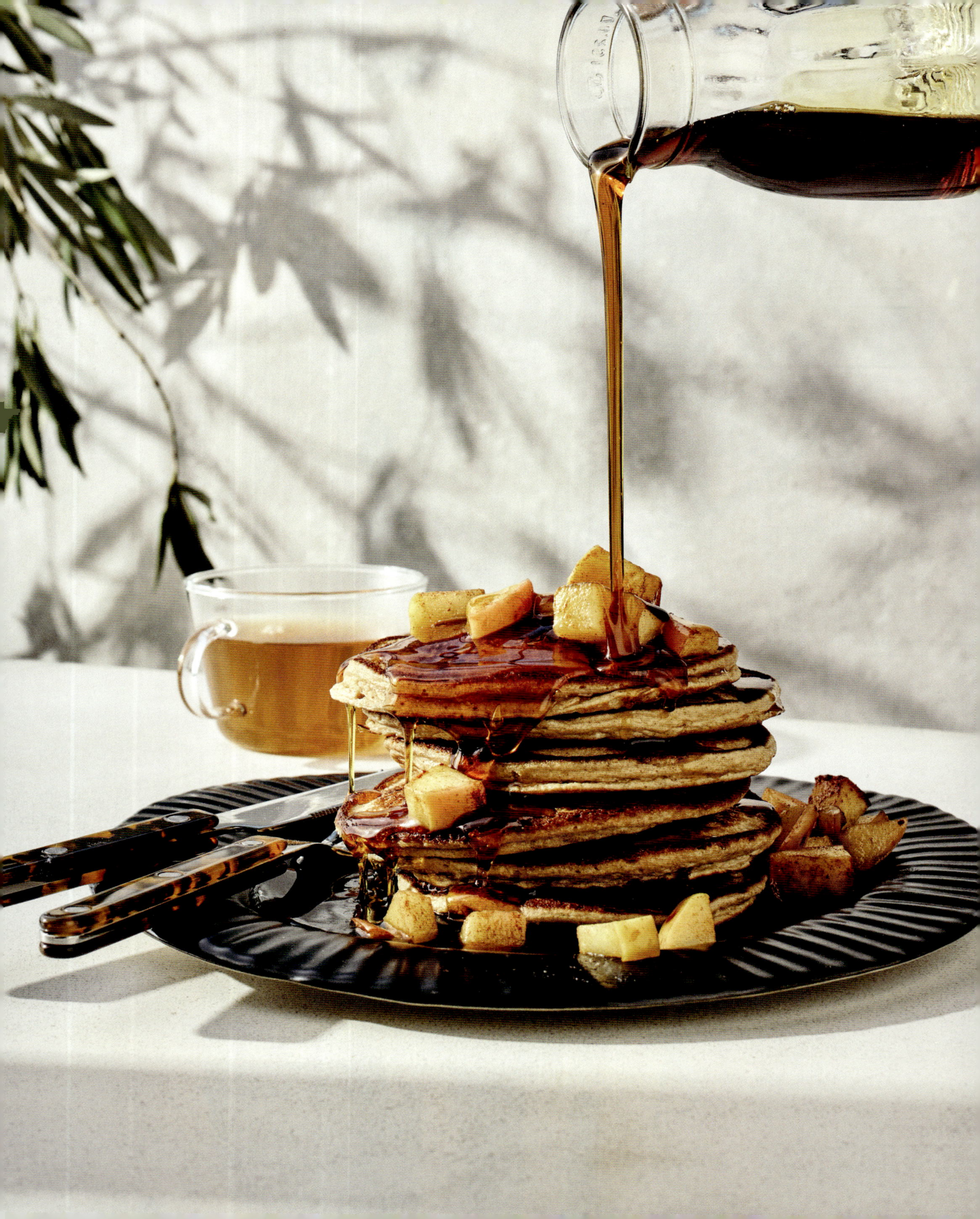

Gluten-Free
**IF MODIFIED:**
Dairy-Free

# Cinnamon-Apple Protein Pancakes

**MAKES 8 TO 10 PANCAKES (2 SERVINGS) • PREP TIME: 10 MINUTES • COOK TIME: 10 MINUTES • TOTAL TIME: 20 MINUTES**

These protein-packed pancakes are light and fluffy and naturally sweetened with apples and a touch of cinnamon—basically, the perfect cozy weekend stack. With fiber-rich oats, omega-loaded hemp seeds, and protein from eggs and cottage cheese, they're a powerhouse meal that actually keeps you full. Bonus: Even kids and picky eaters love them.

**FOR THE PANCAKES**

- 1 cup gluten-free protein oats
- ½ cup applesauce
- 2 large eggs
- ½ cup cottage cheese (for dairy-free, use ⅓ cup vanilla protein powder + ¼ cup almond milk)
- 2 tablespoons hemp seeds
- 1½ teaspoons baking powder
- 1 teaspoon vanilla extract
- 1 teaspoon ground cinnamon
- ¼ teaspoon sea salt

**FOR THE CINNAMON-APPLE TOPPING**

- 2 tablespoons ghee
- 2 crisp apples (such as Fuji), peeled, cored, and diced
- ½ teaspoon ground cinnamon
- Optional toppings: maple syrup, hemp seeds

1. **Make the pancake batter:** In a blender, combine the oats, applesauce, eggs, cottage cheese, hemp seeds, baking powder, vanilla, cinnamon, and salt. Blend for 30 seconds, or until smooth.
2. **Make the cinnamon-apple topping:** Heat a large nonstick skillet over medium-low heat. Melt 1 tablespoon of the ghee, add the apples and cinnamon, and sauté for 5 minutes, stirring occasionally, until the apples soften. Transfer to a small bowl and set aside.
3. **Cook the pancakes:** Wipe out the skillet and return to medium-low heat. Pour in a little bit of the remaining ghee and swirl to coat the pan. Drop ¼-cup portions of the batter into the skillet, spacing them out to avoid overcrowding. Cook for 2 to 3 minutes, until bubbles appear on the surface. Flip and cook for another 2 to 3 minutes, until golden brown. Repeat with the remaining ghee and batter.
4. Serve the pancakes topped with the cinnamon apples, and maple syrup and hemp seeds, if desired.

**STORAGE:** Leftover pancakes will keep in an airtight container in the fridge for up to 3 days or in the freezer for up to 1 month. Reheat in a toaster or skillet for the best texture.

**PER SERVING (4 TO 5 PANCAKES)**
Protein: 25g
Carbohydrates: 50g
Fat: 27g

**MAKE-AHEAD TIP:** *You can prep the topping up to 3 days in advance. Store in an airtight container in the fridge, then quickly reheat in a skillet or microwave before serving. The pancake batter can be blended the night before—just give it a quick stir in the morning before cooking.*

Gluten-Free
**IF MODIFIED:**
Dairy-Free

# Honey-Blackberry Overnight Oats

**SERVES 4 • PREP TIME: 15 MINUTES, PLUS 4 HOURS CHILLING • TOTAL TIME: 4 HOURS 15 MINUTES**

- 2 cups gluten-free protein oats
- 2¼ cups unsweetened almond milk
- ¾ cup vanilla protein powder
- ¼ cup hemp seeds
- 3 tablespoons chia seeds
- ½ cup unsweetened plain Greek yogurt (or coconut yogurt for dairy-free)
- 1 teaspoon vanilla extract
- 1 tablespoon honey, plus more for topping
- ½ teaspoon ground cinnamon
- 3 cups frozen blackberries
- ½ cup slivered almonds, or coarsely chopped pecans or walnuts
- 2 tablespoons almond butter, for topping

Starting your morning with 35 grams of protein gives you a major leg up on the day. During postpartum, this was my hack for making sure I had breakfast ready *STAT*—no thinking required. I'd grab a jar straight from the fridge while holding Hayes, and just like that, I had fuel for the next few hours. I'm a sucker for the honey-berry-oat flavor combo—it's sweet, tart, and comforting all at once, making it perfect any time of year. And you can level it up even more with a higher-protein yogurt like skyr if you like.

1. In a large bowl, combine the oats, almond milk, protein powder, hemp seeds, chia seeds, yogurt, vanilla, honey, and cinnamon. Mix well to combine.
2. Gather four clean 16-ounce jars with tight-fitting lids. In each jar, place 2 tablespoons blackberries on the bottom. Divide the oat mixture evenly among the jars, then top each with 3 more tablespoons blackberries, 2 tablespoons nuts, a drizzle of honey, and 1/2 tablespoon almond butter.
3. Seal the jars and store in the fridge to allow the oats to thicken for at least 4 hours, or up to overnight. Enjoy chilled, straight from the fridge.

---

**PER SERVING**
Protein: 35g
Carbohydrates: 50g
Fat: 22g

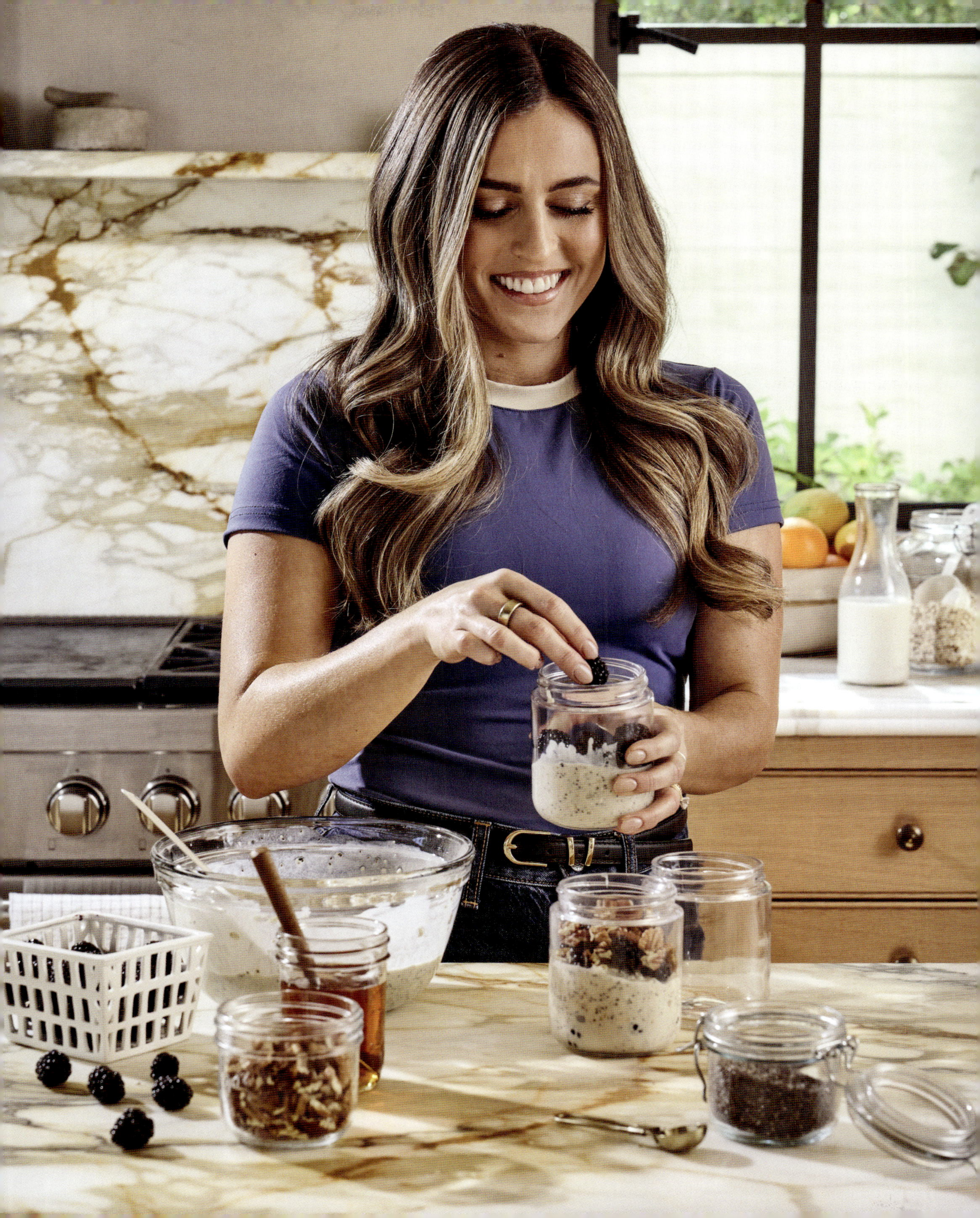

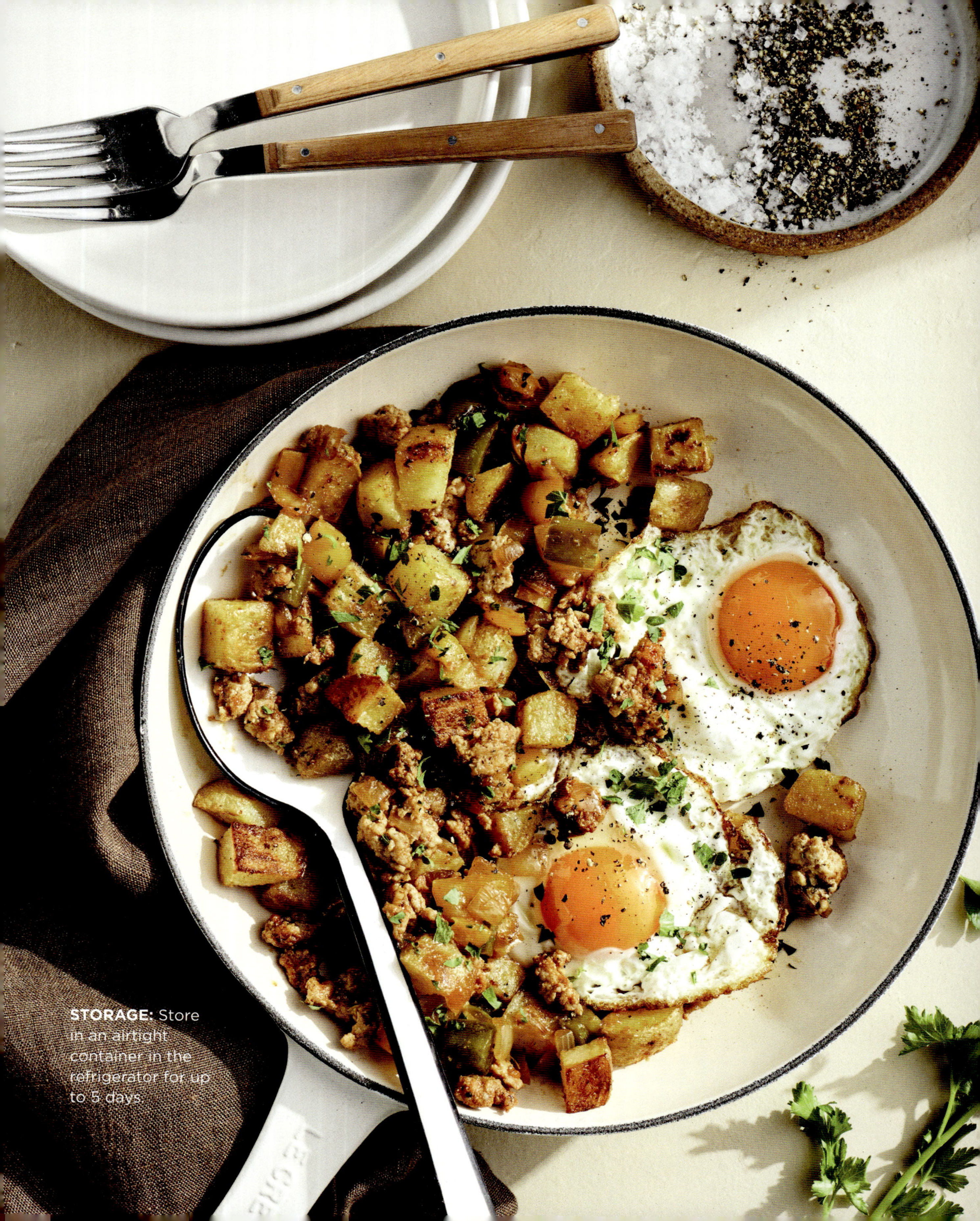

**STORAGE:** Store in an airtight container in the refrigerator for up to 5 days.

Dairy-Free
Gluten-Free
Grain-Free
No Added Sugar
Paleo

# Roasty Breakfast Potato Hash

**SERVES 4 • PREP TIME: 10 MINUTES • COOK TIME: 35 MINUTES • TOTAL TIME: 45 MINUTES**

Golden, crispy potatoes meet perfectly seasoned ground chicken, sweet peppers, and caramelized onions in this hearty breakfast hash. It's the kind of dish that feels like something you'd order at your regular brunch spot, but it's incredibly easy to whip up at home—and almost definitely has more protein than what you'd get at a restaurant. Enjoy the hash on its own or topped with a fried egg—or wrap it up in a warm tortilla for the ultimate breakfast burrito.

**FOR THE POTATOES**

5 cups diced potatoes (Yukon Golds or russets work best)
1 tablespoon avocado oil
1½ teaspoons garlic powder
1½ teaspoons onion powder
1 teaspoon sea salt

**FOR THE HASH**

1½ tablespoons extra-virgin olive oil
1 large green bell pepper, seeded and diced (or sub sliced zucchini, mushrooms, or red onion)
1 large yellow bell pepper, seeded and diced
1 medium yellow onion, diced
1 pound ground chicken
1 teaspoon dried oregano
1 teaspoon smoked paprika
1 teaspoon garlic powder
½ teaspoon onion powder
½ teaspoon chili powder (optional)
1 teaspoon sea salt, or to taste
½ teaspoon freshly ground black pepper
2 tablespoons chopped fresh parsley or cilantro, for garnish
Hot sauce, for garnish (optional)

1. Preheat the oven to 425°F. Line a baking sheet with parchment paper.
2. **Make the potatoes:** On the baking sheet, toss the potatoes with the avocado oil, garlic powder, onion powder, and salt until evenly coated. Spread the potatoes in a single layer. Roast for 30 to 35 minutes, flipping halfway through, until golden brown and crispy. Set aside.
3. **Make the hash:** Meanwhile, in a large skillet, heat 1 tablespoon of the olive oil over medium heat. Add the green bell pepper, yellow bell pepper, and onion and sauté for 5 to 7 minutes, stirring occasionally, until softened and slightly caramelized. Push the sautéed vegetables to the perimeter of the skillet.
4. Add the remaining ½ tablespoon olive oil to the skillet, then add the ground chicken, oregano, paprika, garlic powder, onion powder, chili powder (if using), salt, and pepper. Cook for 6 to 8 minutes, breaking up the chicken with a spatula, until it is browned and fully cooked through. Stir the vegetables and chicken together, mixing well.
5. Add the roasted potatoes and stir to combine, then cook for 2 to 3 minutes, until heated through. Garnish with parsley and a dash of hot sauce, if using. Serve warm.

### *To Reheat:*

- **STOVETOP:** Heat 1 tablespoon olive oil in a large skillet over medium heat. Add the hash and cook for 4 to 5 minutes, stirring occasionally, until heated through and crispy.
- **OVEN:** Preheat the oven to 375°F. Spread the hash on a parchment-lined baking sheet and bake for 10 to 12 minutes, until warmed through and slightly crisp.

**PER SERVING**
Protein: 30g
Carbohydrates: 40g
Fat: 14g

Gluten-Free
Grain-Free
No Added Sugar

# Everything Bagel Egg Wraps

**SERVES 2 • PREP TIME: 5 MINUTES •COOK TIME: 10 MINUTES • TOTAL TIME: 15 MINUTES**

- 4 large eggs
- ½ cup full-fat cottage cheese
- 2 teaspoons everything bagel seasoning
- 1 tablespoon avocado oil
- 2 large tortillas (I prefer Siete brand for a grain-free option)
- 2 ounces smoked wild salmon or 1 slice cooked turkey bacon
- 1 Persian cucumber, thinly sliced
- ½ avocado, thinly sliced

If you love everything bagels but want something lighter and higher in protein, this wrap's your move. Eggs whipped with protein-rich cottage cheese turn fluffy and flavorful, then get wrapped into a tortilla for that perfect soft-yet-toasty bite. Smoked salmon, avocado, and crisp cucumber bring freshness and healthy fats, making this the kind of breakfast (or lunch) you'll want on repeat.

1. In a medium bowl, whisk together the eggs, cottage cheese, and everything bagel seasoning.
2. In a medium nonstick skillet over medium-high heat, heat ½ tablespoon of the oil. Add half the egg mixture, swirling to coat the bottom of the pan, and cook for 1 to 2 minutes, until just set. Place a tortilla directly on top of the eggs and let sit for 30 seconds. Carefully flip the entire egg-tortilla layer so the tortilla is now on the bottom and cook for another 2 to 3 minutes, until the tortilla is toasted and the egg is fully set. Remove from the heat and transfer to a plate. Top with half of the smoked salmon, cucumber, and avocado, then roll up into a wrap.
3. Repeat with the remaining ½ tablespoon oil, the egg mixture, tortilla, and toppings to make the second wrap. Serve immediately.

**PER SERVING**
Protein: 31g
Carbohydrates: 17g
Fat: 34g

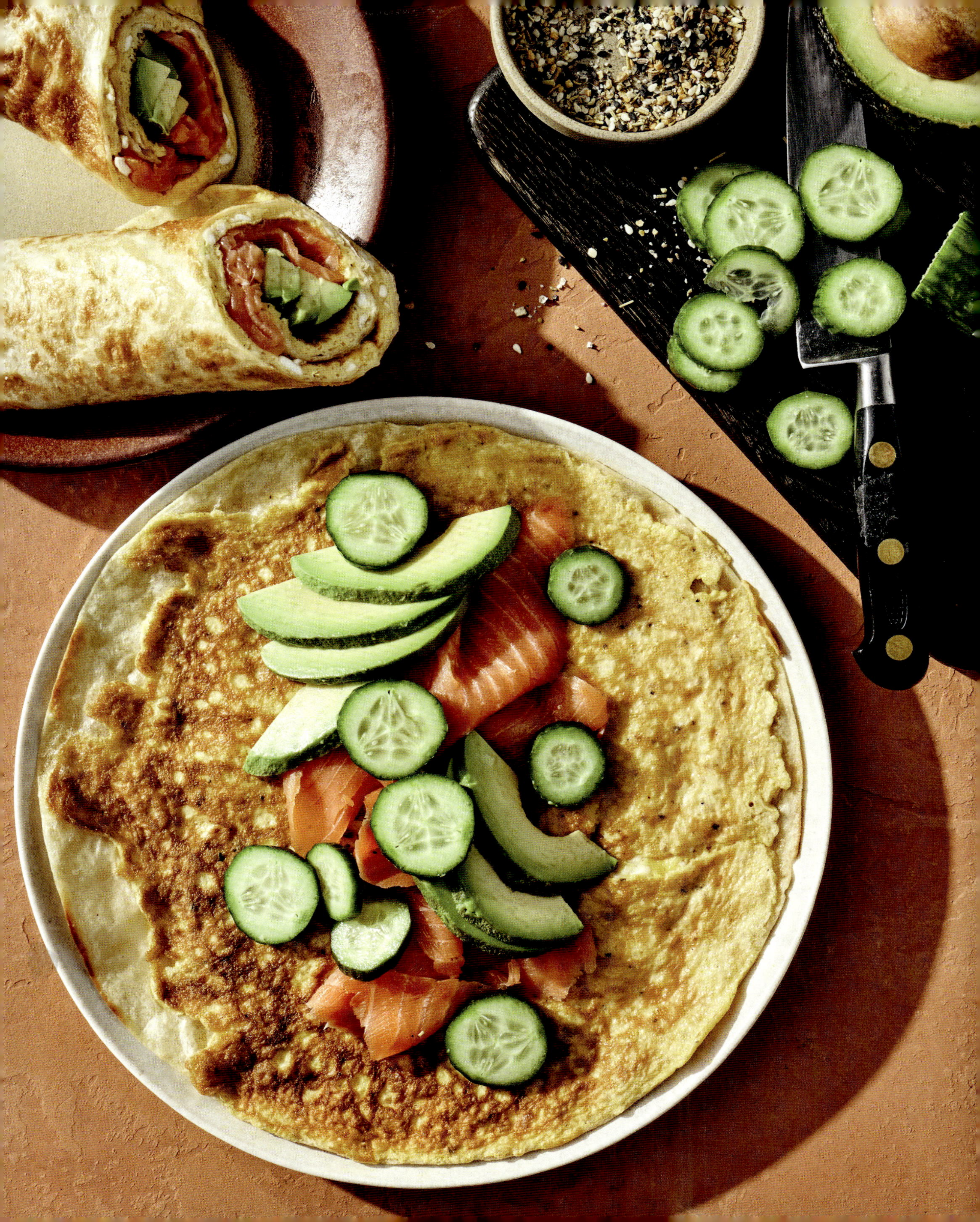

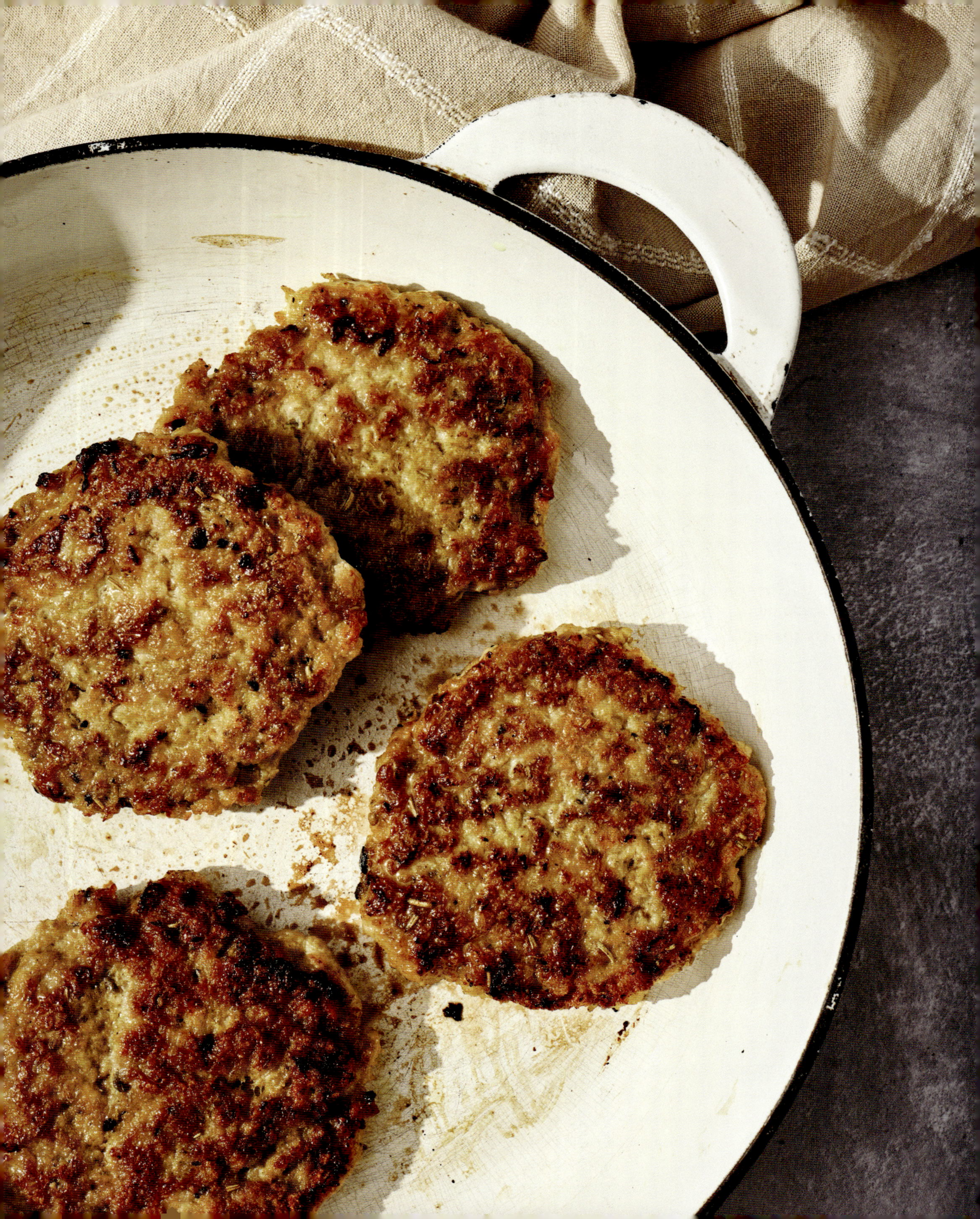

Dairy-Free
Gluten-Free
Grain-Free

# Maple-Chicken Breakfast Patties

**MAKES 18 PATTIES (9 SERVINGS) • PREP TIME: 15 MINUTES • COOK TIME: 20 MINUTES • TOTAL TIME: 35 MINUTES**

- 2 pounds ground chicken
- ¼ cup maple syrup
- 1½ tablespoons dried rosemary, minced
- 2 teaspoons garlic powder
- 2 teaspoons onion powder
- 2 teaspoons Himalayan pink salt
- 1½ teaspoons dried oregano
- ½ teaspoon ground cinnamon
- ½ teaspoon ground turmeric
- ¼ teaspoon freshly ground black pepper
- 3 tablespoons extra-virgin olive oil or avocado oil
- Flaky salt, for garnish

This recipe was born from my addiction to store-bought sausage patties. I ate them for months and months before it finally hit me . . . why not just make my own? But bigger, better (with simple ingredients and no weird preservatives), and in batches I could refrigerate or freeze for the weeks ahead. Now, I can grab a couple for a quick breakfast, or pair one with a few fried eggs and avocado and layer it all into a breakfast sandwich (check out Ready-When-You-Are Breakfast Sandwiches on page 62). Either way, they give me the protein I want in the morning. My family also loves them as part of a big breakfast spread, or just on-the-go.

1. In a medium bowl, use a fork to break up the ground chicken and combine it with the maple syrup, rosemary, garlic powder, onion powder, pink salt, oregano, cinnamon, turmeric, and pepper. Mix gently until well incorporated.
2. Using gloves or wet hands, measure out 2 to 3 tablespoons of the meat mixture and form a ½-inch-thick patty. Repeat to make about 18 patties.
3. In a large skillet over medium heat, heat 1 tablespoon of the oil. Add enough patties to fill the skillet without overcrowding and cook for 4 to 5 minutes, until golden brown. Flip and cook for 4 to 5 minutes more, until the internal temperature reaches 165°F. You can cover the skillet with a lid to speed up cooking.
4. Repeat with the remaining patties, adding more oil as needed. Serve immediately, topped with flaky salt.

**STORAGE:** Store cooked patties in an airtight container in the fridge for up to 5 days. To freeze, let them cool completely, then place individual patties between parchment and store in a freezer-safe bag or container for up to 2 months. To reheat, warm chilled patties in a skillet over medium heat for 2 to 3 minutes per side. For frozen patties, either thaw overnight in the fridge or cook directly from frozen in a skillet over medium-low heat for 4 to 5 minutes per side, until heated through. You can also reheat frozen patties in a 350°F oven for 10 to 12 minutes.

**PER SERVING (2 PATTIES)**
Protein: 26g
Carbohydrates: 6g
Fat: 9g

Dairy-Free
Gluten-Free
Grain-Free
No Added Sugar

# Chorizo-Style Breakfast Tacos

**SERVES 4 • PREP TIME: 10 MINUTES • COOK TIME: 10 MINUTES • TOTAL TIME: 20 MINUTES**

- 1 pound ground turkey (light or dark meat)
- 1 tablespoon apple cider vinegar
- 1 teaspoon smoked paprika
- 1 teaspoon dried oregano
- ½ teaspoon chili powder
- ½ teaspoon ground cumin
- ½ teaspoon garlic powder
- ¼ teaspoon ground cinnamon
- 1 teaspoon sea salt
- ½ teaspoon freshly ground black pepper
- 1 tablespoon avocado oil
- 5 ounces baby spinach, chopped
- 6 large eggs, beaten
- 1 package 6-inch tortillas (I prefer Siete brand for a grain-free option), warmed
- Optional toppings: sliced avocado, pico de gallo, sour cream, hot sauce

These breakfast tacos bring all the smoky, bold flavors of chorizo sausage, but without the extra grease. A mix of lean ground turkey, warm spices, and just the right kick of heat makes them lighter than a usual sausage taco so you won't feel weighed down after breakfast. Best of all, the tacos come together pretty quickly, which makes them great for weekday mornings. Load them up with avocado and pico de gallo or a drizzle of hot sauce, and suddenly breakfast feels like your favorite taco spot.ß

1. In a medium bowl, combine the ground turkey, vinegar, paprika, oregano, chili powder, cumin, garlic powder, cinnamon, salt, and pepper. Mix until well combined.
2. In a large skillet, heat the oil over medium heat. Add the spiced turkey, breaking it up with a spatula, and cook for 6 to 8 minutes, until browned and just cooked through.
3. Add the spinach and cook for 1 to 2 minutes, until wilted. Add the eggs and cook for 1 to 2 minutes, stirring occasionally, until the eggs are almost set. Remove from the heat.
4. Serve the eggs in warm tortillas, topped with your choice of avocado, pico de gallo, sour cream, and/or hot sauce.

---

**PER SERVING**
Protein: 33g
Carbohydrates: 14g
Fat: 19g

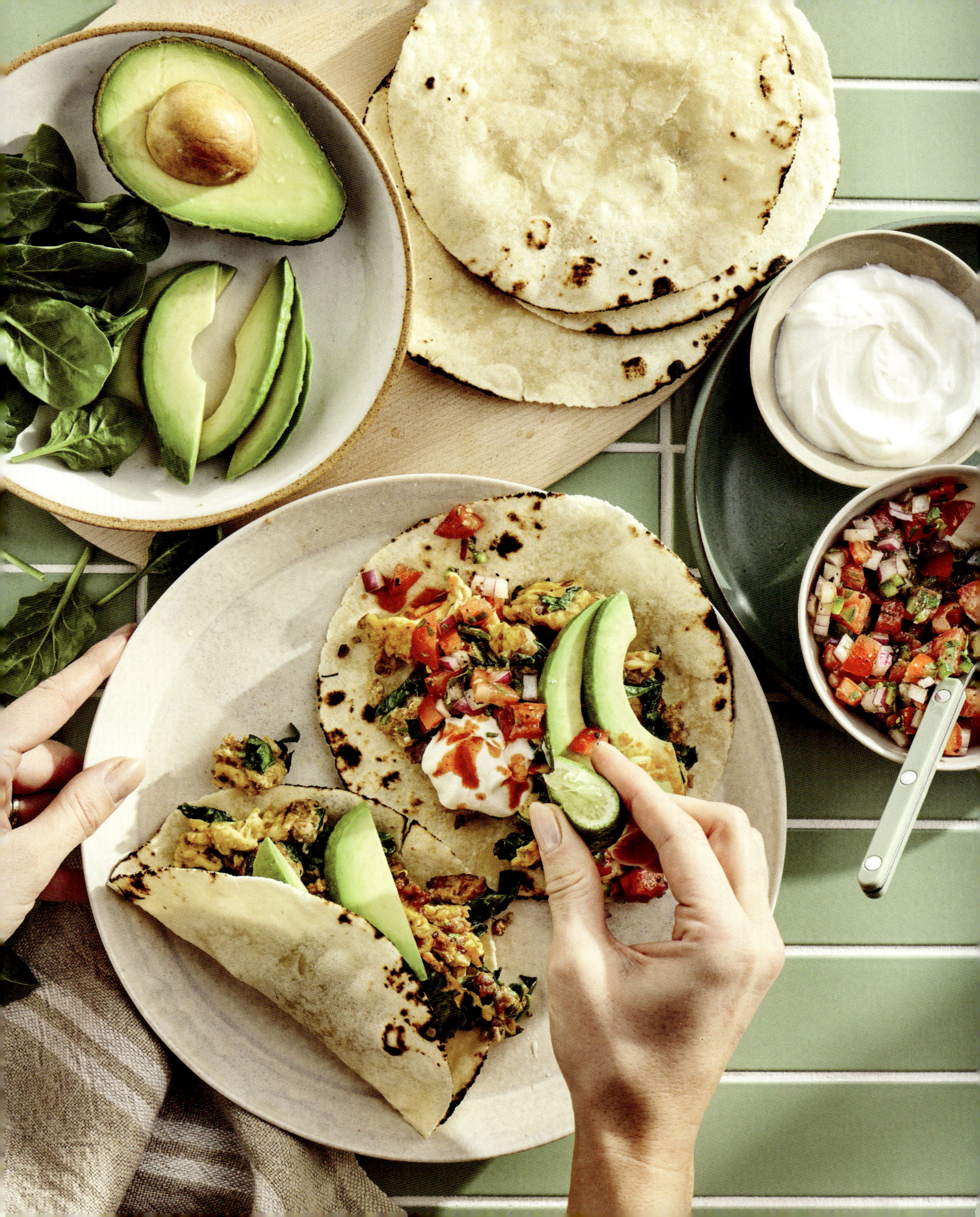

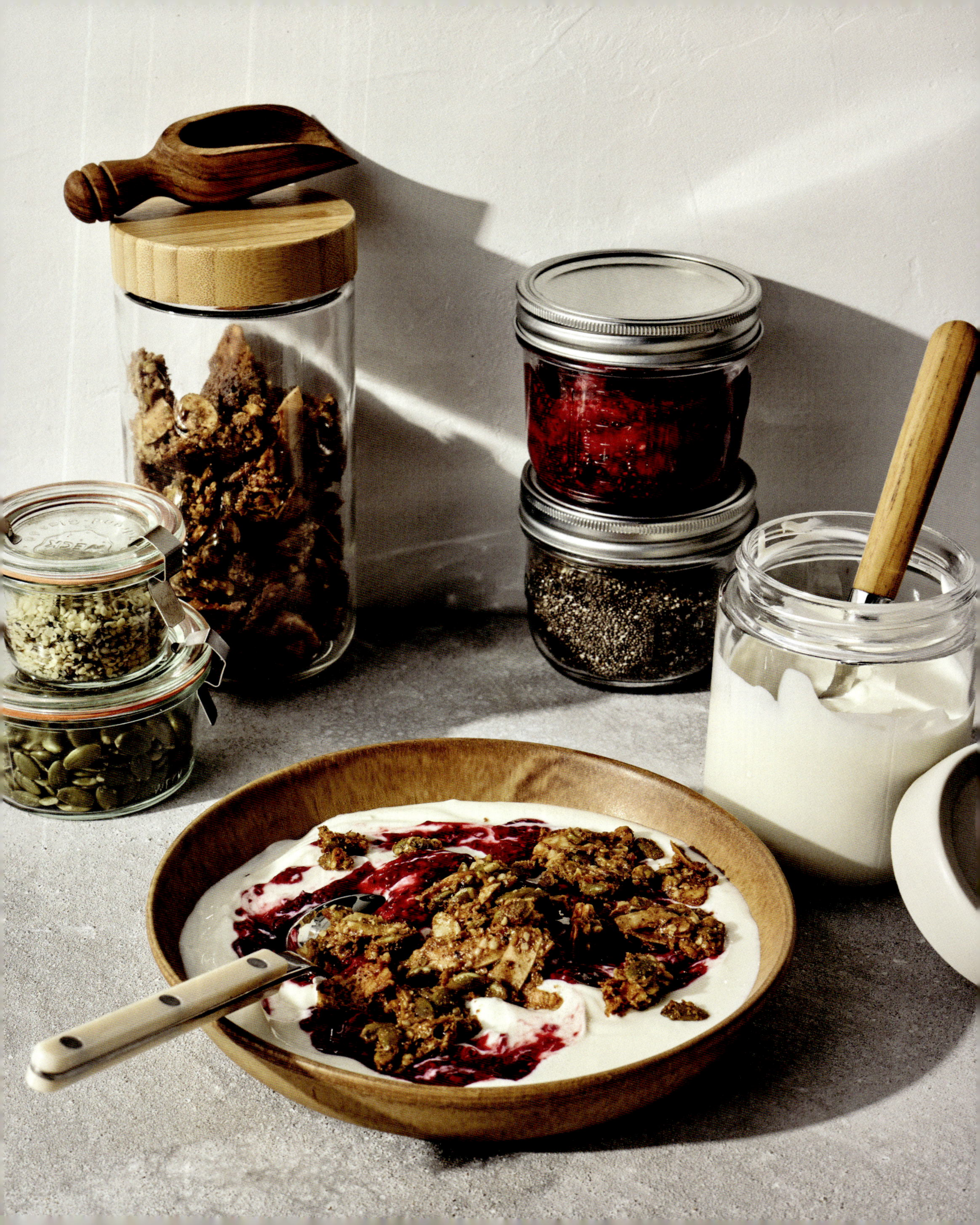

Gluten-Free
Grain-Free
**IF MODIFIED:**
Dairy-Free
No Added Sugar

# Berry Crumble Yogurt Bowls

SERVES 2 (WITH LEFTOVER GRANOLA AND JAM) • PREP TIME: 10 MINUTES • COOK TIME: 20 MINUTES, PLUS 20 MINUTES COOLING • TOTAL TIME: 50 MINUTES

When I need a break from eggs, I switch to yogurt and granola. The trick to making it filling—especially with dairy-free yogurt—is to stir in a scoop of protein powder you love. You can also use Greek yogurt, skyr, or a protein-rich plant-based option for something extra filling. This grain-free granola is crunchy, full of flavor, and makes the perfect no-added-sugar snack too. **Pro tip:** Make a batch of granola (and some jam) ahead of time so you can throw this bowl together in seconds.

FOR THE GRANOLA

¾ cup sliced almonds
½ cup coconut flakes
½ cup pistachios, coarsely chopped
⅓ cup creamy unsweetened almond butter (or preferred nut butter)
⅓ cup pumpkin seeds (often labeled "pepitas")
⅓ cup hemp seeds
2 tablespoons coconut oil, melted
2 tablespoons maple syrup (omit for no added sugar option)
1 teaspoon vanilla extract
½ teaspoon ground cinnamon
¼ teaspoon sea salt

FOR THE JAM

2 cups mixed berries
1 tablespoon chia seeds
1 tablespoon freshly squeezed lemon juice
1 teaspoon vanilla extract
Maple syrup or raw honey (optional)

FOR THE YOGURT BOWLS

2 cups plain Greek yogurt (or coconut yogurt for dairy-free)
1 serving vanilla protein powder

1. **Make the granola:** Preheat the oven to 325°F. Line a baking sheet with parchment paper.
2. In a medium bowl, combine the almonds, coconut, pistachios, almond butter, pumpkin seeds, hemp seeds, coconut oil, maple syrup, vanilla, cinnamon, and salt. Mix until well combined.
3. Spread the mixture onto the baking sheet, pressing it flat. Bake for 20 minutes, or until golden. Let cool for 20 minutes, then break into crumbles and set aside.
4. **Make the jam:** In a medium saucepan over medium heat, cook the berries, stirring occasionally, for 5 minutes, until bubbling and beginning to break down.
5. Stir in the chia seeds, lemon juice, and vanilla. If you'd like it a bit sweeter, stir in up to 1 tablespoon maple syrup or honey. Remove from the heat and let cool for 10 minutes to thicken.
6. In a bowl, mix the yogurt and protein powder until smooth. Top with berry jam and granola.

**STORAGE:** Store leftover jam in an airtight container in the fridge for up to 1 week. Keep leftover granola in an airtight container at room temperature or in the fridge for up to 1 week.

---

**PER SERVING**
Protein: 48g
Carbohydrates: 40g
Fat: 51g

**IF MODIFIED:**
Dairy-Free
Gluten-Free

# Ready-When-You-Are Breakfast Sandwiches

**SERVES 12 • PREP TIME: 20 MINUTES • COOK TIME: 18 MINUTES • TOTAL TIME: 38 MINUTES**

- 2 tablespoons extra-virgin olive oil
- 1 bell pepper, seeded and diced (or sub sliced mushrooms, zucchini, or red onion—whatever you've got on hand)
- 4 cups baby spinach, coarsely chopped
- 12 large eggs
- ¼ cup almond milk
- 1 teaspoon garlic powder
- 1½ teaspoons sea salt
- 1 teaspoon freshly ground black pepper
- ¾ cup pesto
- 12 English muffins (gluten-free if preferred)
- 12 Maple-Chicken Breakfast Patties (page 57)
- 12 slices cheddar (or dairy-free cheese of choice)
- Hot sauce, for topping (optional)

We all love a good breakfast sandwich—they're portable and make waking up so much more worth it. The recipe makes 12 sandwiches—that's 12 potential breakfasts (or snacks) you don't have to think about, which makes life feel a little less chaotic. Even better, the eggs bake on a sheet pan, making them a cinch to batch up.

1. Preheat the oven to 350°F. Grease a 13 x 9-inch rimmed baking sheet with 1 tablespoon of the oil.
2. In a large skillet, heat the remaining 1 tablespoon oil over medium-high heat. Add the bell pepper and sauté for 2 to 3 minutes, until softened. Add the spinach and cook for 1 to 2 minutes, until wilted. Remove from the heat and set aside.
3. In a large bowl, whisk together the eggs, almond milk, garlic powder, salt, and pepper. Add the cooked veggies to the egg mixture and stir to combine.
4. Pour the egg mixture into the baking sheet. Bake for 15 to 18 minutes, until set. Set aside to cool, then cut into 12 squares.
5. To assemble, spread 1 tablespoon pesto on the bottom half of each English muffin. Layer with an egg square, a sausage patty, and a slice of cheese. Place the top halves of the muffins over the fillings and wrap each sandwich in foil.

**STORAGE:** Store the wrapped sandwiches in the fridge for up to 5 days, or freeze for up to 1 month.

### *To Reheat:*

FROM THE FRIDGE

- **OVEN:** Keep wrapped in foil and bake at 350°F for 10 to 15 minutes.
- **MICROWAVE:** Unwrap from foil, wrap in a paper towel, and microwave on defrost (50% power) for 40 to 60 seconds; flip and heat on high for 10 to 30 seconds.

---

**PER SERVING**
Protein: 32g
Carbohydrates: 36g
Fat: 30g

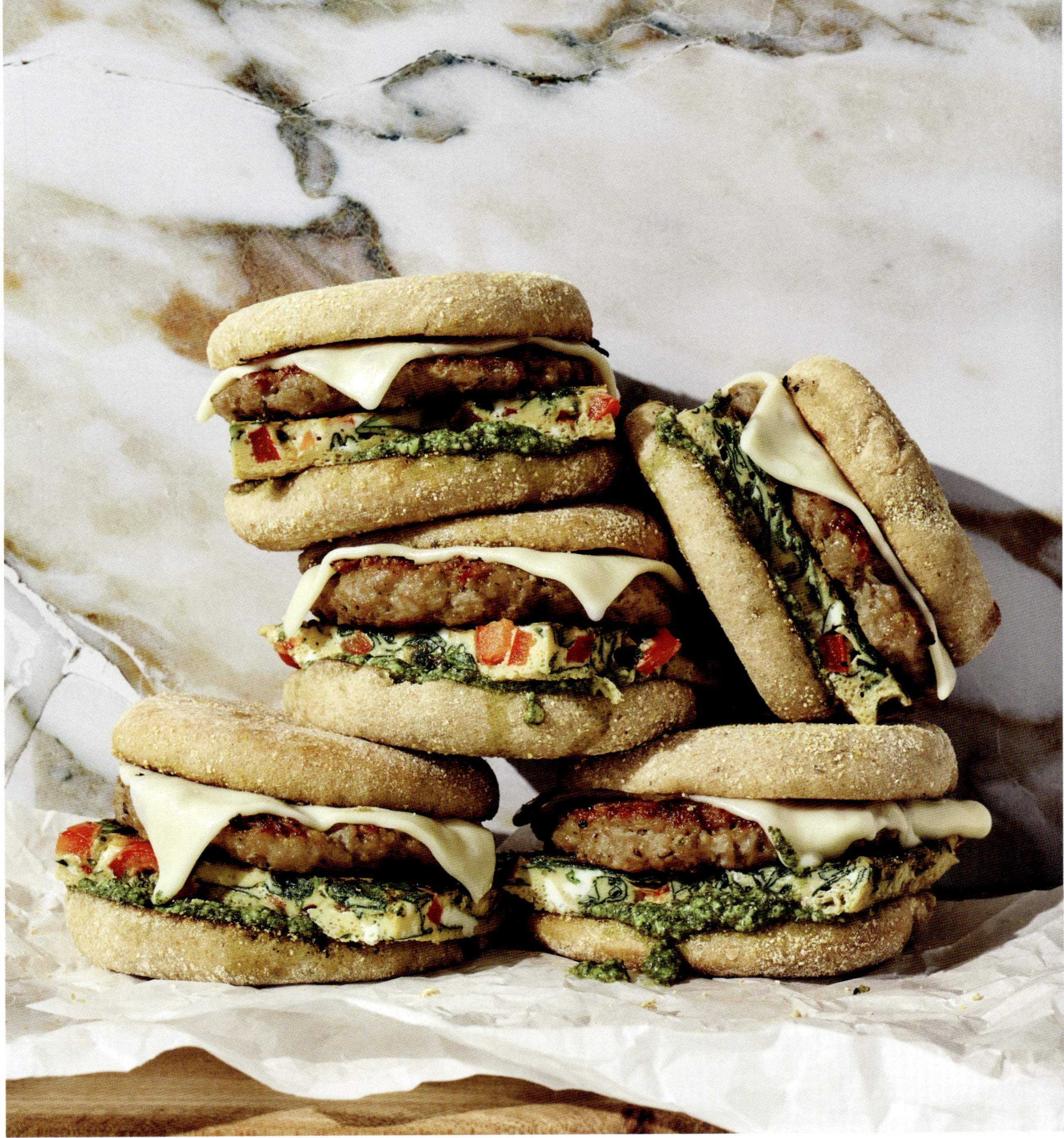

FROM THE FREEZER

- **OVEN:** Unwrap, place on a baking sheet, and bake at 350°F for 30 minutes.
- **MICROWAVE:** Unwrap, wrap in a paper towel, defrost for 1 minute; flip and heat on high for 10 to 30 seconds.
- **AIR FRYER:** Separate the components and air-fry at 350°F—6 to 8 minutes for the egg and sausage and 3 to 5 minutes for the muffin and cheese; reassemble and enjoy.

**TIP:** *For even reheating, thaw overnight in the fridge or separate components when reheating from frozen.*

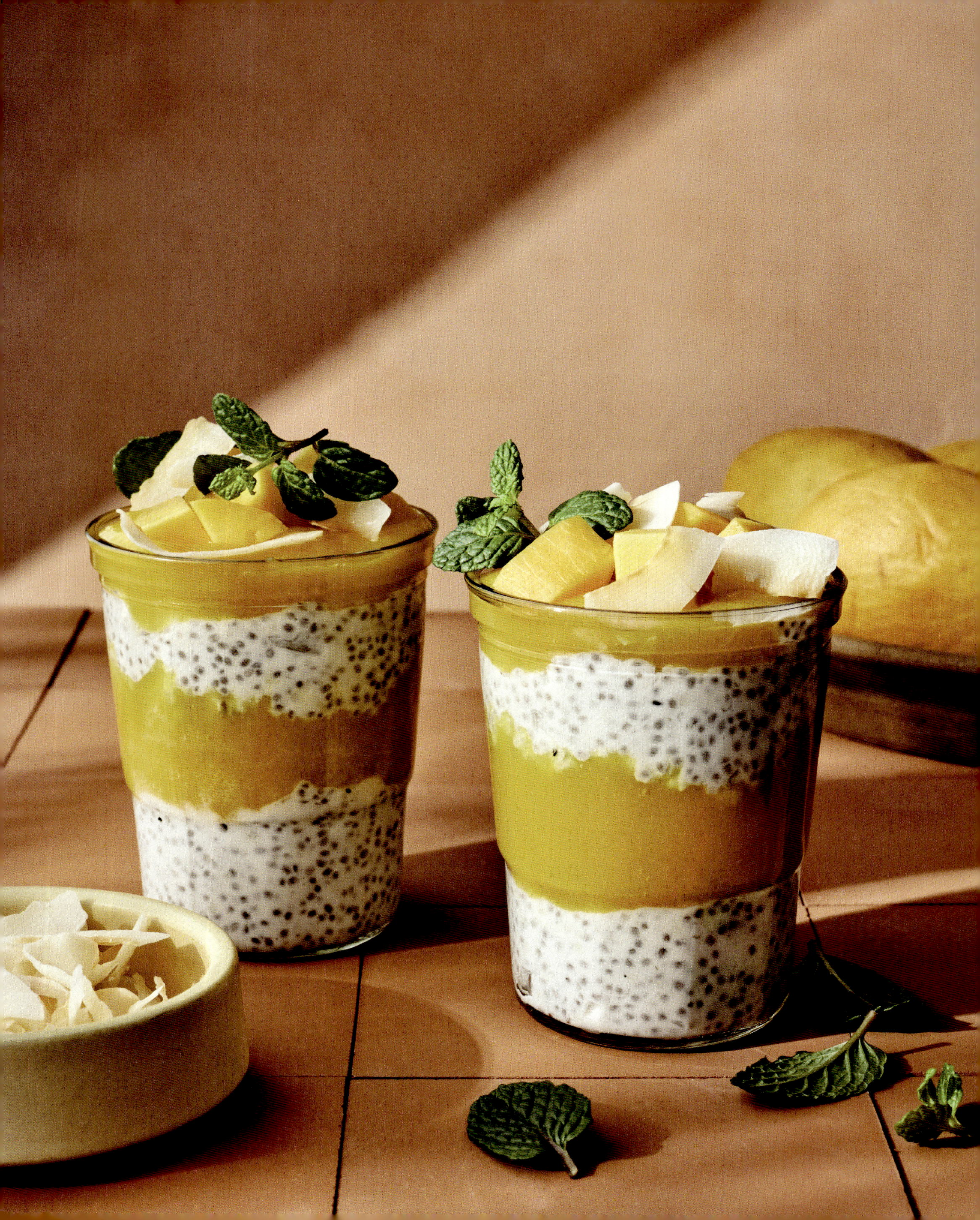

Dairy-Free
Gluten-Free
Grain-Free

# Make-Ahead Coconut-Mango Chia Pudding

**SERVES 2 • PREP TIME: 15 MINUTES • CHILL TIME: 30 MINUTES • TOTAL TIME: 45 MINUTES**

**FOR THE MANGO PUREE**

1 large ripe mango, coarsely chopped

1 teaspoon maple syrup

Juice of ½ lemon

Pinch of sea salt

**FOR THE CHIA PUDDING**

1 (13.5- to 14-ounce) can unsweetened full-fat coconut milk

⅓ cup unsweetened almond milk

1 tablespoon maple syrup

1 teaspoon vanilla extract

½ cup vanilla protein powder

¼ cup chia seeds

3 tablespoons hemp seeds

**FOR THE TOPPINGS**

1 large ripe mango, diced

3 tablespoons unsweetened coconut flakes

Fresh mint leaves, torn or chopped, for garnish

When I first tasted a version of this pudding at Cavallo Point Lodge in the Bay Area I knew I had to re-create it. Light, creamy, and just sweet enough, it's made with coconut milk, mango puree, and a mix of chia and hemp seeds for the perfect balance of flavor and function. Prep it the night before and wake up to something that tastes like a mini vacation.

1. **Make the mango puree:** In a blender, combine the mango, maple syrup, lemon juice, and salt. Blend on high until smooth. Set aside.
2. **Make the chia pudding:** Rinse the blender, then add the coconut milk, almond milk, maple syrup, vanilla, and protein powder and blend until smooth. In a medium airtight container, combine the milk mixture with the chia seeds and hemp seeds. Whisk well, then refrigerate for 30 minutes to 1 hour, until thickened.
3. In two 12- to 16-ounce jars (or larger), layer the chia pudding and mango puree, repeating the layers once more to fill the jars. Just before serving, top with diced mango, coconut, and mint.

**STORAGE:** Store parfaits (without toppings) in the fridge for up to 1 week. Add toppings just before serving for best texture and freshness.

---

**PER SERVING**
Protein: 33g
Carbohydrates: 51g
Fat: 39g

Gluten-Free
Grain-Free
No Added Sugar

# Cheesy Bacon and Chive Egg Muffins

**MAKES 12 EGG MUFFINS (6 SERVINGS) • PREP TIME: 15 MINUTES • COOK TIME: 30 MINUTES • TOTAL TIME: 45 MINUTES**

**Avocado oil spray**
**12 slices bacon (pork or turkey)**
**8 large eggs**
**¼ cup full-fat cottage cheese**
**½ teaspoon sea salt**
**½ teaspoon freshly ground black pepper**
**1 bell pepper, seeded and finely diced (sliced mushrooms, zucchini, or red onion all work great here too)**
**1½ cups shredded cheddar cheese (or preferred cheese)**
**1½ tablespoons minced chives, plus extra for topping**

If there's one thing I love, it's a good fast-food glow-up. These savory egg muffins deliver all the flavors of a classic bacon, egg, and cheese—but in a better-for-you, protein-packed version. Crispy bacon, melty cheese, and fresh chives make every bite super satisfying, while the eggs and cottage cheese keep things light and fluffy. Plus, the recipe is perfect for meal prepping because you can make the muffins ahead of time: make a batch, stash in the fridge or freezer, and you've got an easy, grab-and-go breakfast ready whenever you need one. Just reheat and enjoy!

1. Position one rack in the center of the oven and one directly below it. Fill a rimmed baking sheet with ½ cup water and place on the bottom rack to create steam. Preheat the oven to 300°F. Spray a 12-cup muffin tin with avocado oil.
2. Heat a large skillet over medium heat. Cook the bacon for 8 to 12 minutes, until crisp. Set aside to cool, then crumble or chop into small pieces.
3. In a blender, combine the eggs, cottage cheese, salt, and pepper and blend until smooth. (Alternatively, you can whisk together in a large bowl.)
4. Divide the bacon crumbles, bell pepper, 1 cup of the cheese, and the chives evenly among the cups of the muffin tin, then fill each about three-fourths full with the egg mixture. Bake for 18 minutes, or until the eggs are mostly set. Sprinkle the remaining ½ cup cheese on the tops and continue to bake for 6 minutes, until the muffins are fully set and the cheese is melted. Let cool for 10 minutes before serving. Enjoy immediately, topped with extra chives.

**STORAGE:** Store the muffins in an airtight container in the fridge for up to 4 days, or in the freezer for up to 1 month.

### *To Reheat:*

FROM THE FRIDGE

- Microwave for 20 to 30 seconds, or warm in a toaster oven at 300°F for 5 minutes.

FROM FROZEN

- Microwave for 45 to 60 seconds, or bake in a 325°F oven for about 10 minutes, until heated through.

---

**PER SERVING (2 MUFFINS)**
Protein: 24g
Carbohydrates: 2g
Fat: 22g

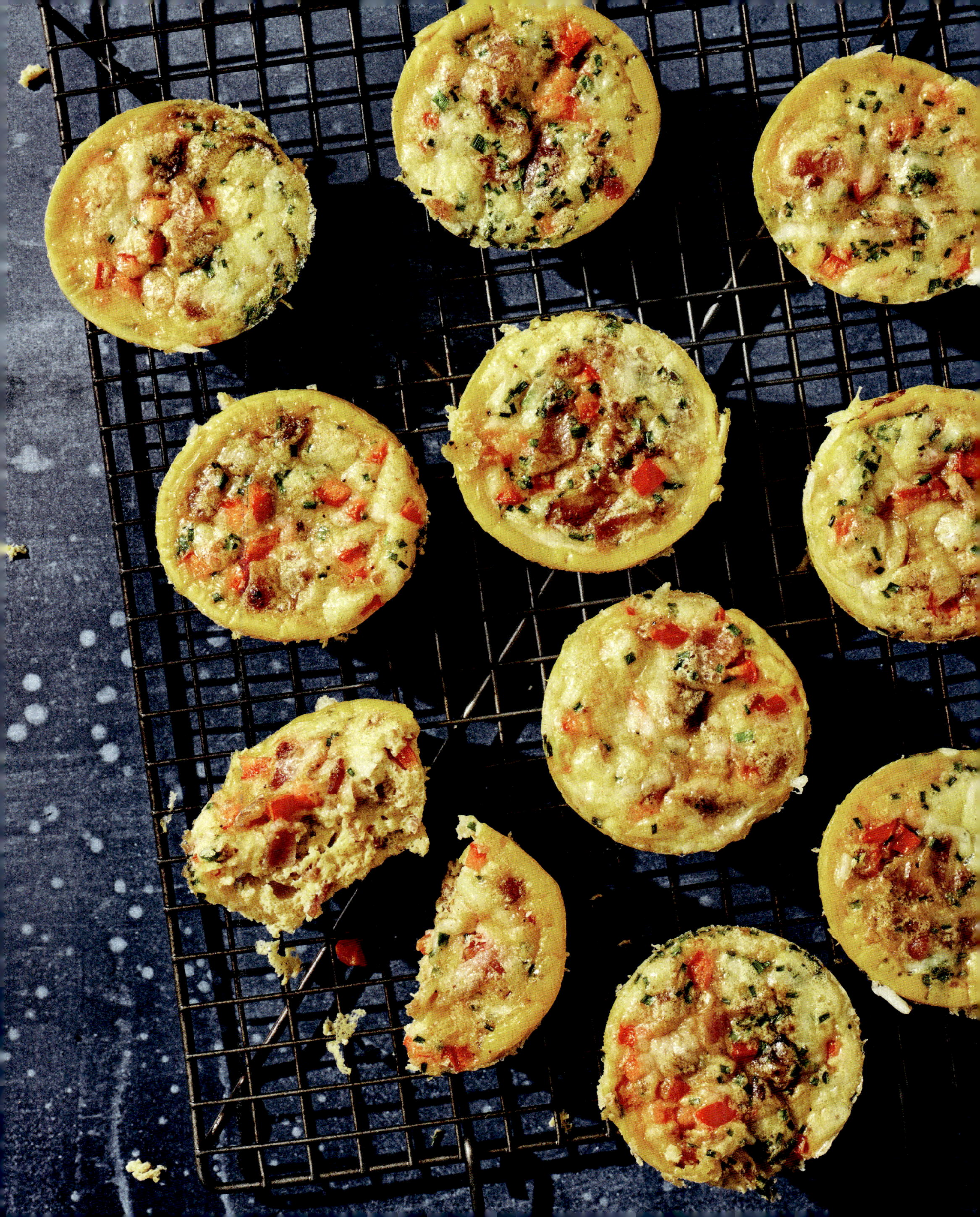

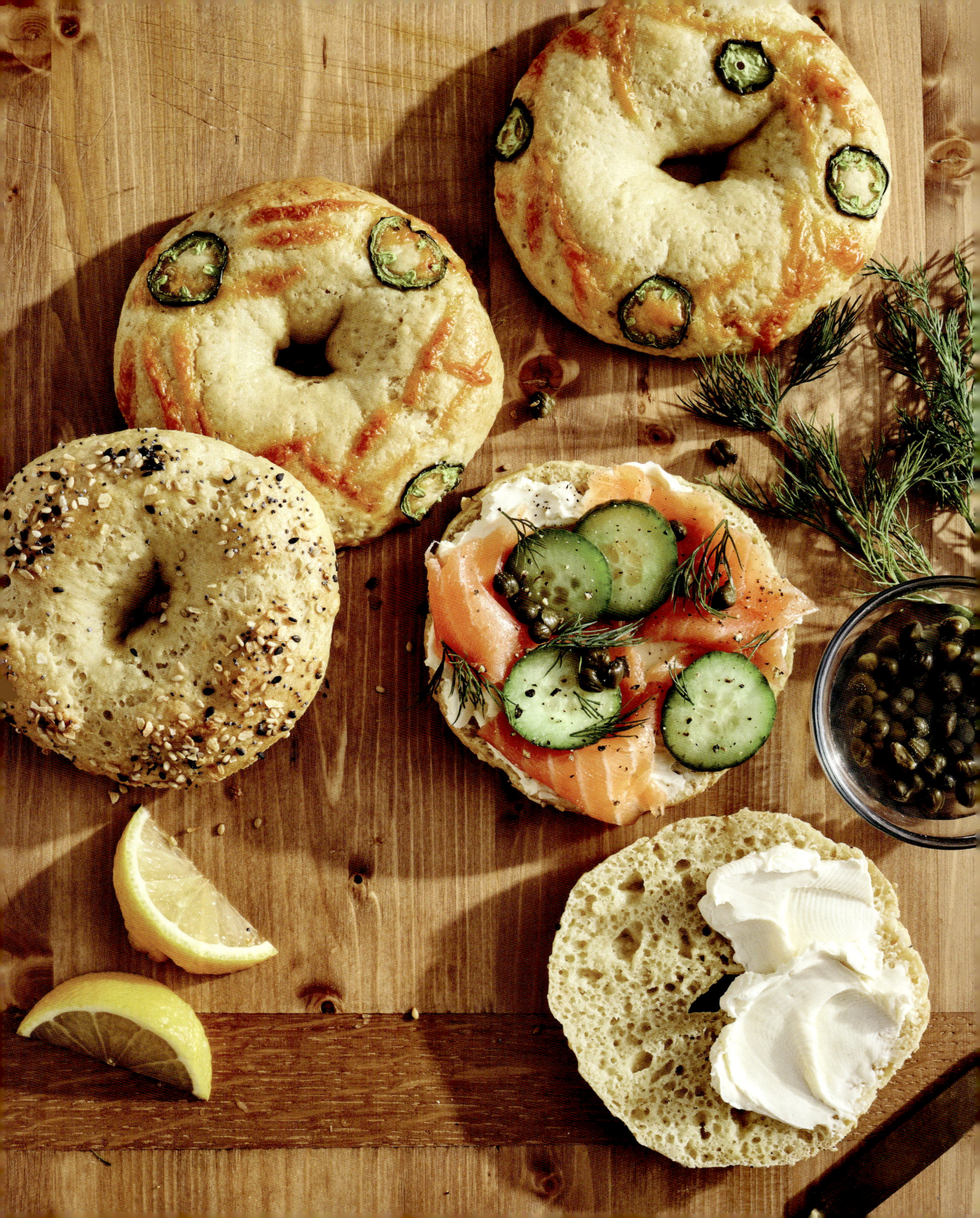

Gluten-Free
No Added Sugar

# Better-than-a-Bagel-Run Bagels

**MAKES 4 BAGELS • PREP TIME: 20 MINUTES • COOK TIME: 20 MINUTES, PLUS 20 MINUTES COOLING • TOTAL TIME: 1 HOUR**

**1 cup full-fat cottage cheese**

**1 cup gluten-free flour**

**1½ teaspoons baking powder**

**¼ teaspoon sea salt**

**1 large egg, beaten**

**Optional toppings: everything bagel seasoning, poppy seeds, shredded cheese, jalapeño, chives**

Who knew homemade bagels could be this easy? With just a handful of ingredients—plus a sneaky protein boost from cottage cheese—these gluten-free bagels have that classic soft, chewy texture you'd expect from the real thing. The best part? You can customize them however you like. Whether you're team everything seasoning, love a little jalapeño kick, or want to melt some cheese on top, these bagels are fully customizable.

1. Preheat the oven to 400°F. Line a baking sheet with parchment paper.
2. In a food processor, blend the cottage cheese until smooth. Set aside.
3. In a large bowl, whisk together the flour, baking powder, and salt. Add the blended cottage cheese and gently stir to combine. Transfer the mixture to a floured surface and knead for 1 to 2 minutes (or 8 to 10 turns), until it forms a semi-smooth ball. Be mindful not to over-knead, which can lead to dense bagels.
4. Divide the dough into four equal portions and roll each into a 6-inch log. Shape each into a circle by bringing the two ends together and pinching the seam to seal. Lightly brush each bagel with the beaten egg.
5. Add desired toppings. Bake for 20 to 25 minutes (no need to flip), until golden. Let cool for 20 minutes, then slice and serve.

**STORAGE:** Store in an airtight container at room temperature for up to 3 days.

---

**PER SERVING (1 BAGEL)**
Protein: 9g
Carbohydrates: 25g
Fat: 4g

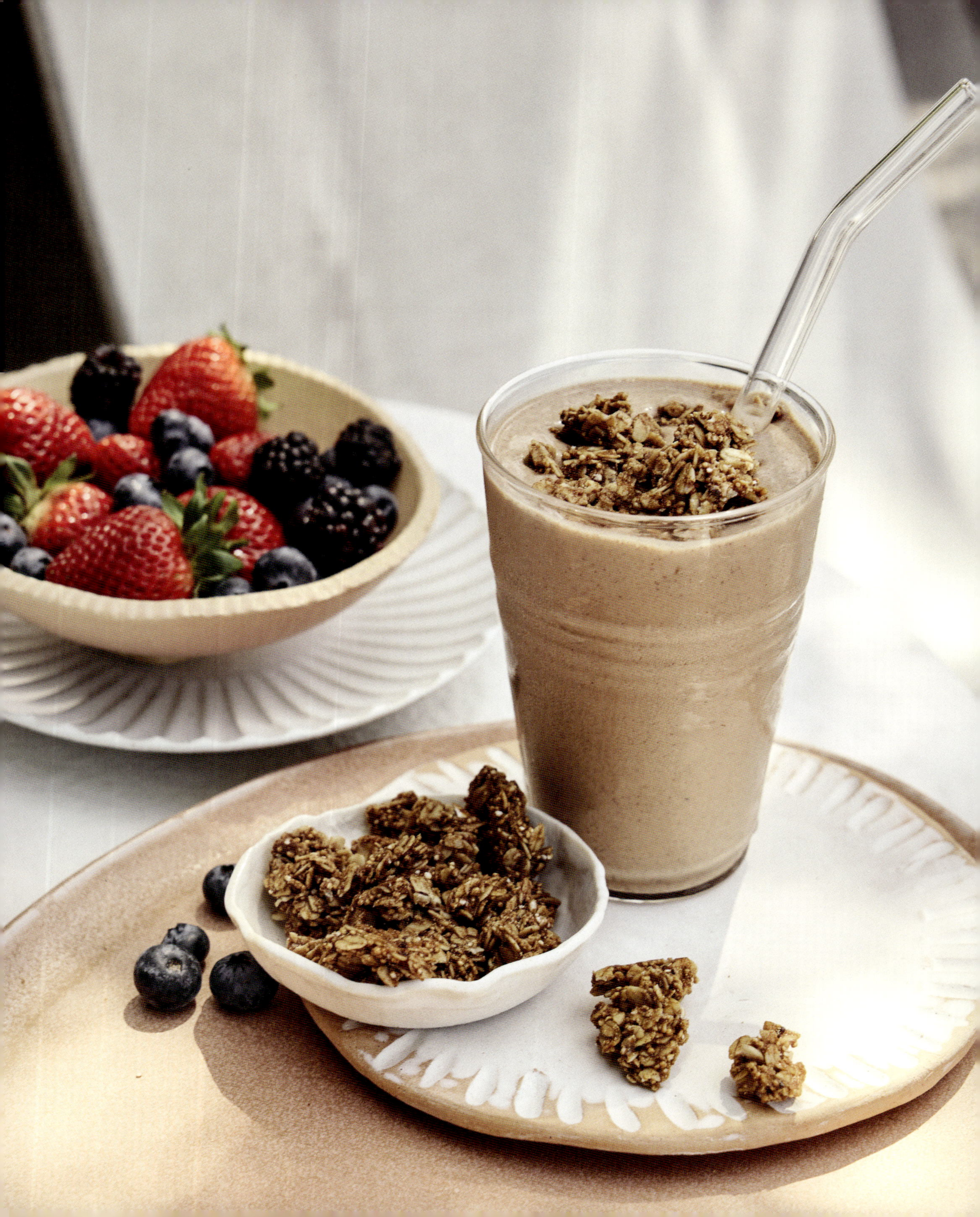

72 Pick-Me-Up Mocha Smoothie
75 Strawberry Shortcake Smoothie
76 Salted Peanut Butter Cup Smoothie
79 Passionberry Smoothie
80 Pumpkin Pie Smoothie

# Smoothies

Dairy-Free
Gluten-Free
Grain-Free
No Added Sugar

# Pick-Me-Up Mocha Smoothie

**SERVES 1 • TOTAL TIME: 5 MINUTES**

- ½ cup almond milk
- ½ cup cold brew coffee
- 1 serving chocolate protein powder (or 1 serving vanilla protein powder + 1 tablespoon cacao powder)
- 2 tablespoons collagen peptides
- 1 tablespoon almond butter (optional, for added healthy fats and longer-lasting energy)
- 1 pinch sea salt
- 1 frozen banana
- 1 pitted Medjool date, frozen
- 1 cup ice
- Optional toppings: cacao nibs, coconut whipped cream

You know the saying, "work smarter, not harder"? This smoothie is exactly that. By combining caffeine and protein in one frosty, chocolatey smoothie, you have the ultimate shortcut for starting your day strong. Cold brew provides caffeine, while protein and healthy fats keep you going. The whole thing tastes like a treat, but works like serious fuel.

In a blender, combine the almond milk, cold brew, protein powder, collagen peptides, almond butter, salt, banana, date, and ice. Blend for 1 minute, or until smooth. Serve immediately, topped with cacao nibs and coconut whipped cream, if desired.

**PER SERVING**
Protein: 32g
Carbohydrates: 49g
Fat: 3g

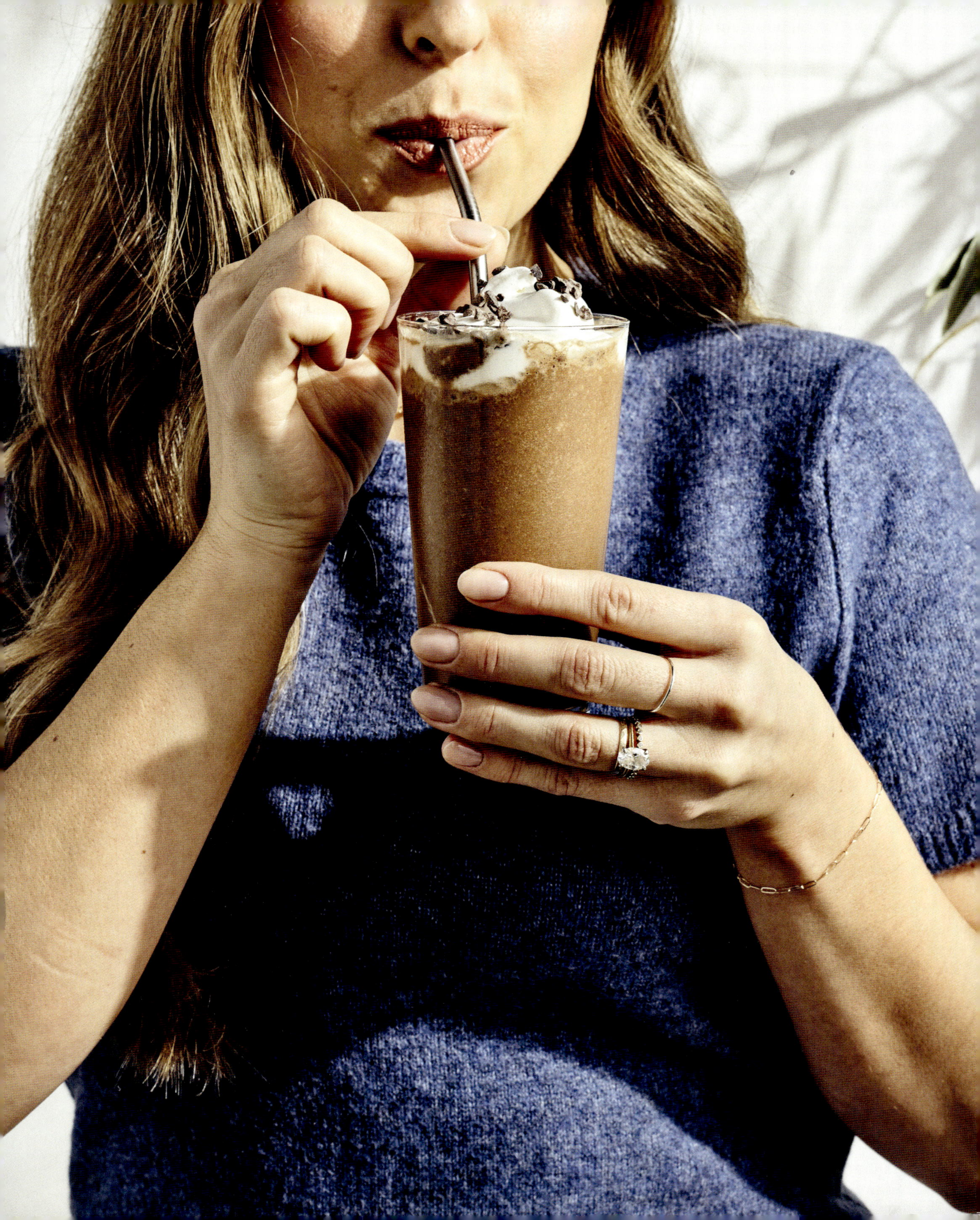

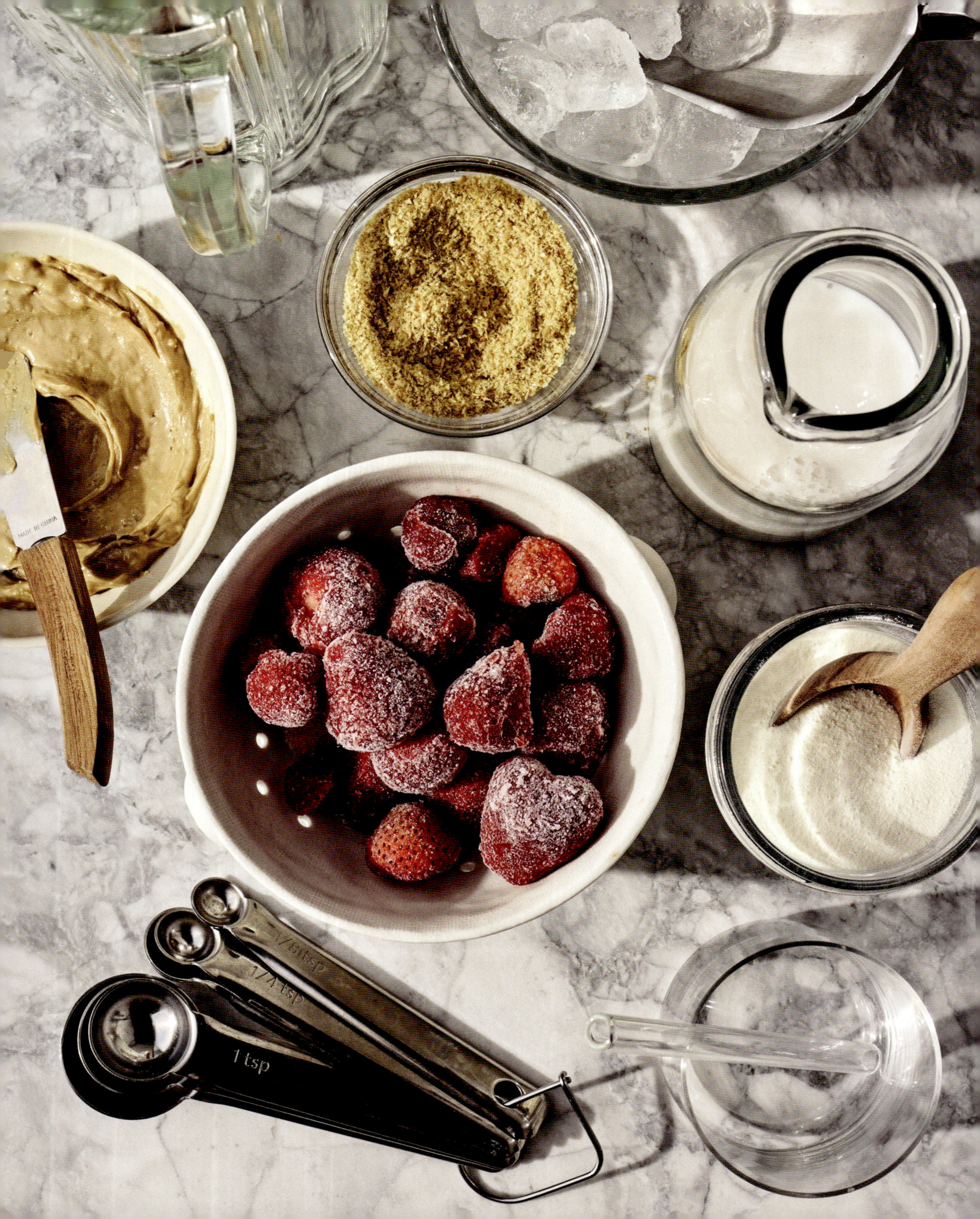
1/8 tsp
1/4 tsp
1 tsp

Dairy-Free
Gluten-Free
Grain-Free
No Added Sugar

# Strawberry Shortcake Smoothie

**SERVES 1 • TOTAL TIME: 5 MINUTES**

- 1½ cups unsweetened almond milk
- 1 teaspoon vanilla extract
- 1 serving vanilla protein powder
- 1 serving collagen peptides
- 1 tablespoon ground flaxseed
- 2 tablespoons cashew butter
- 1 heaping cup frozen strawberries (fresh works, too, just add extra ice for texture)
- ½ cup ice

Strawberry shortcake flavor in a smoothie—sweet, creamy, and just nostalgic enough. Juicy strawberries, cashew butter, and vanilla blend into a treat that tastes indulgent but is full of nutrients. It's the smoothie you'll want for breakfast, a snack, or even dessert.

In a blender, combine the almond milk, vanilla, protein powder, collagen peptides, flaxseed, cashew butter, strawberries, and ice. Blend for 1 minute, or until smooth. Serve immediately.

**PER SERVING**
Protein: 40g
Carbohydrates: 29g
Fat: 21g

Dairy-Free
Gluten-Free
Grain-Free
No Added Sugar

# Salted Peanut Butter Cup Smoothie

**SERVES 1 • TOTAL TIME: 5 MINUTES**

**1 cup unsweetened almond milk (or preferred milk)**
**1 serving vanilla protein powder**
**2 tablespoons peanut butter**
**2 tablespoons hemp seeds**
**1 tablespoon cacao powder**
**1 tablespoon cacao nibs**
**½ teaspoon ground cinnamon**
**Pinch of sea salt**
**1 frozen banana**
**1 pitted Medjool date, frozen**
**1 cup ice**
**Granola, for topping (optional)**

Sometimes you just want chocolate for breakfast. That's totally okay—I'm not here to judge. I love finding ways to turn sweets into something that actually energizes you, and this smoothie does exactly that. With protein powder, hemp seeds, and peanut butter, it gives you a lasting boost while still hitting that sweet, chocolatey craving.

In a blender, combine the almond milk, protein powder, peanut butter, hemp seeds, cacao powder, cacao nibs, cinnamon, salt, banana, date, and ice. Blend for 1 minute, or until smooth. Serve immediately, topped with granola, if using.

---

**PER SERVING**
Protein: 32g
Carbohydrates: 61g
Fat: 25g

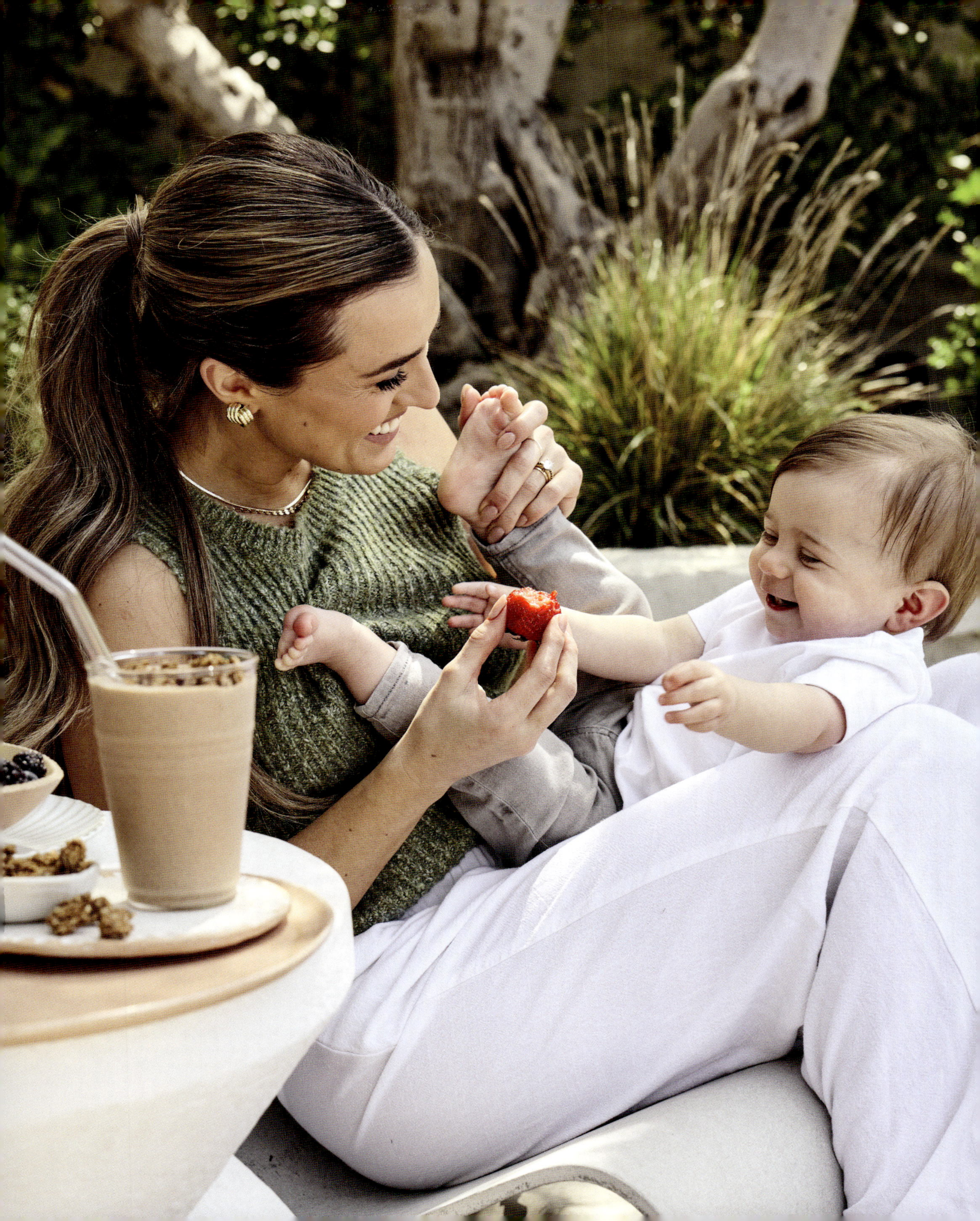

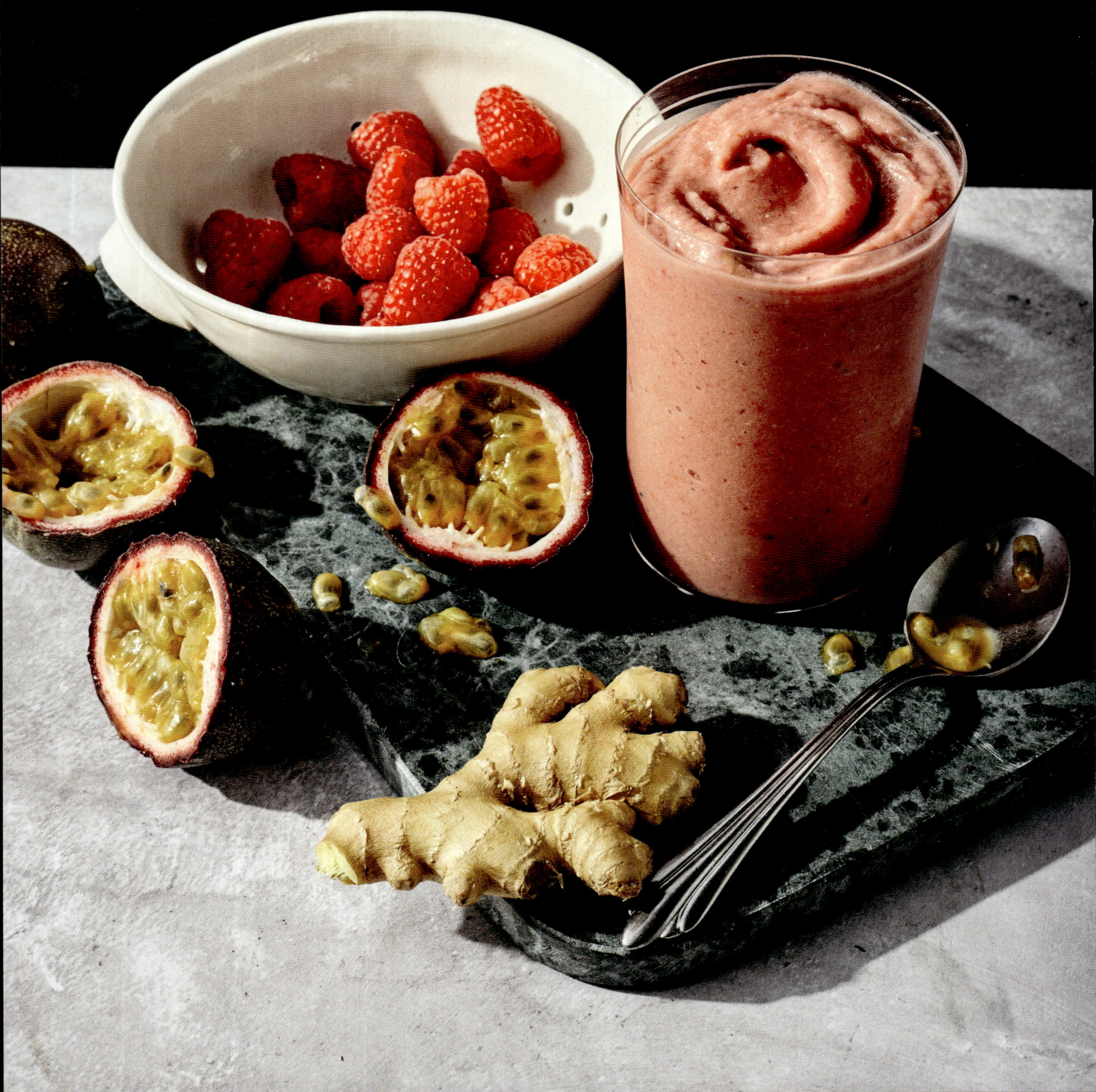

Dairy-Free
Gluten-Free
Grain-Free
No Added Sugar

# Passionberry Smoothie

**SERVES 1 • TOTAL TIME: 5 MINUTES**

- 1 cup coconut water
- 1½ servings vanilla protein powder
- 1 tablespoon hemp seeds
- 1 teaspoon grated peeled fresh ginger
- 1 banana, frozen
- ¼ cup frozen raspberries
- ¼ cup frozen passion fruit cubes
- ½ cup ice

This tropical wake-up call is tart, juicy, and refreshing and boasts passion fruit, raspberries, and a zing of fresh ginger to snap you out of that morning fog. It's also hydrating, energizing, and just the right amount of punchy.

In a blender, combine the coconut water, protein powder, hemp seeds, ginger, banana, raspberries, passion fruit, and ice. Blend for 1 minute, or until smooth. Serve immediately.

---

**PER SERVING**
Protein: 35g
Carbohydrates: 51g
Fat: 7g

Dairy-Free
Gluten-Free
Grain-Free
No Added Sugar

# Pumpkin Pie Smoothie

**SERVES 1 • TOTAL TIME: 5 MINUTES**

**1¼ cups almond milk (or preferred milk)**

**1½ servings vanilla protein powder**

**¼ cup canned pumpkin puree**

**1½ tablespoons almond butter**

**1 tablespoon ground flaxseed**

**1 teaspoon pumpkin pie spice**

**½ frozen banana**

**1 pitted Medjool date, frozen**

**1 cup ice**

**Granola, for topping (optional)**

Here's all the cozy fall flavors you love, but without the sugar crash. It's like pumpkin pie in a glass, only way more functional. Pumpkin, almond butter, and warm spices come together for a creamy, spiced smoothie you'll want on repeat, no matter the season.

In a blender, combine the almond milk, protein powder, pumpkin, almond butter, flaxseed, pumpkin pie spice, banana, date, and ice. Blend for 1 minute, or until smooth. Serve immediately, topped with granola, if using.

**PER SERVING**
Protein: 38g
Carbohydrates: 47g
Fat: 19g

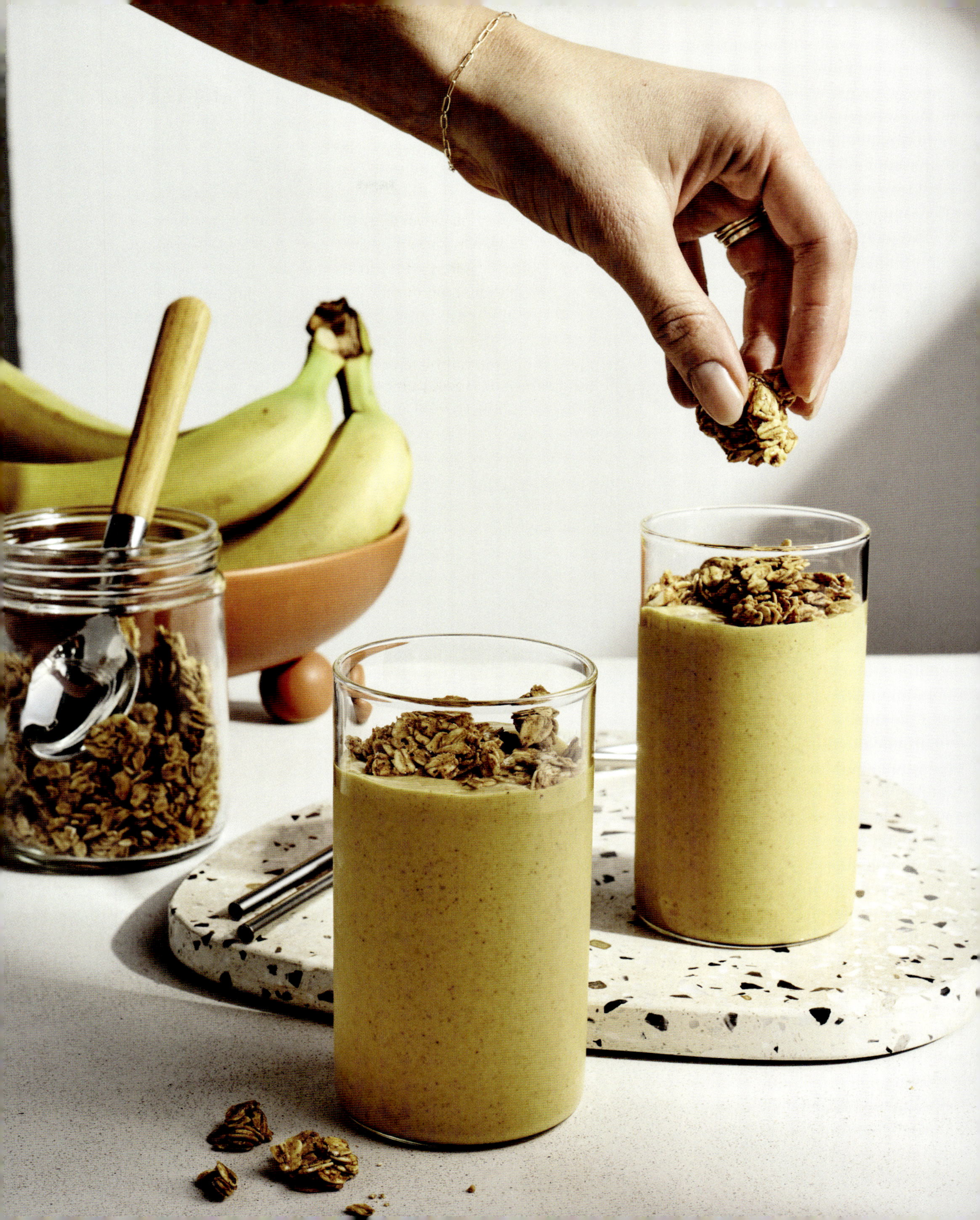

# Everyday Mains

DINNERS WORTH REPEATING 85

30-MINUTES OR LESS MAINS 115

SLOW COOKER MAINS 145

ONE-PAN MEALS 159

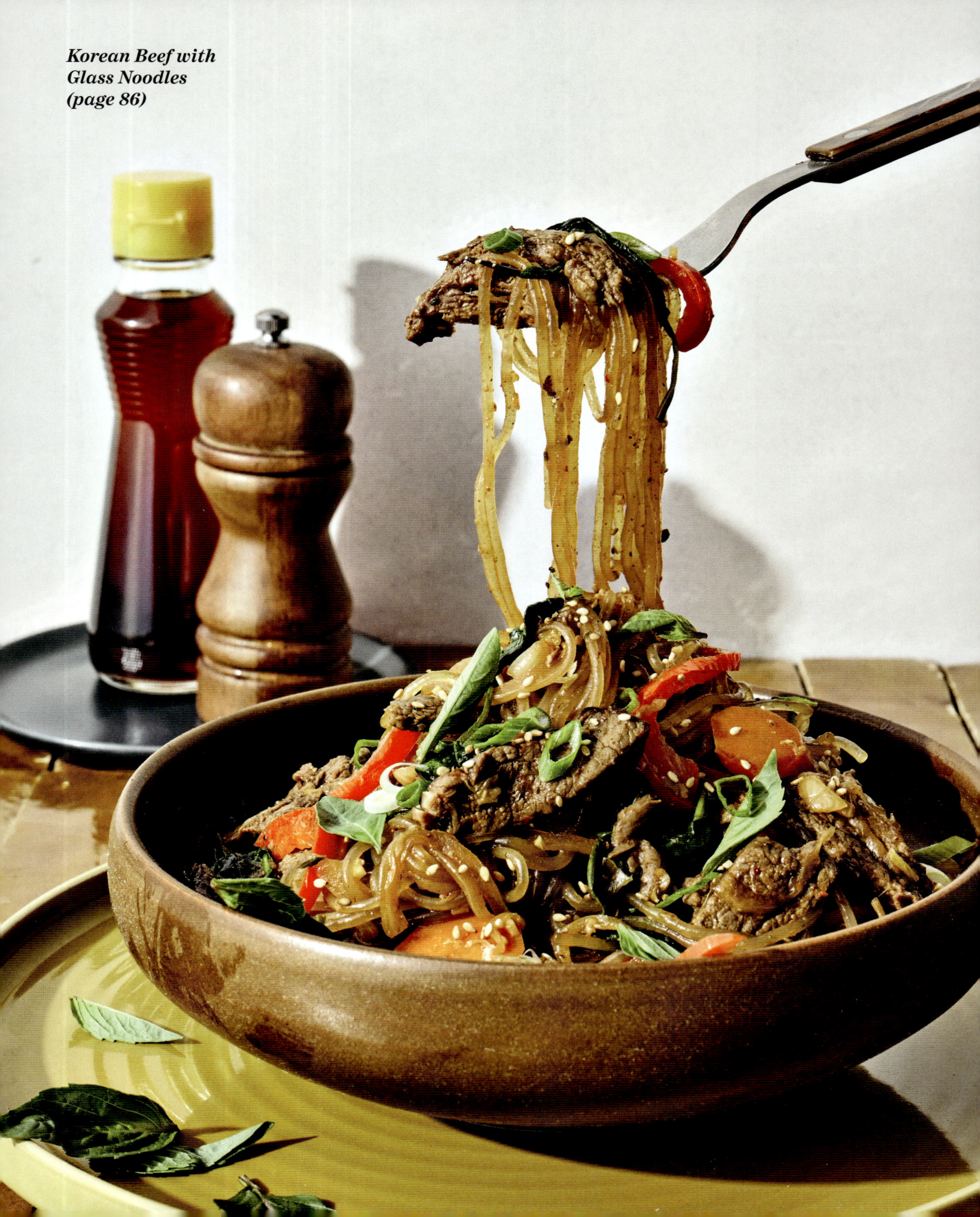

*Korean Beef with Glass Noodles*
*(page 86)*

86 Korean Beef with Glass Noodles

88 Chili-Lime Grilled Steak with Zesty Avocado Salsa

91 Seasoned Crispy Drumsticks

92 Greek-Style Smash Burgers

95 Chicken Milanese with Homemade Alfredo

99 Steak and Chimichurri Baguette Sandwiches

100 Blackened Shrimp Tacos with Pineapple-Avocado Salsa

103 Philly Cheesesteak–Stuffed Poblanos

104 Rosemary-Garlic Lamb Chops with Veggies

107 Szechuan Chicken Lettuce Wraps

108 Beef Bolognese

110 Tomato-Basil Chicken with Spaghetti Squash

112 Seared Halloumi and Chickpea Bowls with Herby Tahini

# Dinners Worth Repeating

Dairy-Free
Gluten-Free
Grain-Free
No Added Sugar

# Korean Beef with Glass Noodles

**SERVES 4 • PREP TIME: 15 MINUTES, PLUS 20 MINUTES MARINATING • COOK TIME: 20 MINUTES • TOTAL TIME: 55 MINUTES**

Bold, savory, and just the right amount of sweet, this dish is everything you love about Korean flavors in a simple, one-pan meal. Juicy, marinated skirt steak, crisp veggies, and glass noodles come together in a rich, garlicky sauce with a hint of sesame. High in protein and naturally gluten-free, it's a weeknight dinner that's just as good meal prepped for later. Don't skip the kimchi—it adds the perfect tangy bite!

**FOR THE MARINADE AND STEAK**

2 tablespoons coconut aminos
1 tablespoon sesame oil
1 clove garlic, minced
1 teaspoon grated fresh ginger
½ teaspoon freshly ground black pepper
1½ pounds skirt steak, thinly sliced

**FOR THE SAUCE**

3 tablespoons coconut aminos
1 tablespoon sesame oil
1 tablespoon rice vinegar
2 cloves garlic, minced
1 teaspoon grated fresh ginger
¼ teaspoon red pepper flakes (optional)
1 tablespoon arrowroot powder

**FOR THE STIR-FRY**

2 tablespoons avocado oil
1 medium onion, thinly sliced
1 large bell pepper, seeded and thinly sliced lengthwise (or snap peas or sliced zucchini)
1 medium carrot, thinly sliced on the diagonal

1. **Marinate the steak:** In a medium bowl, whisk together the coconut aminos, sesame oil, garlic, ginger, and black pepper. Add the steak and toss to coat. Cover and marinate in the fridge for at least 20 minutes, or up to 2 hours.
2. **Make the sauce:** In a small bowl, whisk together the coconut aminos, sesame oil, vinegar, garlic, ginger, red pepper flakes (if using), and arrowroot powder. Set aside.
3. **Stir-fry the veggies, steak, and noodles:** Heat 1 tablespoon of the avocado oil in a large skillet over medium-high heat. Add the onion, bell pepper, and carrot and stir-fry for 6 to 8 minutes, until slightly softened. Remove and set aside.
4. Raise the heat to high and add the remaining 1 tablespoon avocado oil. Add the marinated steak in a single layer and cook for 2 to 3 minutes per side, until browned and caramelized.

---

**PER SERVING**
Protein: 40g
Carbohydrates: 58g
Fat: 34g

**7 ounces sweet potato glass noodles (or preferred noodle), cooked according to package instructions, drained, and rinsed**

**4 cups fresh spinach**

**½ cup kimchi, chopped (optional)**

**FOR GARNISH**

**Fresh Thai basil, chopped (or use regular basil if that's what you have)**

**2 green onions, white and green parts, thinly sliced**

**1 tablespoon sesame seeds**

5. Reduce the heat to medium. Return the vegetables to the skillet and add the cooked noodles, spinach, and kimchi, if using. Sauté for 2 to 3 minutes, until the spinach wilts. Pour in the sauce and toss everything to coat evenly.
6. Remove from the heat and garnish with basil, green onions, and sesame seeds. Serve immediately.

**STORAGE:** Store leftovers in an airtight container in the fridge for up to 4 days. Reheat in a skillet over medium heat or in the microwave, adding a splash of water or broth if the noodles start to stick.

**MEAL-PREP TIP:** *Divide the noodles and beef mixture into 4 airtight containers. Let cool completely before sealing and refrigerating. Reheat in a skillet or microwave with a splash of water or broth to loosen up the sauce and prevent sticking. Garnish with fresh green onion and sesame seeds just before serving for the best texture.*

Dairy-Free
Gluten-Free
Grain-Free
No Added Sugar
Paleo

# Chili-Lime Grilled Steak with Zesty Avocado Salsa

**SERVES 4 TO 6 • PREP TIME: 10 MINUTES, PLUS 1 HOUR MARINATING • COOK TIME: 10 MINUTES • TOTAL TIME: 1 HOUR 20 MINUTES**

Some meals just hit that sweet spot between easy and impressive, and this is one of them. Juicy steak is paired with a creamy, zesty avocado salsa that is rich in heart-healthy fats and antioxidants thanks to the avocado and fresh herbs. The steak brings the protein and iron (hello, energy and strength), while the salsa keeps things feeling light and fresh. Serve with grilled veggies, over a salad, or wrapped up in a tortilla—depending on your mood or what you've got on hand. For dinner, I like to round out the steak with Roasted Japanese Sweet Potatoes (page 183) or Garlicky Roasted Broccolini (page 183).

**FOR THE MARINADE AND STEAK**

2 tablespoons extra-virgin olive oil

2 tablespoons freshly squeezed lime juice (about 1 lime)

½ cup chopped fresh cilantro

2 garlic cloves, minced

1 tablespoon chili powder

1 teaspoon ground cumin

1 teaspoon sea salt

1 teaspoon freshly ground black pepper

1½ pounds flank steak or skirt steak, trimmed of excess fat

**FOR THE SALSA**

3 tomatillos, husks removed

1 avocado, pitted

½ cup fresh cilantro

1 small jalapeño, seeded

2 tablespoons freshly squeezed lime juice (about 1 lime)

1 teaspoon sea salt

For serving: fresh lime wedges, fresh cilantro, flaky salt

1. **Marinate and grill the steak:** In a large bowl, whisk together the oil, lime juice, cilantro, garlic, chili powder, cumin, salt, and pepper. Add the steak and turn to coat. Cover and refrigerate for at least 1 hour, or up to overnight.
2. Preheat the grill (or a 10- to 12-inch grill pan) to medium-high heat.
3. Remove the steak from the marinade, allowing any excess to drip off. Grill for 4 to 5 minutes per side for medium-rare, or longer, if desired. Transfer to a cutting board and let rest for 10 minutes.
4. **Make the salsa:** While the steak rests, combine the tomatillos, avocado, cilantro, jalapeño, lime juice, and salt in a food processor. Blend until smooth.
5. Slice the steak against the grain into ¼-inch-thick strips. Drizzle with the salsa and garnish with lime wedges, cilantro, and flaky salt.

**MAKE-AHEAD TIP:** *The salsa can be made up to 1 day in advance. Store in an airtight container with a piece of plastic wrap pressed directly against the surface to help minimize browning. Give it a quick stir before serving.*

---

**PER SERVING (FOR 4 SERVINGS)**
Protein: 36g
Carbohydrates: 8g
Fat: 29g

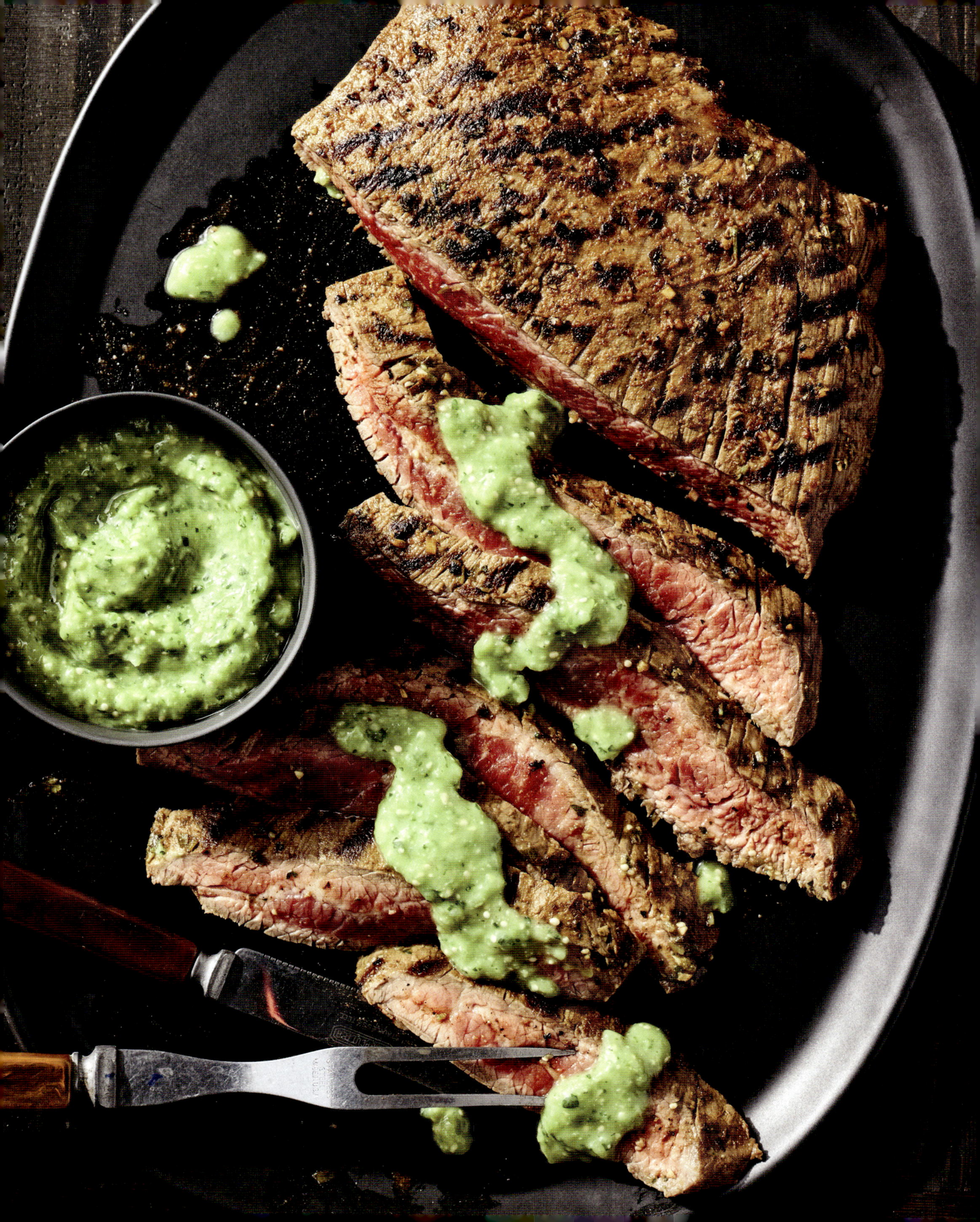

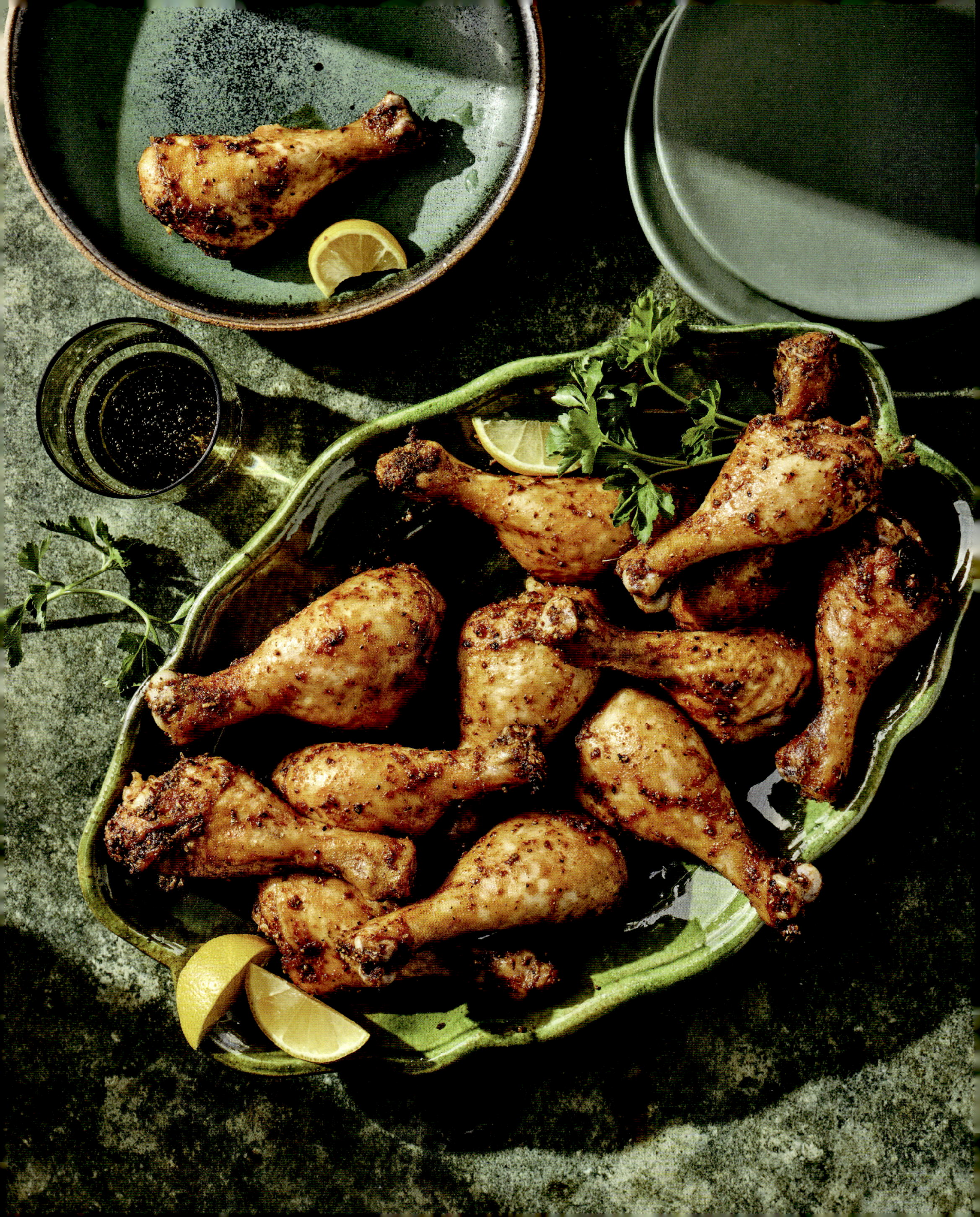

Dairy-Free
Gluten-Free
Grain-Free
No Added Sugar
Paleo

# Seasoned Crispy Drumsticks

**SERVES 5 TO 6 • PREP TIME: 10 MINUTES • COOK TIME: 50 MINUTES • TOTAL TIME: 1 HOUR**

This is one of my most searched and loved recipes, so adding it to the cookbook was a no-brainer. I get why everyone loves the family favorite, originally from my sister and now on weekly rotation in my house. The drumsticks are crispy on the outside, juicy on the inside, and incredibly easy to make. The secret? Drying the chicken well, using a wire rack for airflow in the oven, and roasting at high heat for the perfect golden finish.

- Avocado oil spray
- 5½ pounds (13 to 15) chicken drumsticks
- 3 to 4 tablespoons extra-virgin olive oil
- 2 teaspoons sea salt
- 1 teaspoon freshly ground black pepper
- 2 teaspoons garlic powder
- 2 teaspoons chili powder
- 2 teaspoons dried oregano
- 1 teaspoon paprika

1. Preheat the oven to 420°F. Line a rimmed baking sheet with foil for easier cleanup, then place a wire rack on top. Spray the rack lightly with avocado oil to help prevent sticking and promote crispiness.
2. Pat the drumsticks dry with a paper towel to remove excess moisture. Make sure the skin fully covers each drumstick and isn't folded—this helps the skin get extra crispy in the oven. In a large bowl, toss the drumsticks with the oil, enough to fully coat. Add the salt, pepper, garlic powder, chili powder, oregano, and paprika and mix well to evenly coat.
3. Place a wire rack in the baking sheet, and arrange the drumsticks on the rack in a single layer. Roast for 35 minutes, then flip the drumsticks. Roast for another 15 minutes, until the drumsticks are golden and crispy and the internal temperature reaches 165°F. Set aside to rest for 5 minutes.
4. Serve immediately with Sautéed Greens with Lemon and Olive Oil (page 182) or Cilantro-Lime Rice (page 198).

**STORAGE:** The drumsticks will keep in an airtight container in the fridge for up to 3 to 4 days.

**PER SERVING (FOR 6 SERVINGS)**
Protein: 60g
Carbohydrates: 2g
Fat: 36g

No Added Sugar
**IF MODIFIED:**
Gluten-Free
Grain-Free

# Greek-Style Smash Burgers

**SERVES 3 TO 4 • PREP TIME: 30 MINUTES • COOK TIME: 5 MINUTES • TOTAL TIME: 35 MINUTES**

If you've never tried a smash burger, this is your sign—I promise you'll be hooked after the first bite. These juicy, crispy-edged lamb (or beef) patties are loaded with fresh herbs, za'atar, and feta (which, in my opinion, is what really makes them shine), then smashed into warm pitas for a Mediterranean-inspired handheld meal that hits all the right notes. Topped with homemade tzatziki, crisp veggies, and extra feta, they're bold, fresh, and surprisingly light.

**FOR THE TZATZIKI**

- ¾ cup whole-milk Greek yogurt
- 1 Persian cucumber, grated
- 1 garlic clove, grated
- Juice of ½ lemon
- 2 tablespoons chopped fresh mint
- 2 tablespoons chopped fresh dill
- ½ teaspoon sea salt

**FOR THE BURGERS**

- 1 pound ground lamb or ground beef
- ½ cup finely chopped red onion
- 3 garlic cloves, minced
- 2 tablespoons chopped fresh mint
- 2 tablespoons chopped fresh dill
- ¼ cup crumbled feta
- 1 teaspoon za'atar
- 1 teaspoon sea salt
- ½ teaspoon freshly ground black pepper
- 1 tablespoon avocado oil
- 4 (5- to 6-inch) pita bread rounds (use gluten-free pita, corn tortillas, or lettuce wraps if preferred)
- Optional toppings: sliced Persian cucumber, halved cherry tomatoes, crumbled feta, za'atar, fresh mint, fresh dill

1. **Make the tzatziki:** In a medium bowl, stir together the yogurt, grated cucumber, garlic, lemon juice, mint, dill, and salt until smooth. Cover and refrigerate for at least 15 minutes to let the flavors meld.
2. **Prepare the burgers:** In another medium bowl, mix the ground meat, onion, garlic, mint, dill, feta, za'atar, salt, and pepper until fully combined. Divide into four 5- to 6-ounce (baseball-size) portions and roll into balls.
3. Heat a flattop griddle or large cast-iron skillet over medium-high heat and coat with the oil. Place the meatballs on the hot surface, leaving room between each one. Working one at a time, smash a pita round directly onto each meatball using a burger press or the flat side of a heavy pan until the meat is about ¼ inch thick. Cook for 3 to 4 minutes, until the meat is browned and cooked through. Flip and cook for 1 minute more to toast the pita.
4. Serve the burgers open-faced or folded taco-style, topped with tzatziki, cucumber slices, cherry tomatoes, feta, za'atar, and more fresh mint and dill. Sides can include Garlicky Roasted Broccolini (page 183) and/or Farro (page 182).

**STORAGE:** Store the cooked burger patties and tzatziki separately in airtight containers in the fridge for up to 3 days. The patties can be reheated in a skillet or air fryer to warm through. Tzatziki is best enjoyed chilled and may need a quick stir before serving.

---

**PER SERVING (FOR 4 SERVINGS)**
Protein: 30g
Carbohydrates: 35g
Fat: 26g

**TIP:** *For a gluten-free and grain-free option, serve the burgers wrapped in lettuce leaves instead of pita.*

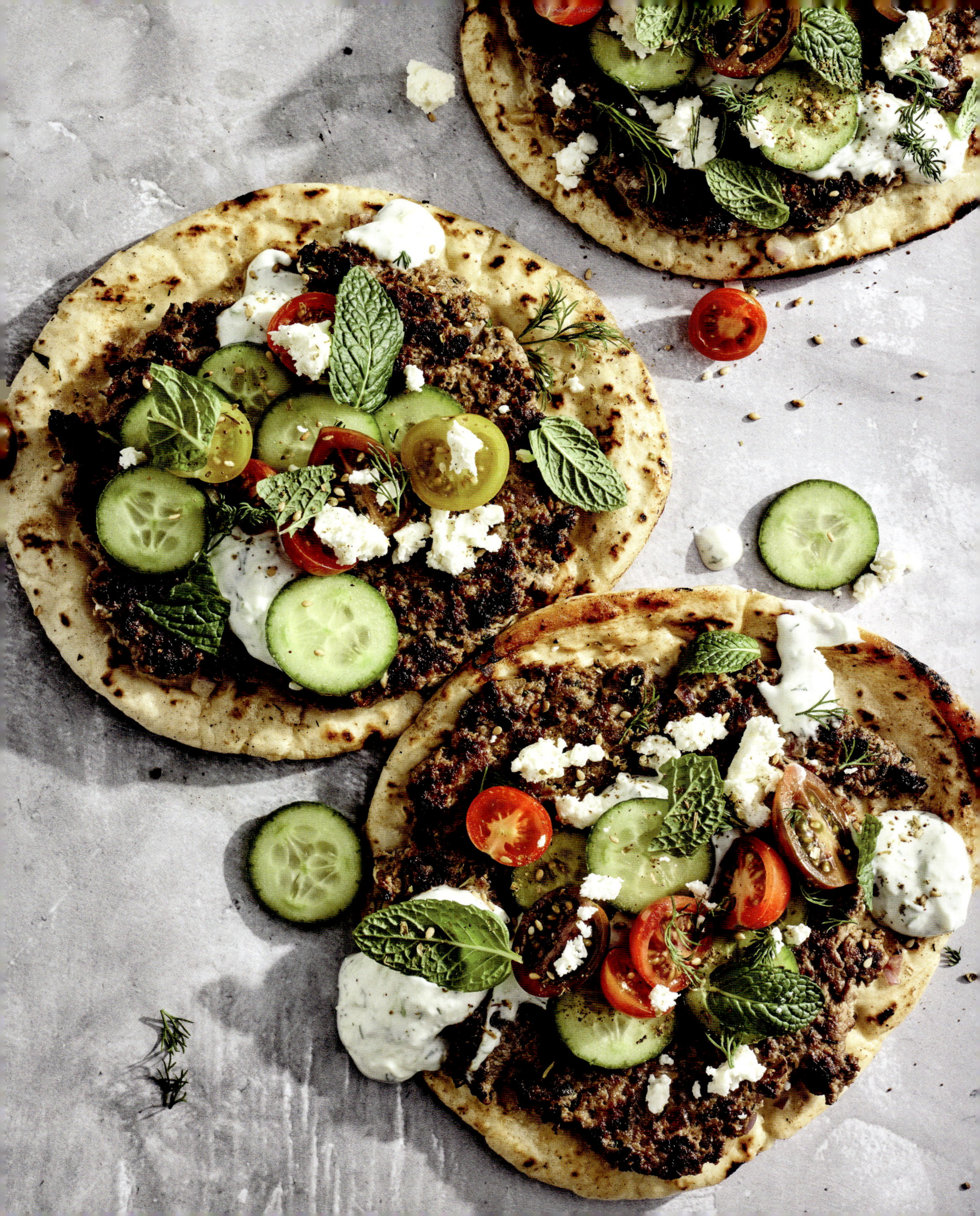

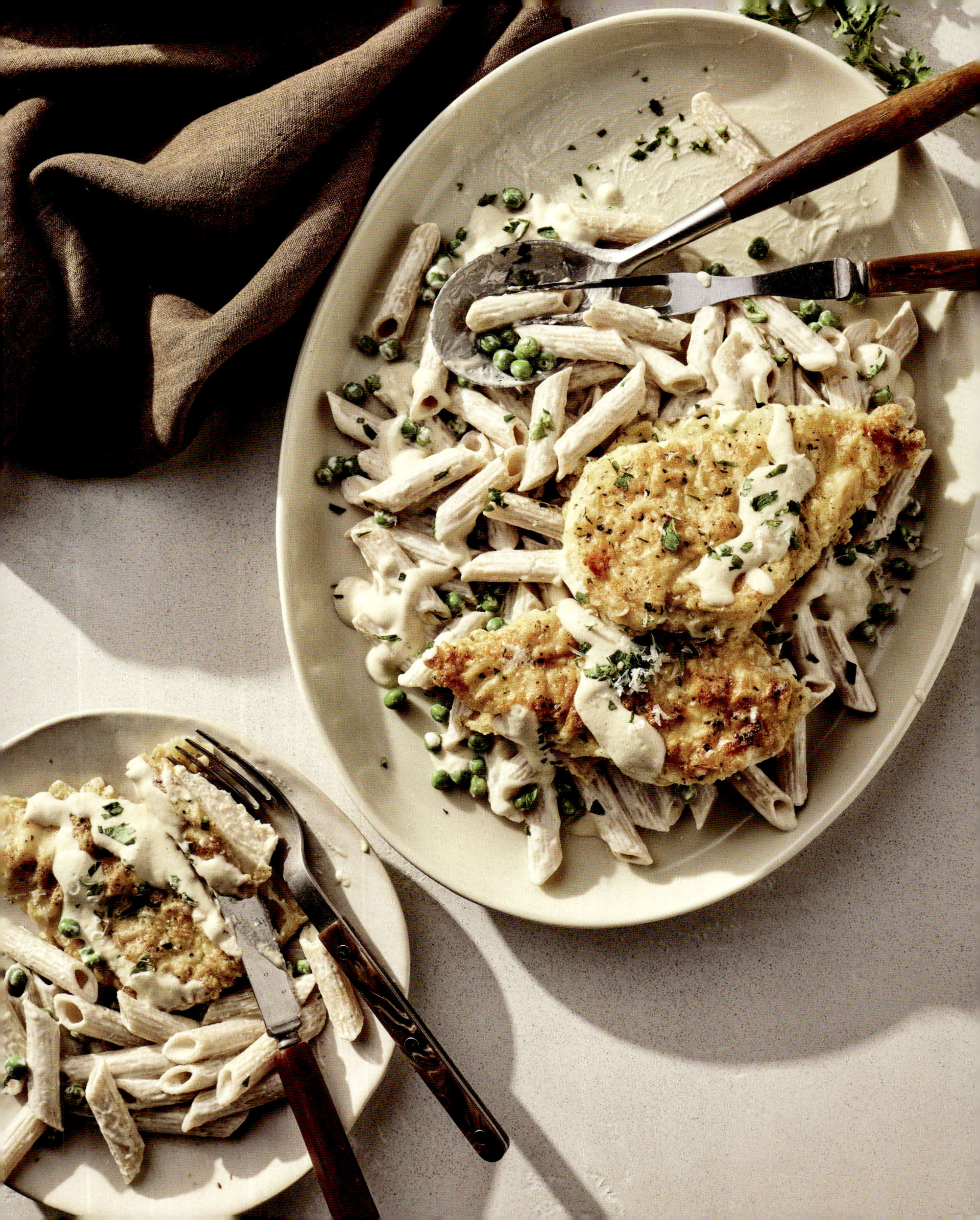

**IF MODIFIED:**
Dairy-Free
Gluten-Free
No Added Sugar

# Chicken Milanese with Homemade Alfredo

SERVES 4 TO 5 • PREP TIME: 25 MINUTES • COOK TIME: 15 MINUTES • TOTAL TIME: 40 MINUTES

Crispy chicken, creamy Alfredo, and a plate of pasta? Say no more. This dish has all the golden, pan-fried crunch you want paired with a rich, velvety sauce that just so happens to be dairy-free and full of protein (but you'd never guess). It's cozy, crave-worthy, and the kind of meal that makes any night feel like a special occasion.

FOR THE ALFREDO SAUCE

- Boiling water, for soaking
- 1 cup raw cashews
- 2 tablespoons extra-virgin olive oil
- ½ small onion, chopped
- 2 tablespoons minced garlic
- ⅓ cup grated Parmesan (or vegan Parmesan for dairy-free)
- 3 tablespoons unflavored collagen peptides
- 1 cup chicken bone broth
- 1 tablespoon lemon juice
- 1½ teaspoons sea salt
- Freshly ground black pepper

FOR THE CHICKEN

- ½ cup arrowroot powder
- 1 teaspoon dried parsley
- 1 teaspoon sea salt
- 1 large egg
- 3 tablespoons milk of choice
- ½ cup gluten-free baking flour, all-purpose flour, or breadcrumbs (fine or panko both work)
- ¼ teaspoon freshly ground black pepper
- 2 large chicken breasts, sliced in half lengthwise
- ¼ cup ghee (or dairy-free butter)

1. **Make the Alfredo sauce:** In a small bowl, pour enough boiling water over the cashews to cover. Soak for 15 to 20 minutes, then drain and set aside.
2. Meanwhile, in a small saucepan over medium heat, heat the oil. Add the onion and garlic and sauté for 3 to 5 minutes, until the onion softens.
3. In a blender, combine the soaked cashews, onion mixture, Parmesan, collagen peptides, broth, lemon juice, salt, and pepper. Blend until smooth and creamy. Set aside.
4. **Prepare the chicken:** Set up your dredging station with three separate shallow bowls: Combine the arrowroot powder, ½ teaspoon of the dried parsley, and ½ teaspoon of the salt in the first bowl. Whisk together the egg and milk in the second bowl. And mix the flour, remaining ½ teaspoon dried parsley, the pepper, and a pinch of salt in the third bowl. Dredge each chicken piece in the arrowroot mixture, then the egg mixture, and finally the flour mixture. Place on a clean plate.
5. In a large skillet, heat the ghee over medium-high heat. Add the chicken and cook for 4 to 5 minutes, until golden and crispy on the bottom. Reduce the heat slightly, flip the chicken, cover, and cook until golden and crispy on the bottom, cooked through, and the internal temp reaches 165°F, 3 to 4 minutes longer. Remove the chicken from the skillet and let rest for 5 minutes. Slice into strips.

(recipe and ingredients continue)

FOR THE PASTA

**1 (12-ounce) box penne pasta (gluten-free if preferred; I like pasta from Jovial Foods)**

**1 cup frozen peas**

**¼ cup chopped fresh parsley**

**Grated Parmesan (or vegan Parmesan for dairy-free), for garnish**

6. **Cook the pasta:** While the chicken is cooking, cook the pasta according to the package instructions. One minute before the pasta is done, add the peas. Drain.
7. Transfer the pasta and peas to a large serving bowl. Add 1½ cups of the Alfredo sauce and toss until fully coated.
8. Top with the chicken and drizzle with additional Alfredo sauce. Garnish with parsley and Parmesan and season with salt and pepper.
9. **Optional:** Serve with a side of Sautéed Greens with Lemon and Olive Oil (page 182).

**MAKE-AHEAD TIP AND STORAGE:** *The sauce can be prepared up to 5 days ahead of time. Leftover sauce can be stored in an airtight container and frozen for up to 3 months. Thaw overnight in the fridge and reheat in a saucepan, adding a splash of water or bone broth if needed.*

*Leftover crispy chicken (preferably unsliced) and plain pasta (without sauce) can be stored separately in airtight containers in the fridge for 3 to 4 days. Toss pasta with a drizzle of olive oil before storing to prevent clumping.*

---

**PER SERVING (FOR 5 SERVINGS)**
Protein: 45g
Carbohydrates: 70g
Fat: 33g

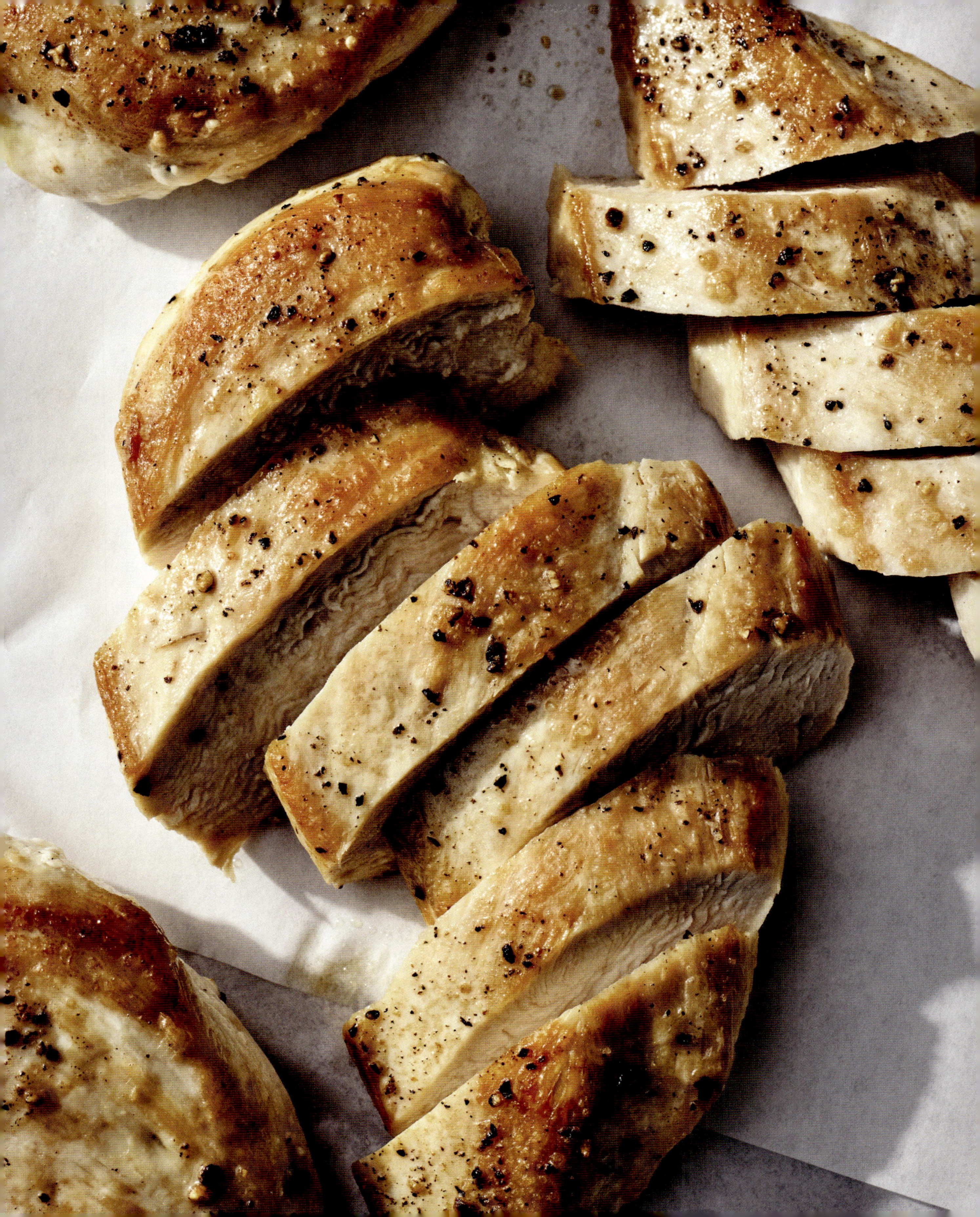

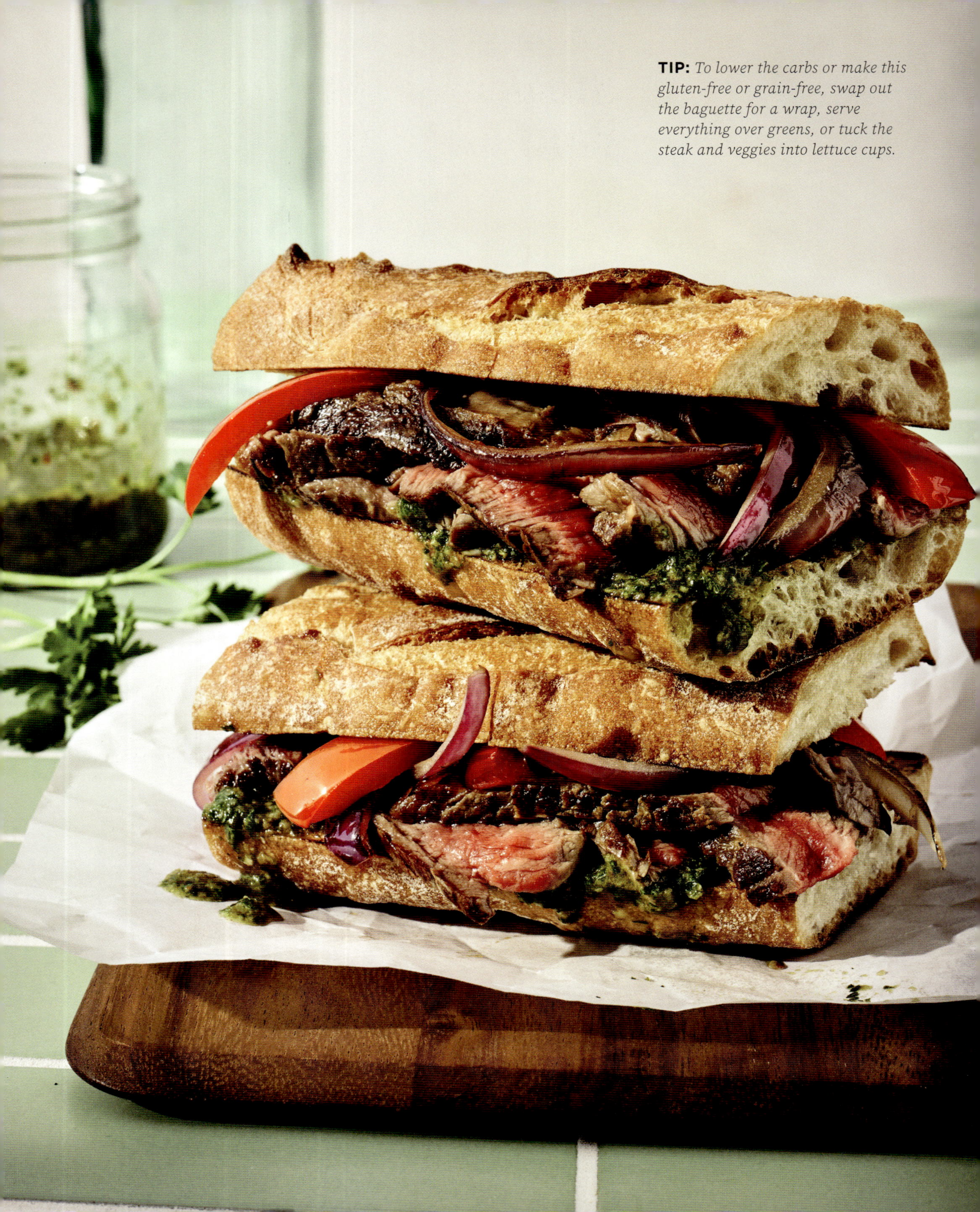

**TIP:** *To lower the carbs or make this gluten-free or grain-free, swap out the baguette for a wrap, serve everything over greens, or tuck the steak and veggies into lettuce cups.*

No Added Sugar
**IF MODIFIED:**
Dairy-Free
Gluten-Free
Grain-Free

# Steak and Chimichurri Baguette Sandwiches

**SERVES 2 TO 4 • PREP TIME: 10 MINUTES • COOK TIME: 18 TO 31 MINUTES • TOTAL TIME: 28 TO 41 MINUTES**

My husband, Bridger, inspired this recipe. After a round of golf (classic), he raved about a steak chimichurri sandwich he'd had. Naturally, I took it as a challenge to re-create it. And here we are. With a crunchy baguette, juicy rib eye, sautéed peppers and onions, and that vibrant chimichurri, this sandwich delivers on all fronts. Simple, bold, and seriously satisfying.

**FOR THE STEAK**

- 1 (10-ounce) sirloin or rib eye steak
- Sea salt and freshly ground black pepper
- 3 tablespoons avocado oil
- 1 red bell pepper, seeded and thinly sliced
- ½ red onion, thinly sliced
- ½ teaspoon sea salt

**FOR THE CHIMICHURRI**

- ½ cup packed fresh cilantro leaves
- ½ cup packed fresh parsley leaves
- ⅓ cup extra-virgin olive oil
- 3 tablespoons chopped red onion
- 2 tablespoons red wine vinegar
- 1 clove garlic
- ½ teaspoon sea salt
- ¼ teaspoon ground cumin
- Pinch of red chili flakes
- Freshly ground black pepper

**FOR THE SANDWICH**

- 1 (20- to 26-inch) baguette (or gluten-free roll)
- 2 tablespoons ghee (or vegan butter for dairy-free)

1. **Cook the steak:** Season the steak generously with salt and pepper on both sides, pressing the seasoning into the meat.
2. In a medium skillet, heat 2 tablespoons of the avocado oil over medium-high heat. Sear the steak for 4 to 8 minutes per side, depending on thickness and desired doneness. Transfer to a cutting board and let rest for at least 5 minutes. Slice into ½-inch-thick strips, cutting against the grain.
3. In the same skillet, heat the remaining 1 tablespoon avocado oil over medium-high heat. Add the bell pepper and sliced onion and sauté for 8 to 10 minutes, tossing every few minutes, until slightly charred and tender. Cover the skillet if you want to speed up the cooking. Season with the salt and set aside.
4. **Make the chimichurri:** In a food processor, combine the cilantro, parsley, olive oil, chopped onion, vinegar, garlic, salt, cumin, chili flakes, and black pepper. Pulse until smooth.
5. **Make the sandwich:** Preheat the oven to broil (high heat). Slice the baguette in half lengthwise and spread the ghee on the cut sides. Place cut side up on the center oven rack and broil for 2 to 5 minutes, until golden and crisp. Watch closely to prevent burning.
6. Layer the steak onto the baguette, followed by the chimichurri, then the sautéed peppers and onions. Close the sandwich and slice diagonally into smaller pieces for serving.

**MAKE-AHEAD TIP:** *The chimichurri can be made up to 5 days in advance. The flavor actually gets even better after a day or two. Store in a sealed jar in the fridge—just give it a good stir before using.*

---

**PER SERVING (FOR 2 SERVINGS)**
Protein: 51g
Carbohydrates: 47g
Fat: 79g

Dairy-Free
Gluten-Free
Grain-Free

# Blackened Shrimp Tacos with Pineapple-Avocado Salsa

**SERVES 4 • PREP TIME: 15 MINUTES, PLUS 30 MINUTES MARINATING • COOK TIME: 5 MINUTES • TOTAL TIME: 50 MINUTES**

Smoky spicy shrimp meets sweet juicy pineapple-avocado salsa in the ultimate taco night upgrade. Quick to cook and rich in protein, these tacos are fresh, vibrant, and downright delicious. Shrimp is one of the leanest protein sources out there—and when it's wild-caught you're getting even more nutrition and flavor in every bite.

**FOR THE SHRIMP AND MARINADE**

1½ pounds wild-caught shrimp, peeled, deveined, and tails removed

1 tablespoon extra-virgin olive oil, plus more for the pan

2 teaspoons smoked paprika

1 teaspoon garlic powder

½ teaspoon chili powder

1 teaspoon sea salt

1 teaspoon coconut sugar

**FOR THE SALSA**

1 cup diced fresh pineapple (or canned pineapple in unsweetened juice, drained)

1 avocado, diced

¼ small red onion, finely chopped

3 tablespoons fresh cilantro leaves, minced

½ jalapeño, seeded and minced

1 tablespoon lime juice

1 tablespoon extra-virgin olive oil

½ teaspoon sea salt

¼ teaspoon freshly ground black pepper

For serving: 4 grain-free tortillas (I prefer Siete brand) or butter lettuce leaves

Optional toppings: shredded cabbage, extra cilantro, lime wedges, dairy-free crema

1. **Marinate the shrimp:** In a large bowl, toss the shrimp with the oil, paprika, garlic powder, chili powder, salt, and coconut sugar until evenly coated. Set aside to marinate for 30 minutes.
2. **Make the salsa:** While the shrimp marinates, stir together the pineapple, avocado, onion, cilantro, jalapeño, lime juice, oil, salt, and pepper in a medium bowl. Cover and refrigerate to chill.
3. If using tortillas, heat them in a dry sauté pan over medium heat for 30 to 60 seconds per side, until slightly charred. Keep warm wrapped in a towel.
4. **Cook the shrimp:** In the same pan, heat a small drizzle of oil over medium heat. Add the shrimp in a single layer and cook for 5 to 6 minutes, flipping halfway through, until opaque and lightly blackened around the edges.
5. Add the shrimp to the tortillas. Top with the salsa and your favorite toppings.

---

**PER SERVING**
Protein: 41g
Carbohydrates: 22g
Fat: 24g

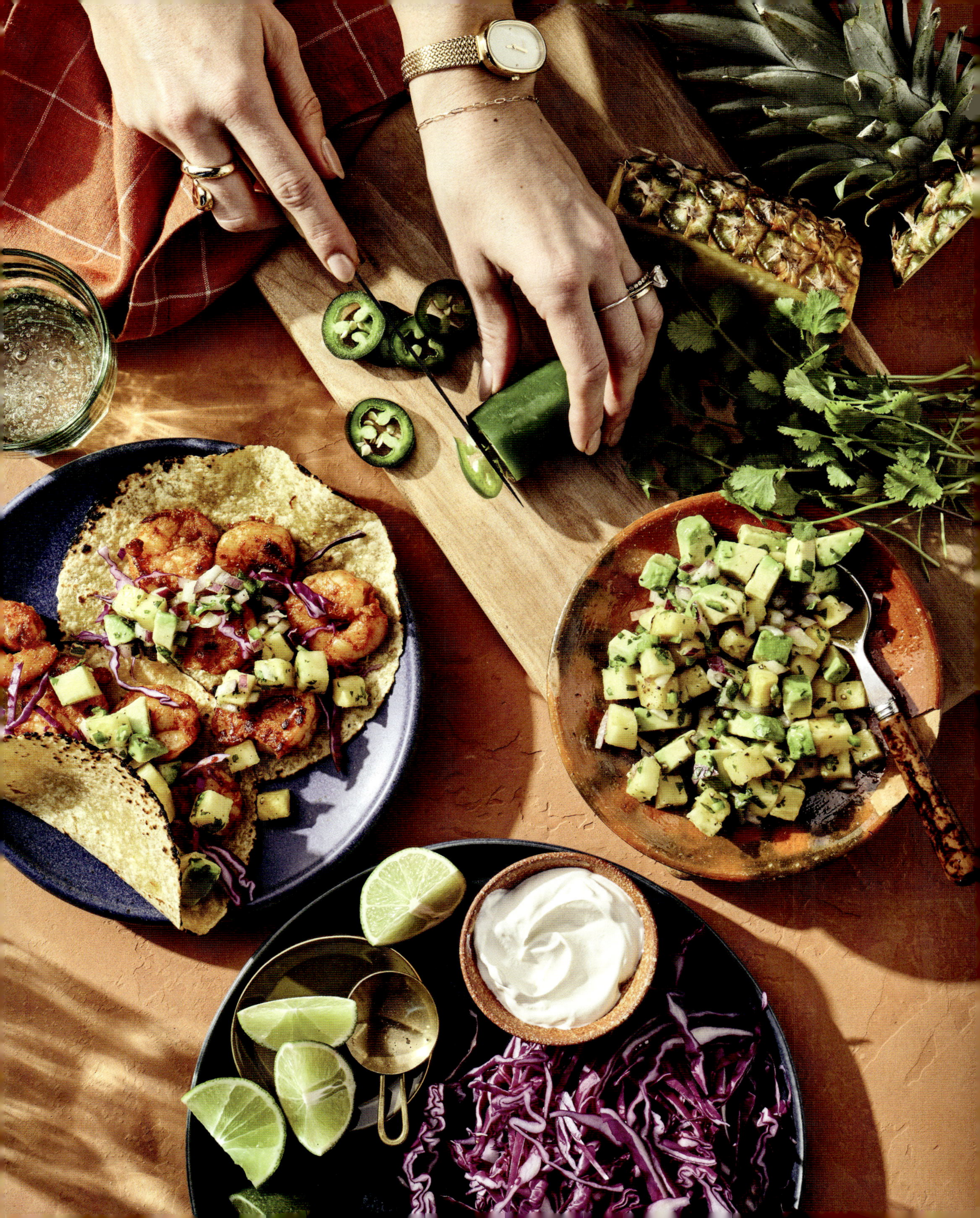

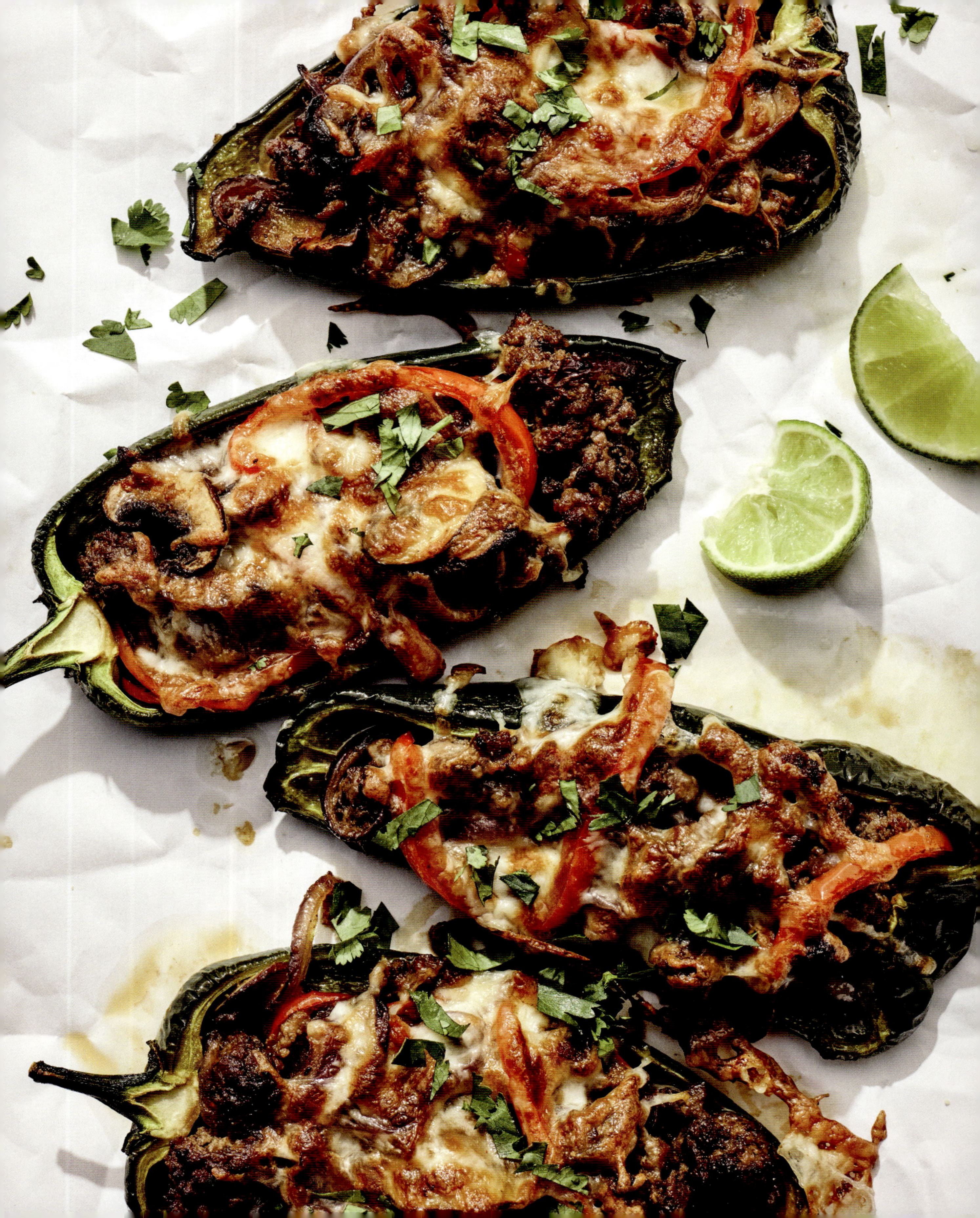

Gluten-Free
Grain-Free
No Added Sugar

# Philly Cheesesteak–Stuffed Poblanos

SERVES 4 TO 6 • PREP TIME: 20 MINUTES • COOK TIME: 30 MINUTES • TOTAL TIME: 50 MINUTES

Craving a Philly cheesesteak but want a lower-carb option instead? These stuffed poblanos bring all the flavor of the classic sandwich, but in a more nutrient-dense package than the traditional hoagie roll. Juicy steak (or ground beef), sautéed peppers, onions, and mushrooms, plus plenty of melted cheese, makes for a filling, high-protein meal that comes together quickly enough for a weeknight dinner.

FOR THE PEPPERS

4 large poblano peppers, halved and seeded

1 tablespoon extra-virgin olive oil, for brushing

Sea salt and freshly ground black pepper

FOR THE STEAK AND VEGGIE FILLING

2 tablespoons extra-virgin olive oil or ghee

1 pound thinly sliced sirloin steak (or ground beef)

½ medium red onion, thinly sliced

1 medium bell pepper (red, green, yellow, or orange), seeded and thinly sliced

1 cup sliced mushrooms

2 cloves garlic, minced

1 tablespoon coconut aminos

½ teaspoon smoked paprika

½ teaspoon garlic powder

½ teaspoon onion powder

Sea salt and freshly ground black pepper

TO STUFF THE POBLANOS AND SERVE

1½ cups shredded mozzarella cheese (or 4 ounces crumbled mozzarella + ½ cup shredded)

Chopped fresh cilantro or parsley, for garnish

Lime wedges, for serving (optional)

1. **Roast the poblanos:** Preheat the oven to 400°F. Line a baking sheet with parchment paper.
2. Brush each poblano half with oil and season with salt and pepper. Place cut side up on the baking sheet and roast for 8 to 10 minutes, until slightly softened. Set aside.
3. **Make the steak and veggie filling:** In a large skillet, heat 1 tablespoon of the oil over medium-high heat. Add the steak and cook for 4 to 5 minutes, until browned. Remove from the skillet and drain excess grease if needed.
4. In the same skillet, heat the remaining 1 tablespoon oil. Add the onion, bell pepper, and mushrooms and sauté for 6 to 8 minutes, until softened and caramelized. Stir in the garlic and cook for 1 minute more.
5. Return the steak to the skillet and stir in the coconut aminos, paprika, garlic powder, onion powder, salt, and pepper. Cook for 2 minutes more, until everything is well combined.
6. **Stuff and bake the poblanos:** Fill each poblano half with the filling, adding about half of the cheese throughout to create cheesy pockets in each. Top with the remaining cheese.
7. Bake for 15 minutes, until the cheese is melted and bubbling. If you like, broil for 1 to 2 minutes for a golden top—watch closely to avoid burning. Sprinkle with cilantro or parsley and serve with lime wedges, if desired.

**STORAGE:** Store leftovers in an airtight container in the fridge for up to 4 days. Reheat in a 350°F oven for 10 to 15 minutes, or in the microwave until warmed through.

---

**PER SERVING (FOR 4 SERVINGS)**
Protein: 36g
Carbohydrates: 12g
Fat: 26g

Dairy-Free
Gluten-Free
Grain-Free
No Added Sugar
Paleo

# Rosemary-Garlic Lamb Chops with Veggies

SERVES 4 • PREP TIME: 15 MINUTES, PLUS 1 HOUR MARINATING • COOK TIME: 10 MINUTES • TOTAL TIME: 1 HOUR 25 MINUTES

Whether you're hosting or just want another reason to grill something (because let's be honest, grilled food is superior), this dish comes together fast. A quick rosemary-garlic marinade makes the lamb chops tender and juicy, while grilled veggies dressed with an easy garlic dressing add the perfect fresh balance. Simple, flavorful, and guaranteed to impress.

FOR THE LAMB

¼ cup extra-virgin olive oil

4 cloves garlic, minced

1 tablespoon fresh rosemary, minced

1 teaspoon sea salt

1 teaspoon freshly ground black pepper

2 pounds (about 8 total) lamb rib chops

FOR THE VEGGIES AND DRESSING

2 bell peppers (red, yellow, or orange), seeded and cut into thick slabs

2 medium zucchini, cut lengthwise into ¼-inch-thick slabs

1 red onion, sliced into ½-inch-thick rounds

4 tablespoons extra-virgin olive oil

Sea salt and freshly ground black pepper

2 tablespoons red wine vinegar

1 clove garlic, minced

2 tablespoons coarsely chopped fresh parsley

1. **Marinate the lamb:** In a small bowl, whisk together the oil, garlic, rosemary, salt, and black pepper. Place the lamb chops in a large resealable bag, pour in the marinade, seal, and shake to coat. Refrigerate for at least 1 hour, or overnight for deeper flavor.
2. **Prep the veggies and dressing:** In a medium bowl, toss the bell peppers, zucchini, and onion with 2 tablespoons of the oil and season with salt and black pepper.
3. In a small bowl, whisk together the remaining 2 tablespoons oil, the vinegar, garlic, and parsley. Set the dressing aside.
4. **Grill the lamb and veggies:** Preheat the grill or a grill pan to medium-high heat.
5. Add the lamb chops and veggies to the grill. Cook the chops for 4 to 5 minutes per side, until the internal temp reaches 135°F for medium-rare. Grill the veggies for 4 to 5 minutes per side, until slightly charred and tender. Remove everything from the grill and let the lamb rest for 5 minutes.
6. Toss the grilled veggies in the dressing until evenly coated. Plate the lamb chops alongside the vegetables and serve immediately. Optional side: the Farro on page 182.

**STORAGE:** Store leftover lamb and veggies separately in airtight containers in the fridge for up to 3 days. Reheat lamb gently in a skillet, or the oven at 325°F, until warmed through; the veggies can be enjoyed warm or cold.

---

**PER SERVING**
Protein: 43g
Carbohydrates: 12g
Fat: 62g

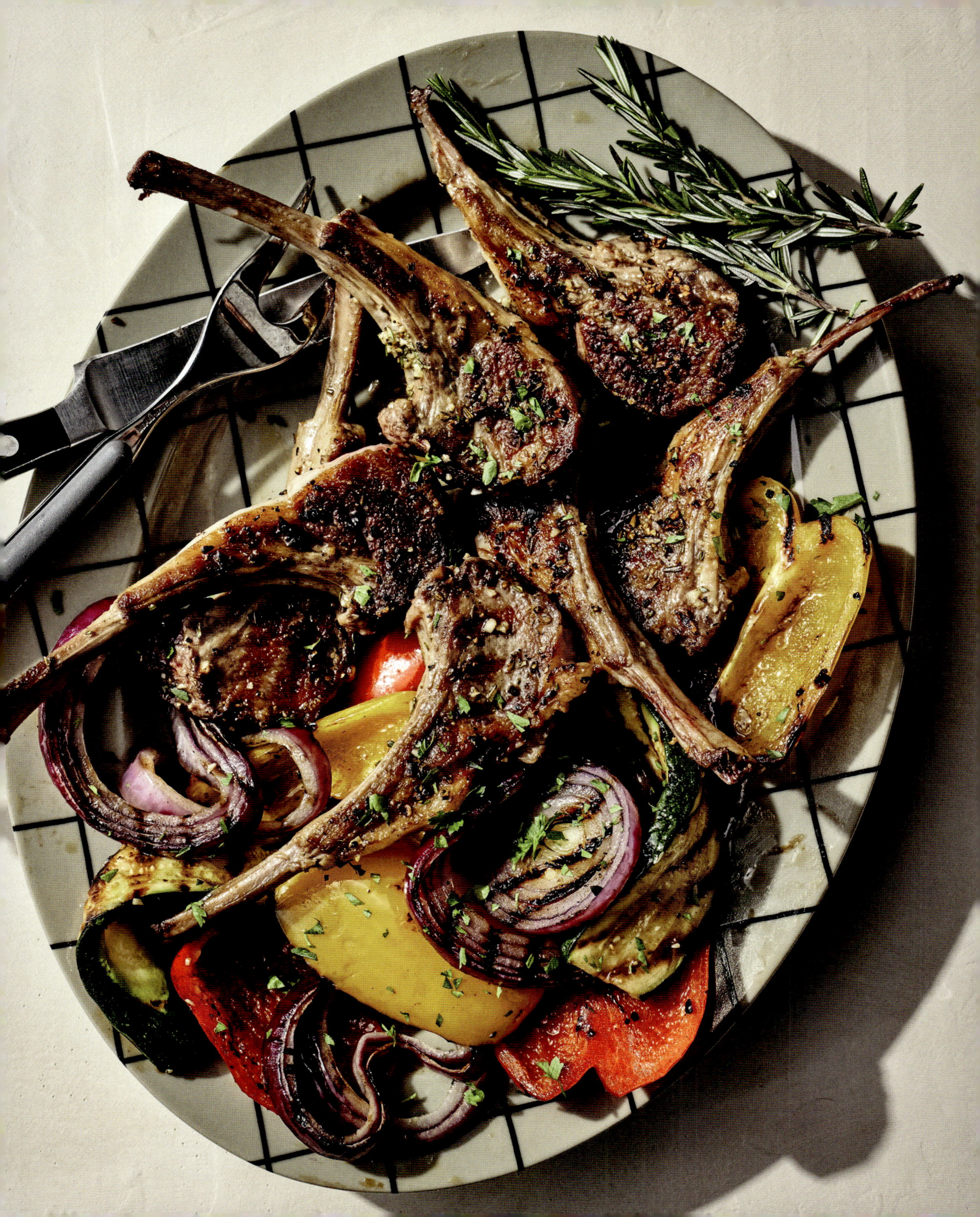

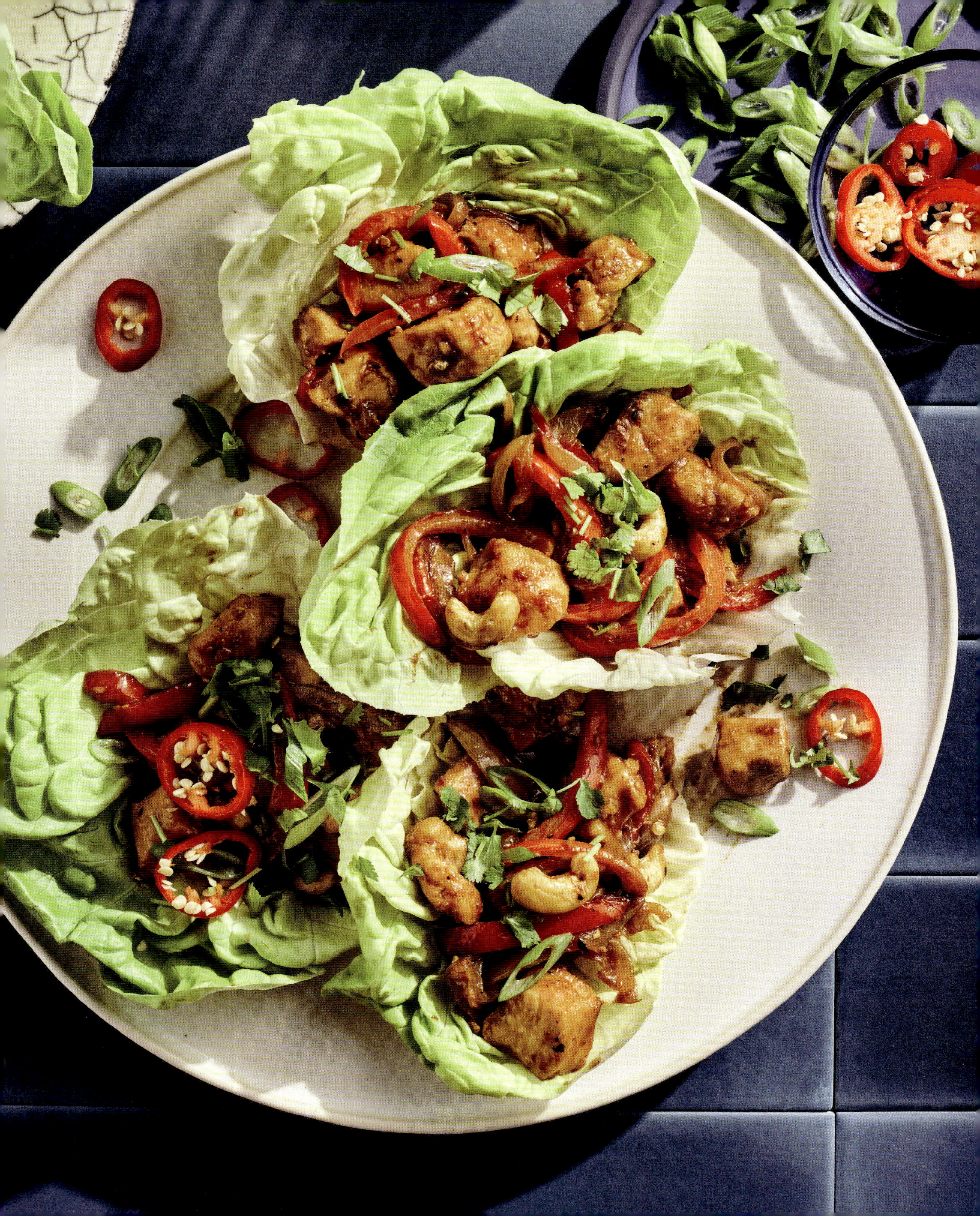

Dairy-Free
Gluten-Free
Grain-Free

# Szechuan Chicken Lettuce Wraps

SERVES 4 TO 5 • PREP TIME: 15 MINUTES • COOK TIME: 17 MINUTES • TOTAL TIME: 32 MINUTES

This is one of those dinners you'll want to put into regular rotation. Juicy chicken, sautéed veggies, crunchy cashews, and the most delicious slightly sweet and spicy Szechuan sauce. It's quick, bold, and way better than takeout because you're in control of every ingredient. Serve in crisp lettuce cups or over rice for a heartier option—either way, it's a winner. Bonus: This one's naturally gluten-free and dairy-free and easy to switch up depending on the veggies you have on hand.

FOR THE SAUCE

¼ cup coconut aminos

2 tablespoons freshly squeezed lime juice (1 lime)

2 tablespoons rice vinegar

2 teaspoons toasted sesame oil

1 tablespoon coconut sugar

FOR THE CHICKEN

2 tablespoons arrowroot powder

1½ teaspoons sea salt

1 teaspoon garlic powder

¼ teaspoon freshly ground black pepper

1½ pounds boneless, skinless chicken breasts, cut into 1-inch cubes

2 tablespoons avocado oil

1 large red bell pepper, seeded and thinly sliced (or try broccoli florets, sugar snap peas, or green beans)

1 small white onion, thinly sliced

1 tablespoon freshly grated ginger

4 garlic cloves, minced

1½ teaspoons ground Szechuan peppercorns

½ cup dry roasted cashews

FOR SERVING

1 head butter lettuce, leaves removed and cleaned

4 green onions, white and green parts, thinly sliced

¼ cup chopped fresh cilantro

1 Fresno chili pepper, thinly sliced (optional)

1. **Make the sauce:** In a small bowl, whisk together the coconut aminos, lime juice, vinegar, sesame oil, and coconut sugar. Set aside.
2. **Cook the chicken:** In a medium bowl, mix the arrowroot powder, salt, garlic powder, and black pepper. Add the chicken and toss to coat.
3. In a large nonstick skillet, heat 1 tablespoon of the avocado oil over medium-high heat. Add the chicken in a single layer (work in batches if needed). Cook undisturbed for 4 minutes, then toss and cook for another 3 to 4 minutes, until the pieces are golden and cooked through. Transfer to a plate.
4. Reduce the heat to medium and add the remaining 1 tablespoon avocado oil. Add the bell pepper and onion, toss to coat, and cook for 4 minutes, until softened. Stir in the ginger, garlic, and Szechuan peppercorns, and cook for 1 to 2 minutes, until fragrant.
5. Return the chicken to the skillet and pour in the sauce. Stir and cook uncovered for 5 to 8 minutes, until the sauce thickens and coats the chicken. In the final few minutes, stir in the cashews. Remove from the heat and let cool slightly.
6. Layer two lettuce leaves together and fill with the chicken mixture. Repeat to use all the filling. Top the wraps with green onions, cilantro, and Fresno chili, if using. Or serve over rice for a heartier option.

**STORAGE:** Store the chicken filling in an airtight container in the fridge for up to 4 days. Keep lettuce leaves separate and assemble just before serving for the best texture. Reheat the filling in a skillet or microwave until warmed through.

---

**PER SERVING (FOR 4 SERVINGS)**
Protein: 56g
Carbohydrates: 10g
Fat: 21g

No Added Sugar
**IF MODIFIED:**
Dairy-Free
Gluten-Free
Grain-Free

# Beef Bolognese

**SERVES 4 TO 5 • PREP TIME: 10 MINUTES • COOK TIME: 1 HOUR 35 MINUTES • TOTAL TIME: 1 HOUR 45 MINUTES**

There's nothing quite like a slow-simmered Bolognese—rich, hearty, and full of depth. This version uses bone broth to add body and extra protein, plus a mix of tomatoes, garlic, and sautéed veggies that make the flavor feel slow-cooked and comforting. I like to use grass-fed beef when I can, but any ground beef will do the trick. Toss the sauce with tagliatelle or a pasta you have on hand for a warm, family-style dinner that's always a hit.

2 tablespoons extra-virgin olive oil
1 white onion, finely diced
3 long carrots, finely diced
3 celery sticks, finely diced
2 to 4 garlic cloves, finely minced
2 pounds ground beef
1 cup beef bone broth
1 tablespoon white wine vinegar
2 (14-ounce) cans crushed tomatoes
1 (8-ounce) can tomato paste
1 tablespoon dried oregano
½ teaspoon dried parsley
½ teaspoon garlic powder
2 teaspoons sea salt
Freshly ground black pepper
½ cup milk of choice (optional, to add a touch of creaminess)
1 (9-ounce) package egg tagliatelle noodles (or other long pasta; gluten-free if preferred)
Fresh basil, for garnish
Freshly grated Parmesan, for garnish (omit for dairy-free)

1. In a large skillet, heat the oil over medium heat. Add the onion, carrots, celery, and garlic and sauté for 10 to 12 minutes, until softened. Add the ground beef to the center of the skillet and break it into small pieces using a wooden spoon. Cook for 7 to 10 minutes, until it is no longer pink.
2. Pour in the broth and vinegar. Reduce the heat to medium-low, cover, and simmer for 30 minutes. Stir in the tomatoes, tomato paste, oregano, parsley, garlic powder, salt, and pepper. Reduce the heat to low and simmer uncovered for 45 minutes, stirring occasionally, until thickened. Stir in the milk, if using, and let the sauce simmer for an additional 5 minutes.
3. Meanwhile, cook the tagliatelle according to package instructions. Reserve ½ cup of the pasta water and drain.
4. Add the pasta to the skillet and toss to coat in the sauce, adding a splash of reserved pasta water if needed to loosen. Serve topped with basil and Parmesan.

**STORAGE:** Store the sauce in an airtight container in the fridge for up to 5 days, or freeze for up to 3 months. Thaw overnight in the fridge, then reheat on the stovetop over low heat, adding a splash of water or broth if needed. Store pasta separately for best texture.

---

**PER SERVING (FOR 5 SERVINGS)**
Protein: 48g
Carbohydrates: 55g
Fat: 22g

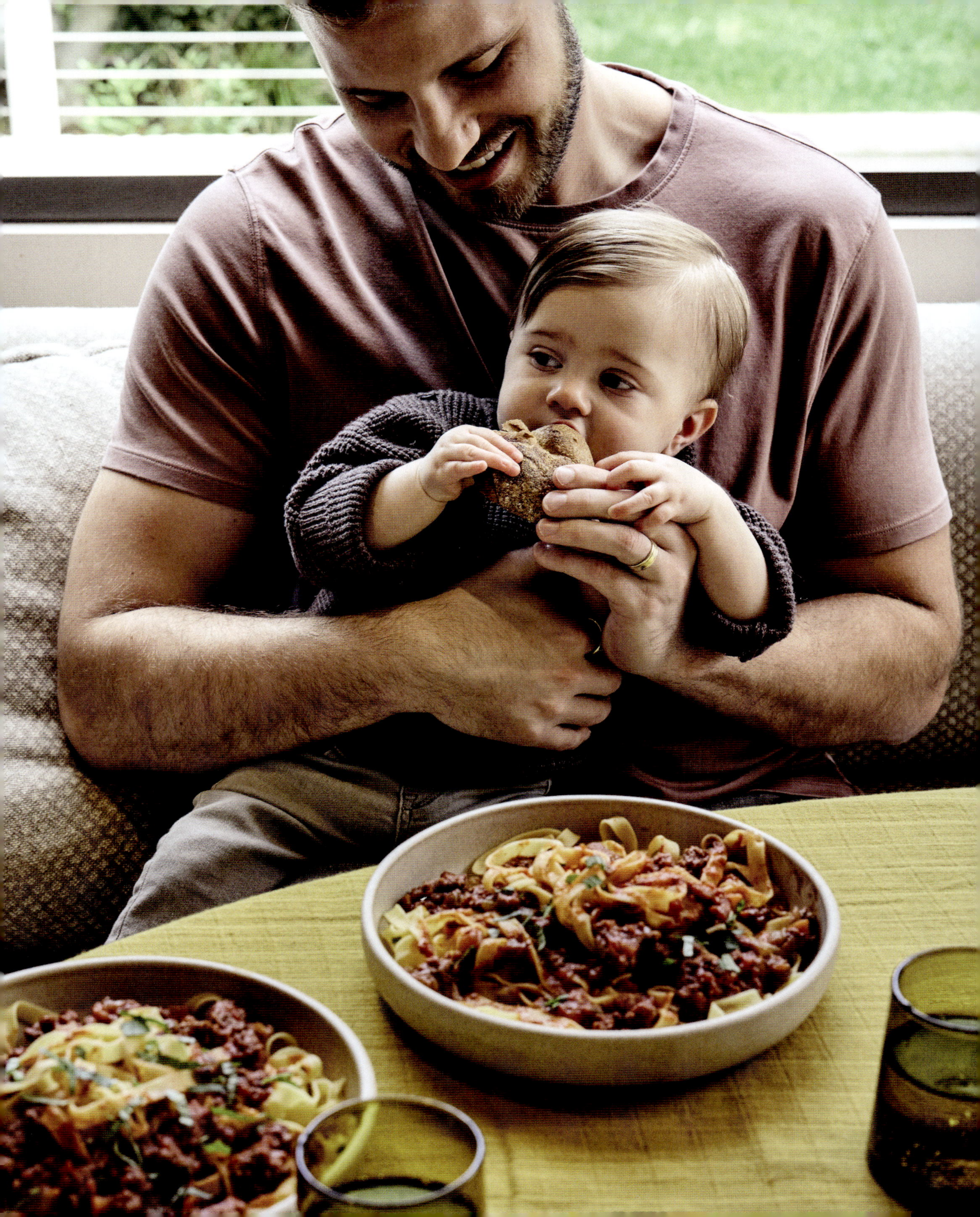

Gluten-Free
Grain-Free
No Added Sugar
**IF MODIFIED:**
Dairy-Free

# Tomato-Basil Chicken with Spaghetti Squash

**SERVES 4 • PREP TIME: 15 MINUTES • COOK TIME: 1 HOUR 15 MINUTES • TOTAL TIME: 1 HOUR 30 MINUTES**

If you struggle to figure out what to eat for lunch during the week like I do, this recipe might just change your life. You can prep the squash, chicken, and sauce separately at the top of the week, and then reheat easily whenever you're hungry. Spaghetti squash keeps it light but satisfying—and it's a great source of fiber and vitamin C. Trust me, future-you will be thrilled.

**FOR THE SPAGHETTI SQUASH**

2 medium spaghetti squash

2 tablespoons extra-virgin olive oil

½ teaspoon kosher salt

**FOR THE CHICKEN**

1½ pounds boneless, skinless chicken breasts, cut into 1-inch cubes

2 tablespoons extra-virgin olive oil

2 tablespoons freshly squeezed lemon juice (1 lemon)

2 teaspoons garlic powder

1½ teaspoons dried oregano

½ teaspoon dried thyme

1½ teaspoons kosher salt

½ teaspoon freshly ground black pepper

**FOR THE SAUCE**

2 tablespoons extra-virgin olive oil

1 cup diced yellow onion (about ½ large)

4 cloves garlic, minced

¼ teaspoon kosher salt

½ teaspoon crushed red pepper flakes

1 tablespoon freshly squeezed lemon juice (½ lemon)

1½ cups marinara sauce (like from Primal Kitchen or Rao's)

½ cup chicken bone broth

1. **Roast the spaghetti squash:** Preheat the oven to 375°F. Line a baking sheet with parchment paper.
2. Cut the squash in half lengthwise and scoop out the seeds. Place flesh side up on the baking sheet, drizzle with the oil, and season with the salt. Flip cut side down, then roast for 35 to 45 minutes, until fork-tender. Let cool slightly, then shred into noodles using a fork. Set aside.
3. **Cook the chicken:** In a medium bowl, toss the chicken with the oil, lemon juice, garlic powder, oregano, thyme, salt, and black pepper. Heat a large skillet over medium-high heat. Working in batches, add the chicken in a single layer and sear for 8 to 10 minutes, flipping halfway, until golden and cooked through. Transfer to a plate and set aside.
4. **Make the sauce:** In the same skillet, heat the oil over medium heat. Add the onion and sauté for 4 minutes, until translucent. Add the garlic, salt, and red pepper flakes and cook for 2 minutes more. Add the lemon juice to deglaze the skillet, scraping up any browned bits. Stir in the marinara, broth, and half the goat cheese. Let simmer gently for 10 minutes, stirring occasionally. Stir in half the basil and reduce the heat to low. Continue simmering, uncovered, for another 10 minutes to let the flavors come together.
5. Add the spaghetti squash noodles to the sauce and toss to coat. Stir in the cooked chicken and the peas and cook over low heat for 2 minutes, until everything is warmed through. Stir in the lemon zest and remaining basil. Serve topped with the remaining goat cheese (crumbled) and the toasted pine nuts.

---

**PER SERVING**
Protein: 47g
Carbohydrates: 29g
Fat: 26g

5 ounces goat cheese (omit for dairy-free)

1 cup julienned fresh basil

1½ cups frozen peas

1 teaspoon grated lemon zest

¼ cup toasted pine nuts, for serving

**MEAL-PREP TIPS:** *Divide the spaghetti squash topped with sauce and chicken into four portions and transfer to airtight glass containers. Let cool before adding toppings. Store in the fridge for up to 4 days. To reheat, microwave (covered with a paper towel) in 30-second increments until warmed through, or warm in a skillet over medium-low heat, covered, stirring occasionally.*

*The spaghetti squash, chicken, and/or sauce can all be cooked up to 4 days in advance and stored separately in airtight containers in the fridge. When you're ready to eat, just toss everything together and reheat. (***Pro tip:** *Keep the goat cheese, pine nuts, and extra basil separate until serving for the best texture and flavor.)*

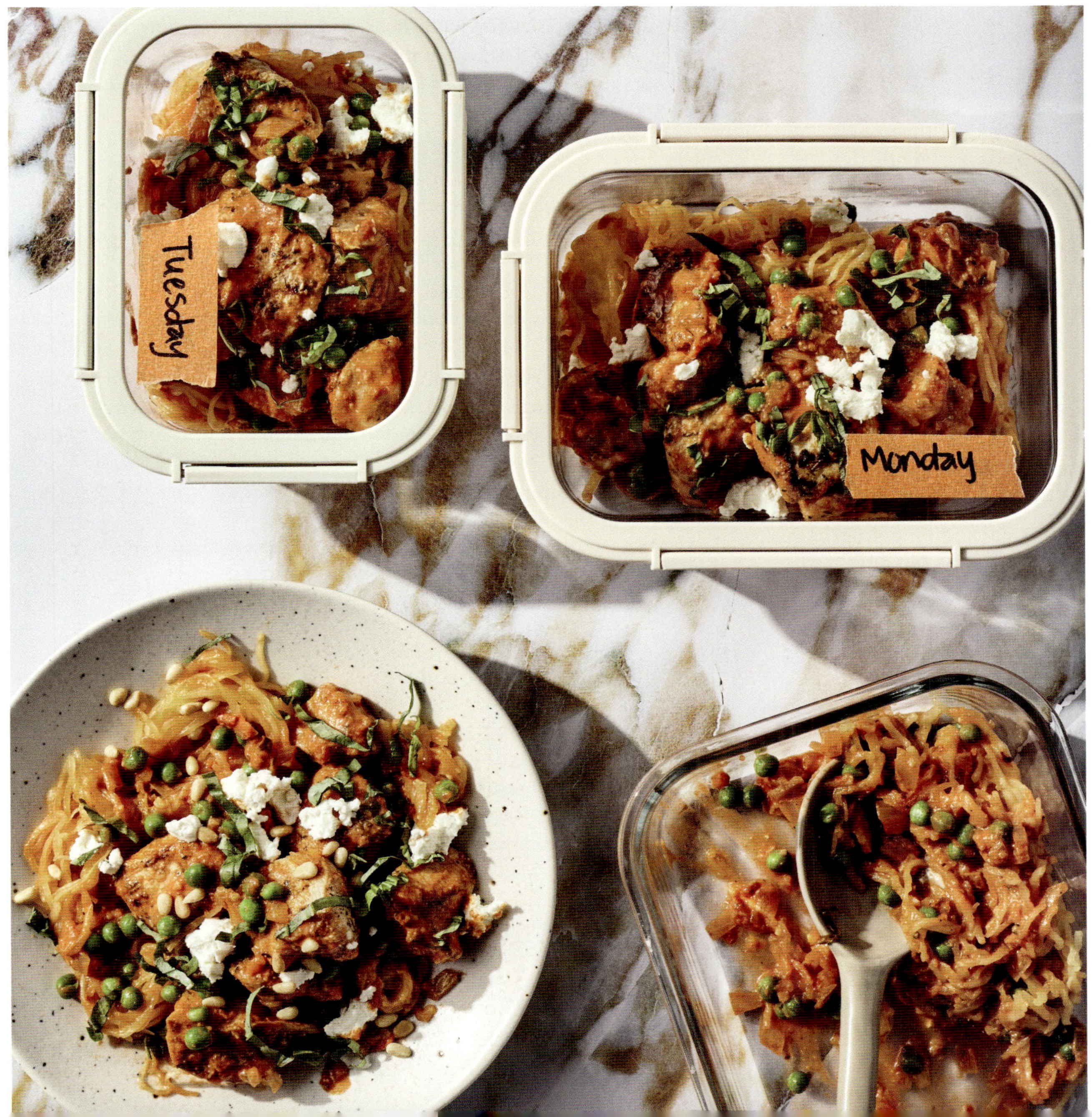

Gluten-Free
No Added Sugar

# Seared Halloumi and Chickpea Bowls with Herby Tahini

**SERVES 3 • PREP TIME: 15 MINUTES • COOK TIME: 25 MINUTES • TOTAL TIME: 40 MINUTES**

Let's talk about halloumi—the firm, salty, grill-able cheese that gets perfectly golden and crispy when seared. It's the kind of ingredient that instantly levels up any dish, and it's the star in this bowl. Paired with roasted chickpeas, caramelized veggies, fluffy quinoa, and a smooth herby tahini sauce, this meal is crunchy, creamy, salty, and straight-up delish.

**FOR THE VEGGIES AND CHICKPEAS**

1 large sweet potato, peeled and cut into ½-inch dice

1 red onion, sliced into ½-inch-thick wedges

1 fennel bulb, trimmed and sliced into ½-inch-thick wedges (reserve fennel fronds for garnish)

1 (15-ounce) can chickpeas, drained, rinsed, and patted dry

2 tablespoons extra-virgin olive oil

1 teaspoon paprika

1 teaspoon garlic powder

1 teaspoon sea salt

1 teaspoon freshly ground black pepper

**FOR THE QUINOA**

1 cup quinoa, rinsed

2 cups bone broth or water

1 teaspoon sea salt

**FOR THE SAUCE**

¼ cup extra-virgin olive oil

¼ cup tahini

2 tablespoons lemon juice

2 cups packed tender herbs (dill, cilantro, parsley, or chives—mix and match!)

1 garlic clove

1 teaspoon sea salt

**FOR THE HALLOUMI**

1 tablespoon extra-virgin olive oil

1 (8-ounce) package halloumi cheese, sliced into ¼-inch-thick slabs

1. **Roast the veggies and chickpeas:** Preheat the oven to 425°F. On a baking sheet, toss the sweet potato, onion, fennel, and chickpeas with the oil, paprika, garlic powder, salt, and pepper. Roast for 25 minutes, stirring halfway through, until golden and tender.
2. **Cook the quinoa:** Meanwhile, in a small saucepan, bring the quinoa, broth, and salt to a boil. Reduce the heat to low, cover, and cook for 15 minutes, or until fluffy.
3. **Make the sauce:** In a blender or food processor, combine ¼ cup water with the oil, tahini, lemon juice, herbs, garlic, and salt. Blend until smooth and creamy.
4. **Sear the halloumi:** Heat a nonstick skillet over medium-high heat. Pour in the oil and heat until hot. Add the halloumi slices and sear for 2 minutes per side, until golden and crisp.
5. **Assemble the bowls:** Divide the quinoa, vegetables, and chickpeas among three bowls. Top with halloumi and drizzle with tahini sauce. Top with reserved fennel fronds, sesame seeds, and lemon wedges.

**STORAGE:** Store components separately in airtight containers in the fridge for up to 4 days. Reheat veggies and halloumi in a skillet or oven for the best texture. Sauce may thicken in the fridge—just stir in a splash of water before using.

**PER SERVING**
Protein: 25g
Carbohydrates: 49g
Fat: 38g

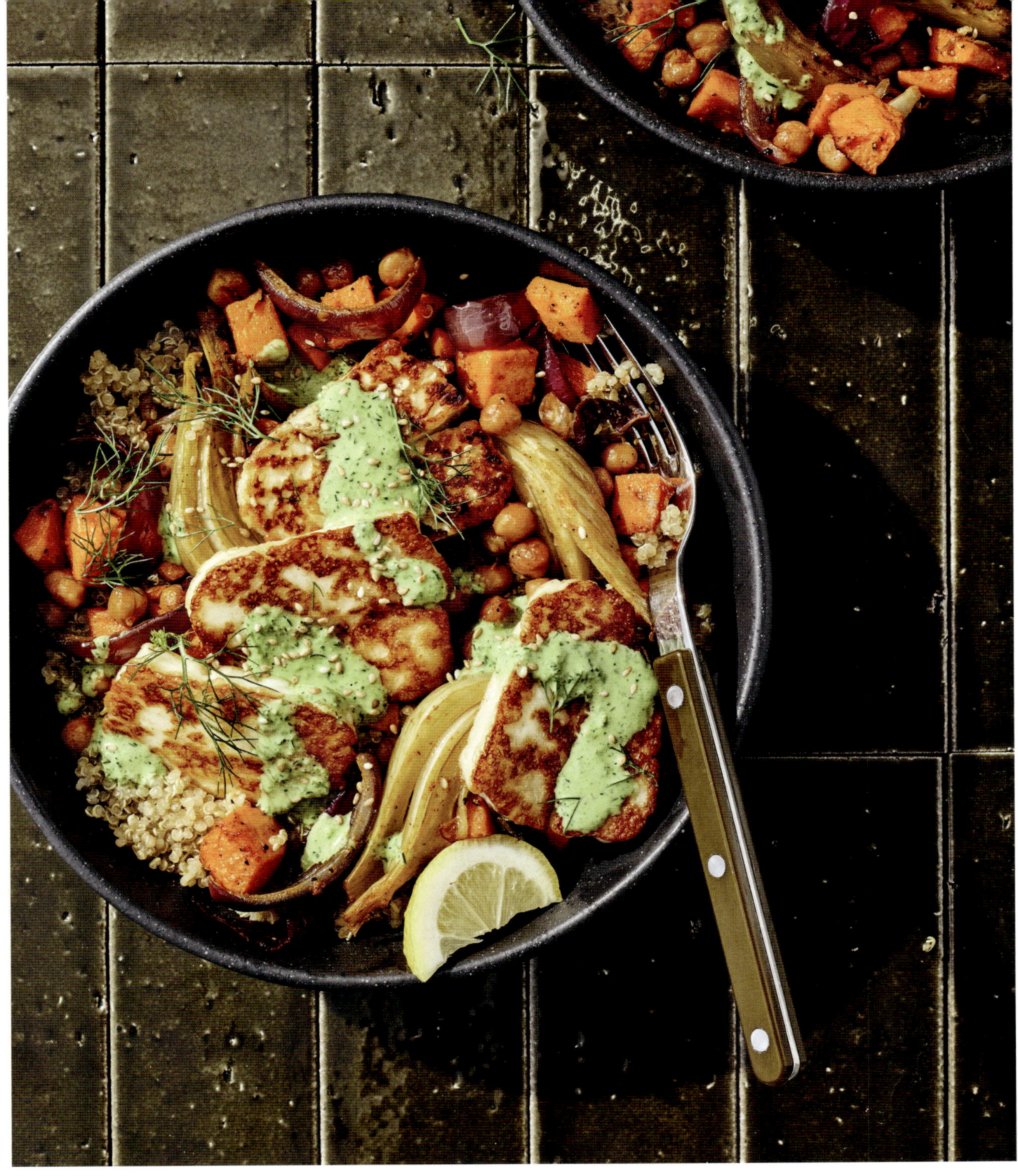

Optional toppings: reserved fennel fronds, toasted sesame seeds, lemon wedges

**MAKE-AHEAD TIP:** *Roast the veggies and chickpeas, cook the quinoa, and blend the herby tahini sauce up to 3 days ahead. Store each component separately. When you're ready to eat, all you'll need to do is quickly sear the halloumi and assemble the bowls.*

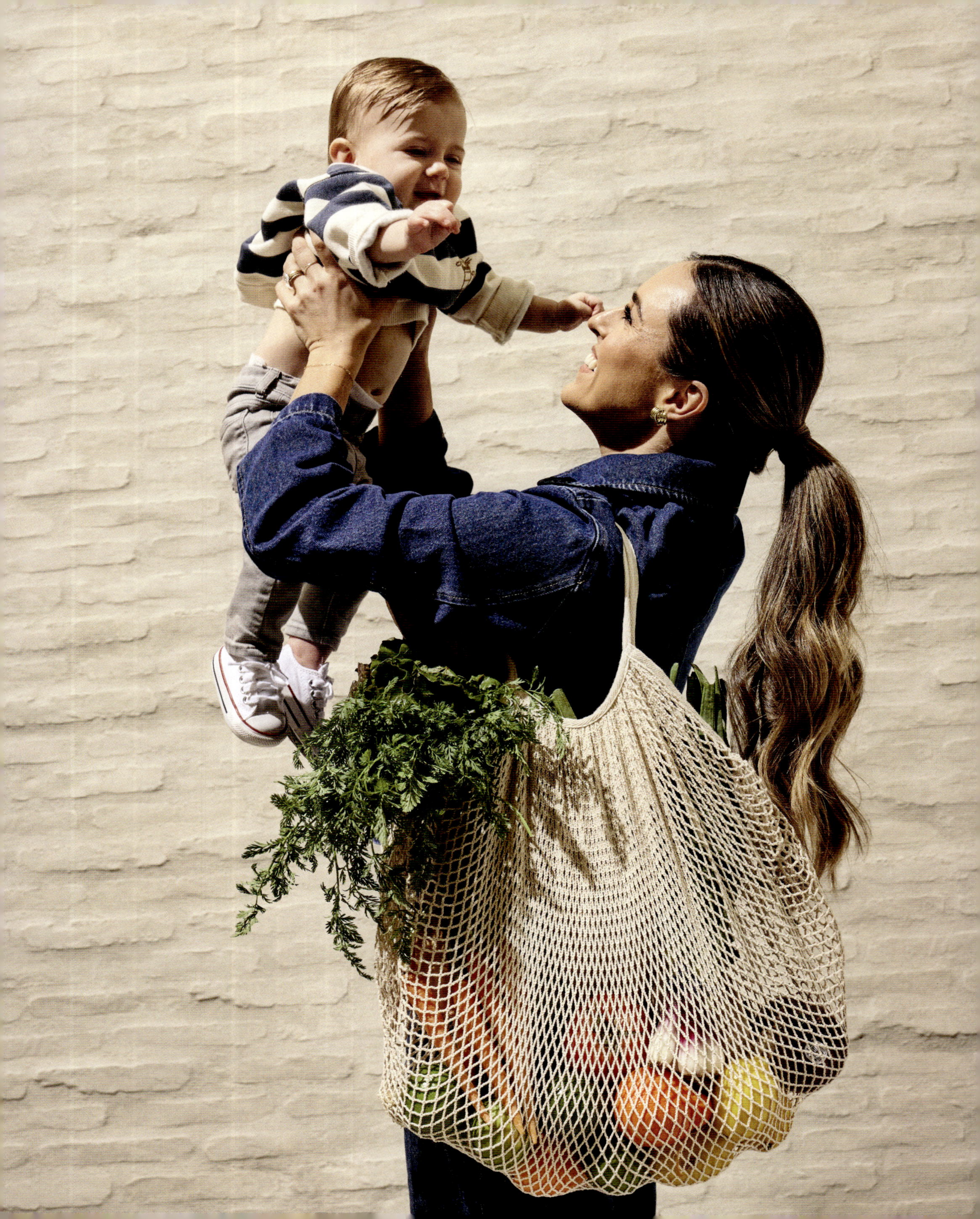

117 Honey-Harissa Salmon with Asparagus

118 Super Crispy Chicken Tenders with Homemade BBQ Sauce

121 Chipotle Chicken and Avocado Bowls

122 Saucy Coconut-Curry Turkey Meatballs

125 Air-Fryer Garlic-Butter Salmon Bites

126 Oven-Baked Beefy Burritos

129 Chili Crisp Tofu and Quinoa Power Bowls

130 Chicken and Peanut Pad Thai Bowls

133 20-Minute Shredded Chicken Verde

134 Grilled Mahi Mahi with Mango Salsa

137 Mexican Meatballs in Creamy Enchilada Sauce

138 Shredded Chicken Quesadillas

141 Loaded Chicken Pesto Panini

142 My Weeknight Hero: Ginger-Garlic Turkey Skillet

# 30-Minutes or Less Mains

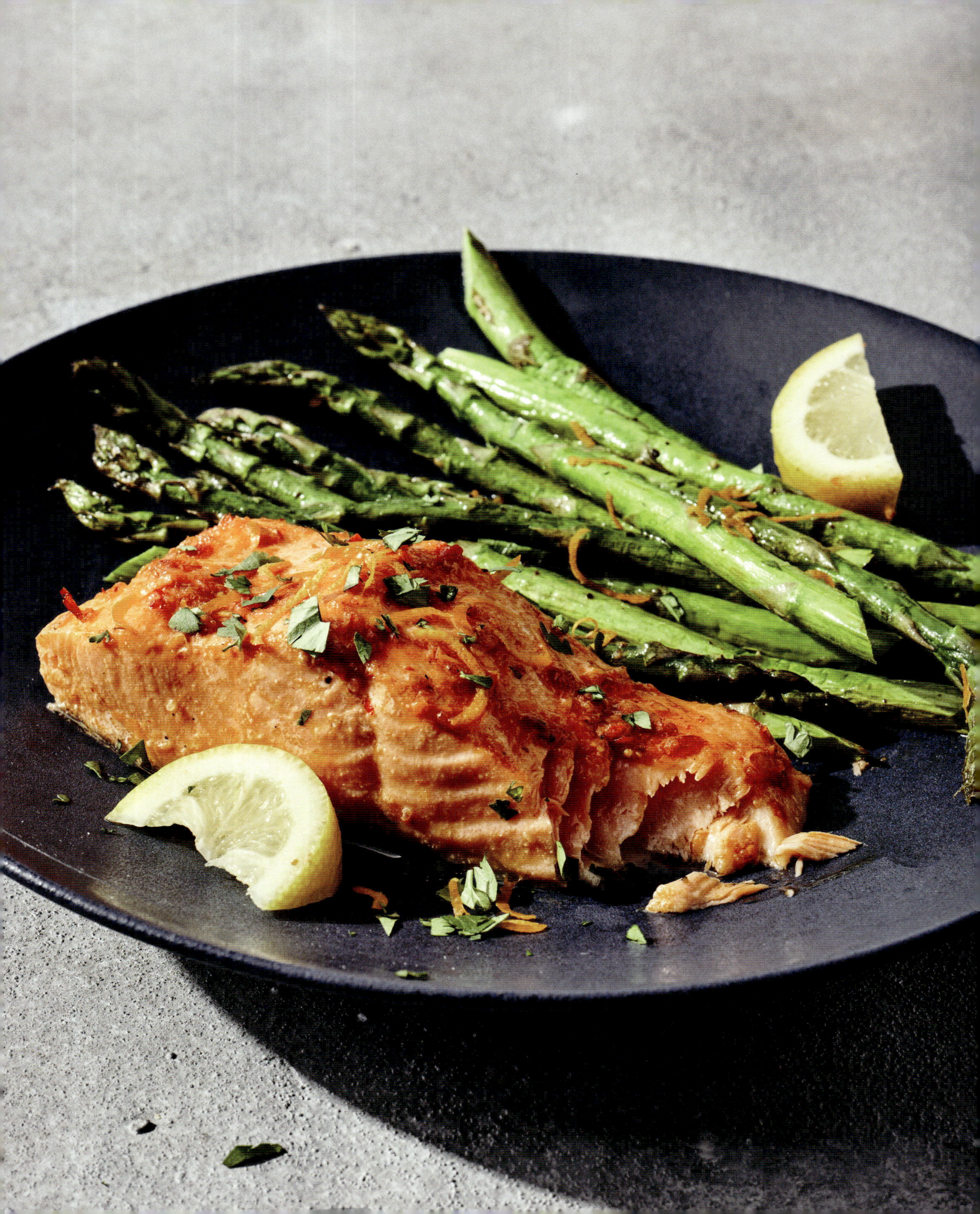

Dairy-Free
Gluten-Free
Grain-Free

# Honey-Harissa Salmon with Asparagus

**SERVES 4 • PREP TIME: 10 MINUTES, PLUS 10 MINUTES MARINATING • COOK TIME: 10 MINUTES • TOTAL TIME: 30 MINUTES**

- Grated zest of 1 orange
- ¼ cup freshly squeezed orange juice
- 2 tablespoons extra-virgin olive oil
- 2 tablespoons harissa paste
- 1 tablespoon honey
- 1 garlic clove, grated
- ½ teaspoon sea salt
- ½ teaspoon freshly ground black pepper
- 4 (6-ounce) wild salmon fillets, skin on
- 1 pound asparagus, ends trimmed
- For serving: chopped fresh cilantro, lemon wedges (optional)

I love making salmon in the oven for easy cleanup, but the real magic here is in the honey-harissa marinade. It's sweet, spicy, and brightened with a splash of citrus that cuts through the richness of the salmon and makes every bite more vibrant. With more than 35 grams of protein per serving and a total cook time under 30 minutes, it's a weeknight win. Serve on its own, or pair with Bone Broth Jasmine Rice (page 198) for a simple, well-rounded meal that delivers on flavor and ease.

1. Preheat the oven to 450°F. Line a baking sheet with parchment paper.
2. In a shallow bowl, whisk together the orange zest, orange juice, 1 tablespoon of the oil, the harissa paste, honey, garlic, ¼ teaspoon salt, and ¼ teaspoon pepper. Add the salmon fillets, turning to coat on both sides. Let the salmon marinate at room temperature for 10 minutes.
3. Place the asparagus on the baking sheet, drizzle with the remaining 1 tablespoon oil, and season with the remaining ¼ teaspoon salt and ¼ teaspoon pepper. Toss to coat. Nestle the salmon fillets among the asparagus on the baking sheet.
4. Roast for 8 to 10 minutes, until the salmon is opaque and flakes easily and the asparagus is fork-tender. Turn on the broiler. Broil the salmon and asparagus together for 1 to 2 minutes, until the salmon is lightly caramelized and the asparagus has a bit of char.
5. Plate the salmon with the asparagus and top with cilantro. Serve with lemon wedges, if desired.

**PER SERVING**
Protein: 37g
Carbohydrates: 13g
Fat: 16g

Gluten-Free
Grain-Free

# Super Crispy Chicken Tenders with Homemade BBQ Sauce

**SERVES 4 • PREP TIME: 15 MINUTES • COOK TIME: 10 TO 20 MINUTES • TOTAL TIME: 30 MINUTES**

**FOR THE BBQ SAUCE**

1 cup unsweetened ketchup (such as Primal Kitchen)

3 tablespoons apple cider vinegar

3 tablespoons coconut aminos

2 tablespoons maple syrup

2 tablespoons yellow mustard

1 teaspoon garlic powder

1 teaspoon smoked paprika

1 teaspoon onion powder

**FOR THE CHICKEN TENDERS**

1 pound chicken tenders

Sea salt and freshly ground black pepper

½ cup arrowroot starch

¾ cup almond flour

¼ cup plus 2 tablespoons grated pecorino romano cheese

½ teaspoon paprika

½ teaspoon garlic powder

2 large eggs

Avocado oil spray

Forget fast food—these homemade tenders are on another level. Ultra crispy on the outside, juicy on the inside, and served with a smoky, tangy BBQ sauce that Bridger could probably survive on alone if I let him. The secret is a double dip in an almond flour coating that creates golden, crunchy perfection that's basically guaranteed to disappear in minutes. Make the BBQ sauce while the tenders bake or air-fry, and you'll have dinner on the table in 30 minutes or less.

1. **Make the BBQ sauce**: In a small saucepan, combine the ketchup, vinegar, coconut aminos, maple syrup, mustard, garlic powder, smoked paprika, and onion powder. Bring to a simmer over medium heat. Reduce the heat to low and simmer, stirring often, for about 15 minutes, until slightly thickened. If baking the tenders, start the sauce while they cook to save time. Set aside to cool.
2. **Make the chicken tenders:** Season the chicken tenders with salt and pepper. Place the arrowroot starch in one shallow bowl. In a second bowl, whisk the eggs. In a third bowl, stir together the almond flour, pecorino, paprika, garlic powder, and ½ teaspoon salt. Working one at a time, dredge each chicken tender first in the arrowroot starch, then into the egg wash, and finally coat in the almond flour mixture. Press the coating on to help it stick.
3. **To bake in the oven:** Preheat the oven to 400°F. Place a wire rack in a rimmed baking sheet, spray the rack with avocado oil, and arrange the tenders on top. Spray the tops with avocado oil. Bake for 15 to 20 minutes, until golden and cooked through.
4. **To air-fry:** Line the air fryer basket with parchment paper and spray with avocado oil. Arrange the tenders in a single layer (you may need to work in batches). Spray the tops with avocado oil. Air fry at 375°F for 10 minutes, until crispy and cooked through.
5. Serve the tenders hot with the BBQ sauce.

**STORAGE:** Store leftover chicken tenders in an airtight container in the fridge for up to 3 days. Reheat in a 375°F oven for 8 to 10 minutes or air fryer for 5 to 6 minutes to bring back that crispy texture.

**PER SERVING**
Protein: 40g
Carbohydrates: 18g
Fat: 22g

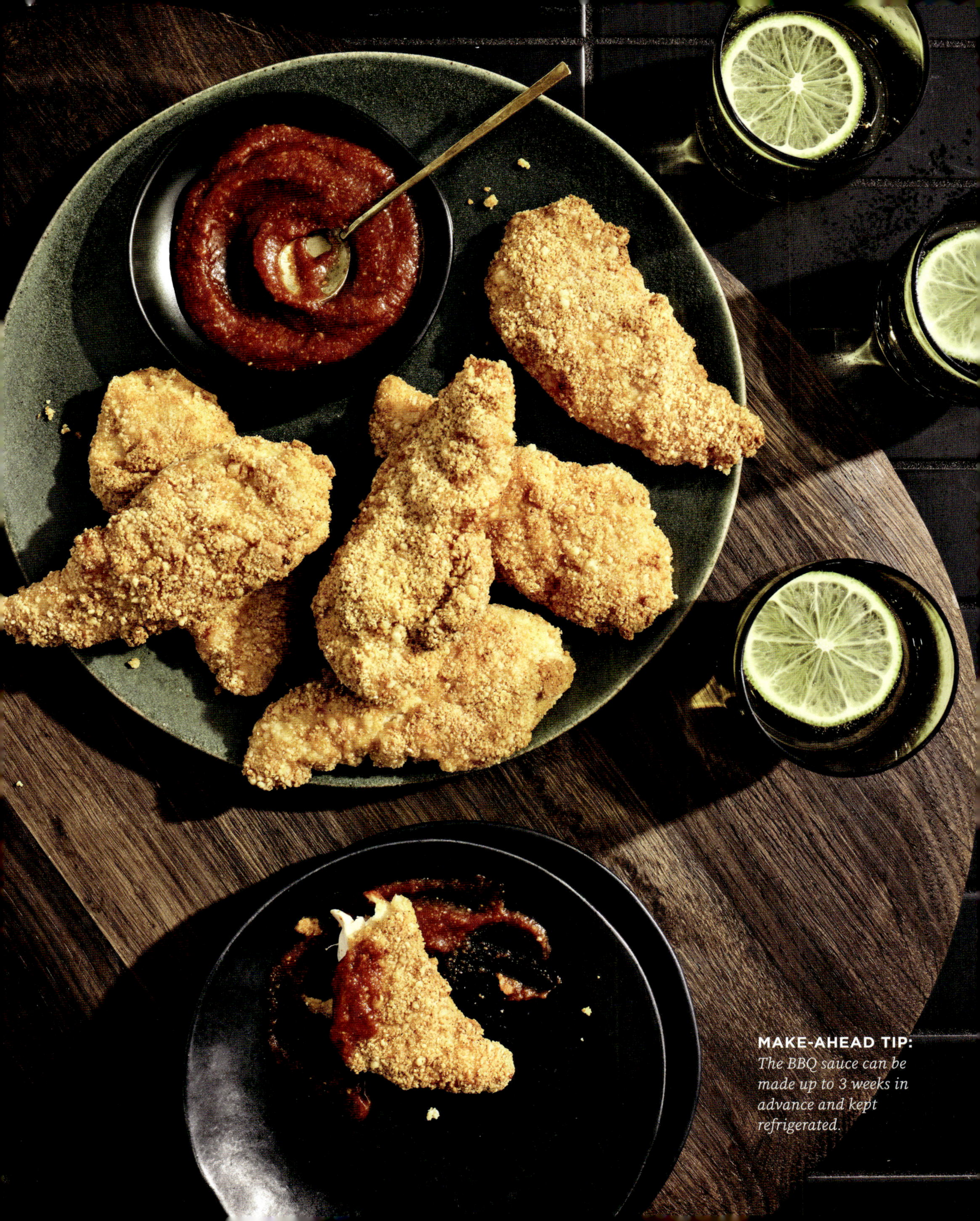

**MAKE-AHEAD TIP:**
*The BBQ sauce can be made up to 3 weeks in advance and kept refrigerated.*

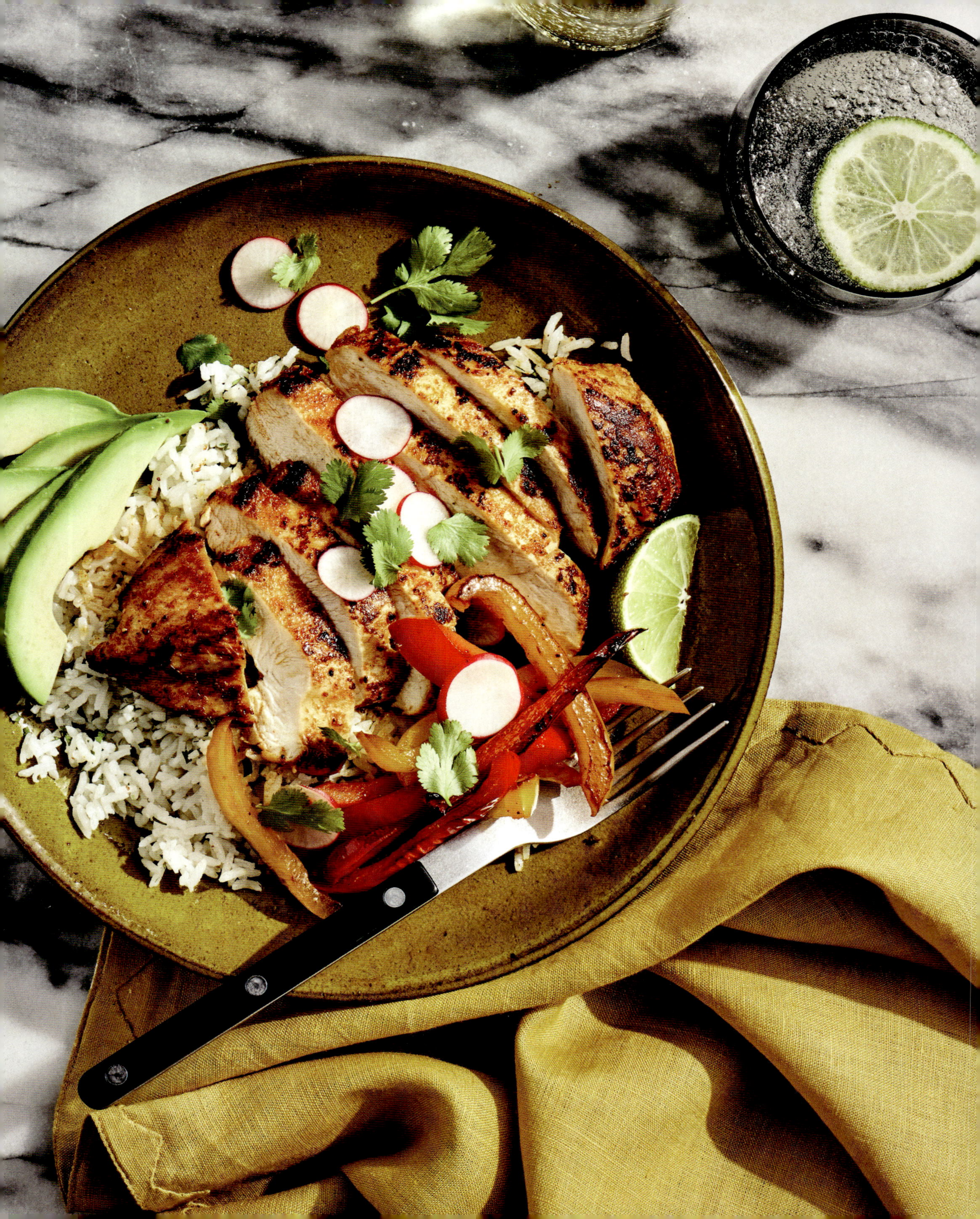

Dairy-Free
Gluten-Free
No Added Sugar

# Chipotle Chicken and Avocado Bowls

**SERVES 4 • PREP TIME: 15 MINUTES • COOK TIME: 15 MINUTES • TOTAL TIME: 30 MINUTES**

This is one of our go-to weeknight dinners when we're craving bold, Mexican-inspired flavor but don't feel like hovering over the stove. The chipotle chicken brings the heat, while creamy avocado and lime cool things down just right. With fluffy cilantro-lime rice, sautéed peppers, and all those textures, this bowl does the most—without asking much from you.

**FOR THE RICE**

1½ cups chicken bone broth

1 cup jasmine rice, rinsed

¼ cup coarsely chopped fresh cilantro

2 tablespoons lime juice

½ teaspoon sea salt

**FOR THE CHICKEN AND BELL PEPPERS**

2 tablespoons extra-virgin olive oil

1 tablespoon lime juice

1½ teaspoons ground cumin

1½ teaspoons smoked paprika

1 teaspoon garlic powder

½ teaspoon chipotle chili powder

½ teaspoon sea salt

½ teaspoon freshly ground black pepper

4 boneless, skinless chicken breasts, pounded ½ inch thick

2 bell peppers (I like a mix of red and yellow), seeded and sliced

Optional toppings: sliced avocado, additional cilantro, store-bought salsa, sour cream, cherry tomatoes, black beans, sliced radish, lime wedges, salt

1. **Cook the rice:** Bring the broth and rice to a boil in a medium saucepan. Reduce the heat to low, cover, and simmer for 12 minutes, or until the liquid is absorbed. Remove from the heat, fluff with a fork, and stir in the cilantro, lime juice, and salt. Cover to keep warm.
2. **Cook the chicken and bell peppers:** Meanwhile, in a large bowl, whisk together the oil, lime juice, cumin, paprika, garlic powder, chipotle powder, salt, and black pepper. Add the chicken and toss to coat evenly.
3. Heat a large cast-iron skillet over medium heat. Add the chicken and cook undisturbed for 4 to 5 minutes. Flip, cover, and cook for another 5 to 6 minutes, until no longer pink. Remove from the heat and let rest for 5 minutes before slicing.
4. In the same skillet, sauté the bell peppers over medium heat for 4 to 5 minutes, stirring occasionally, until softened and lightly charred.
5. Divide the rice, chicken, and bell peppers among four bowls. Top with avocado, cilantro, and any other desired toppings.

**STORAGE:** Store leftover chicken, rice, and veggies in separate airtight containers in the fridge for up to 4 days. Reheat gently in a skillet or microwave before assembling. Add fresh toppings just before serving.

**PER SERVING**
Protein: 42g
Carbohydrates: 45g
Fat: 12g

**MAKE-AHEAD TIP:** *The rice and sautéed peppers can be prepped up to 2 or 3 days ahead and stored separately in airtight containers in the fridge. For the best flavor and texture, cook the chicken fresh just before serving. Then all that's left is quick assembly with your favorite toppings.*

Dairy-Free
Gluten-Free
Grain-Free
No Added Sugar
Paleo

# Saucy Coconut-Curry Turkey Meatballs

**SERVES 4 • PREP TIME: 10 MINUTES • COOK TIME: 15 MINUTES • TOTAL TIME: 25 MINUTES**

These quick and easy meatballs are light, tender, and packed with 30 grams of protein per serving, making them a solid heavy-hitter when you want something filling that doesn't weigh you down. The creamy coconut-curry sauce is rich and comforting, with healthy fats and antioxidants in every bite. My family absolutely loves this one. Serve over rice or with extra veggies for a no-fuss meal that feels indulgent (but totally isn't).

**FOR THE MEATBALLS**

Avocado oil spray
1 pound ground turkey
1 large egg
½ cup almond flour
2 cloves garlic, minced
3 green onions, white and green parts, minced
1 teaspoon coconut aminos
¼ teaspoon ground ginger
½ teaspoon sea salt
⅛ teaspoon freshly ground black pepper

**FOR THE COCONUT CURRY**

1 tablespoon avocado oil
2 cloves garlic, minced
1½ tablespoons red curry paste
1 (14-ounce) can full-fat organic coconut milk
1½ tablespoons coconut aminos
2 long carrots, sliced into ½-inch-thick rounds
1 red bell pepper, seeded and thinly sliced (or sub sliced zucchini or snap peas for a similar texture and flavor)
2 cups fresh spinach
Lime juice
2 tablespoons coarsely chopped fresh cilantro
White or brown rice, for serving (optional)

1. **Make the meatballs:** Preheat the oven to 400°F. Spray a large baking sheet with avocado oil.
2. In a medium bowl, mix the ground turkey, egg, almond flour, garlic, green onions, coconut aminos, ginger, salt, and black pepper. Scoop heaping tablespoons of the mixture and roll into 1-inch meatballs, making about 24 total. Arrange evenly on the baking sheet and bake for 15 minutes, until cooked through.
3. **Make the coconut curry:** While the meatballs bake, heat the oil in a large sauté pan over medium heat. Add the garlic and curry paste and sauté for 1 minute, until fragrant. Stir in the coconut milk, coconut aminos, carrots, and bell pepper. Reduce the heat to medium-low and simmer for 10 minutes, or until the vegetables are tender. Add the spinach and stir until wilted. Add the cooked meatballs to the sauce and gently stir to coat.
4. Season with lime juice, top with cilantro, and serve as is or over rice.

**STORAGE:** Store meatballs and sauce together in an airtight container in the fridge for up to 4 days, or freeze for up to 2 months. Reheat gently on the stovetop or in the microwave. If the sauce thickens, add a splash of coconut milk or broth to loosen.

---

**PER SERVING**
Protein: 30g
Carbohydrates: 8g
Fat: 24g

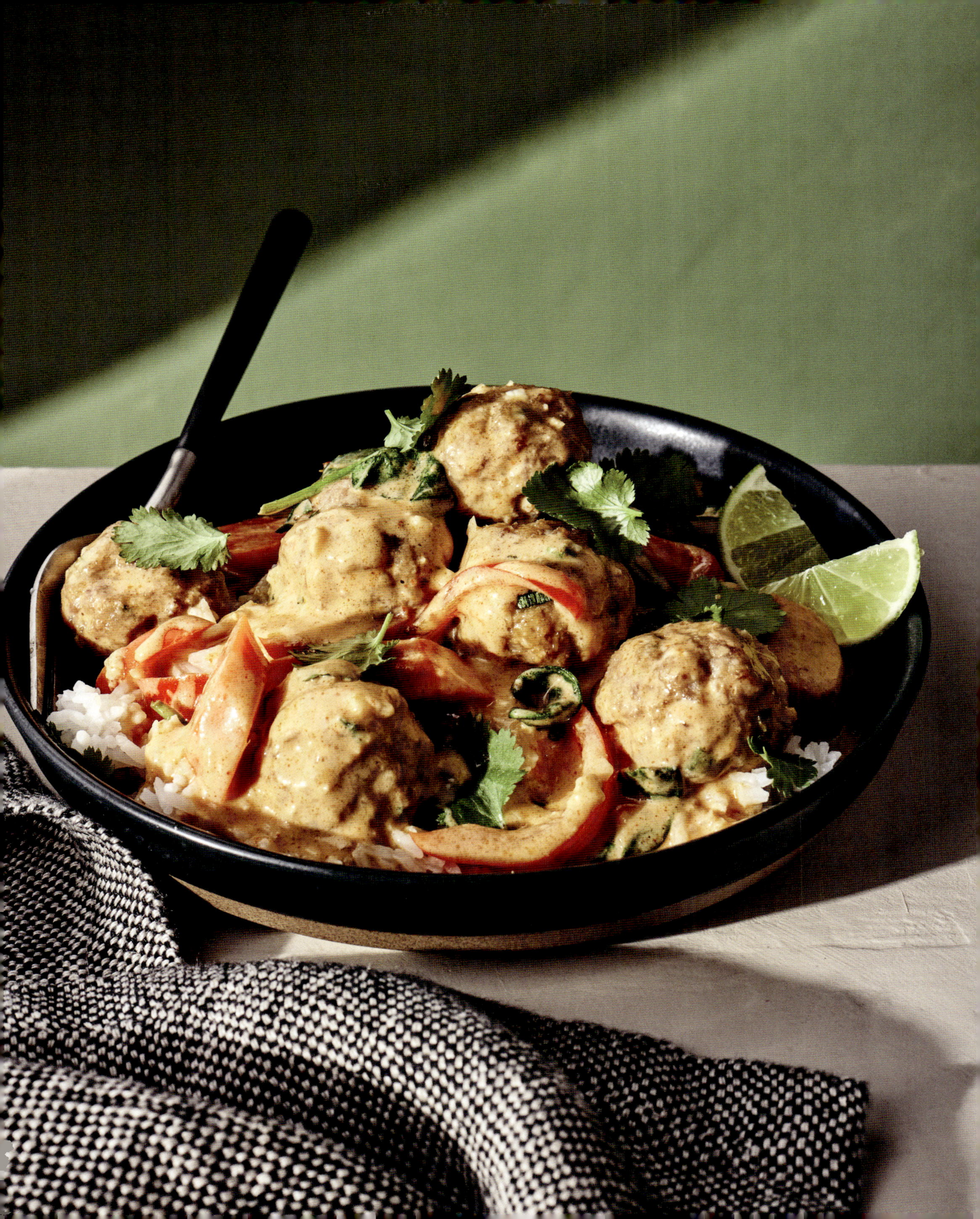

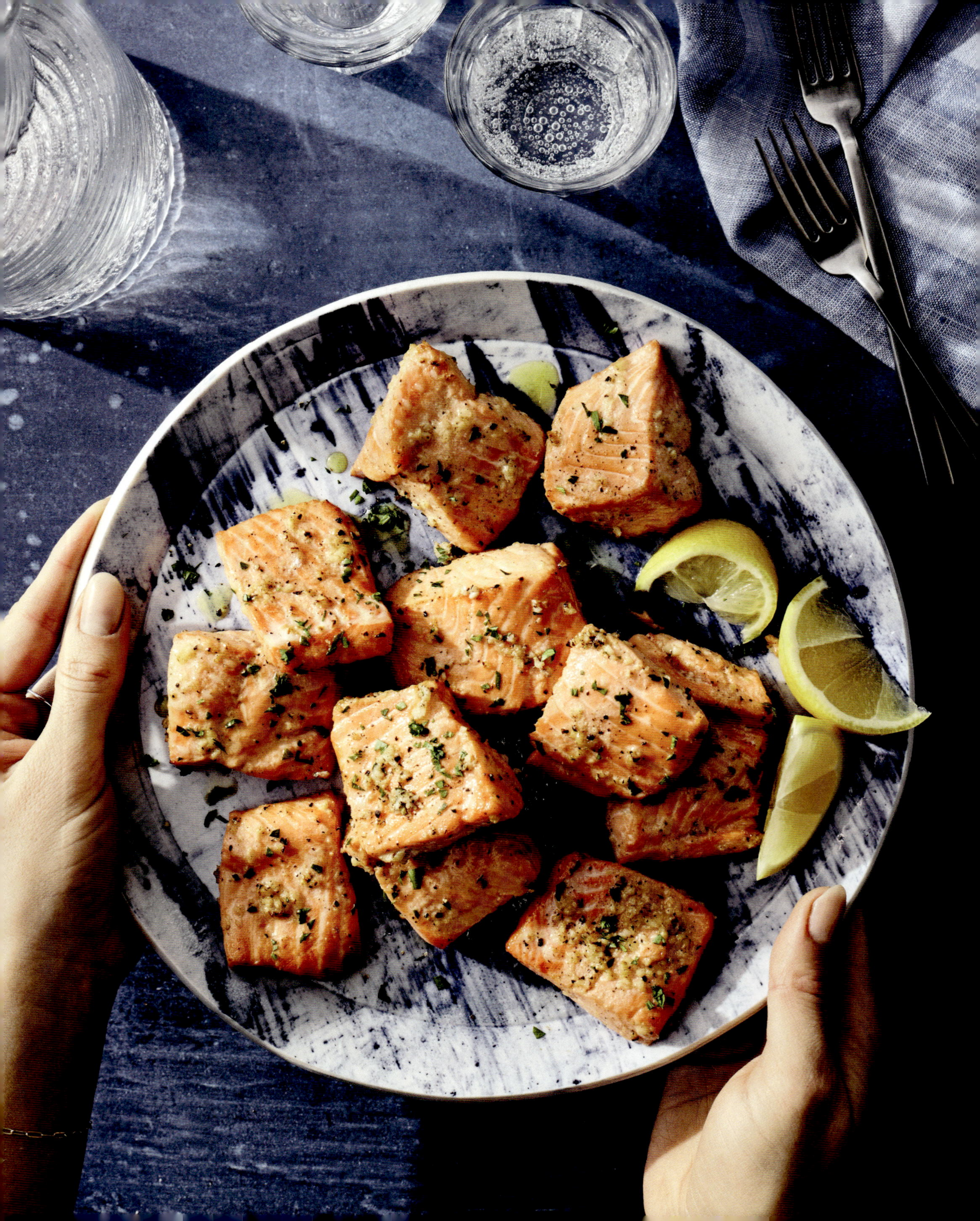

Gluten-Free
Grain-Free
No Added Sugar
**IF MODIFIED:**
Dairy-Free

# Air-Fryer Garlic-Butter Salmon Bites

**SERVES 5 • PREP TIME: 5 MINUTES, PLUS 15 MINUTES MARINATING • COOK TIME: 7 MINUTES • TOTAL TIME: 27 MINUTES**

¼ cup ghee, melted (or vegan butter for dairy-free)
4 cloves garlic, minced
2 tablespoons lemon juice
½ teaspoon sea salt
½ teaspoon freshly ground black pepper
2 pounds wild salmon fillets, skin removed and cut into 1½-inch pieces
2 tablespoons finely chopped fresh parsley, for garnish
Lemon wedges, for serving (optional)

These rich and garlicky salmon bites are my answer to those days when I need something fast and delish—without trashing the kitchen. They're juicy, rich, and full of garlicky-lemony goodness, plus they come together in under 10 minutes in the air fryer or oven. I love adding them to salads, bowls, or veggies for a quick weeknight dinner that feels a little elevated, but couldn't be easier.

1. If using the oven, preheat it to 400°F. (If using a traditional air fryer or an air fryer setting on your oven, there's no need to preheat.)
2. In a large bowl, mix the ghee, garlic, lemon juice, salt, and pepper. Add the salmon pieces and toss to coat. Let marinate at room temperature for 15 minutes (it's normal for the ghee to firm up slightly).
3. **To air-fry:** Place the salmon pieces in a single layer in the air fryer basket. Air-fry at 375°F, shaking the basket halfway through, 7 to 8 minutes.
4. **To bake in the oven:** Line a baking sheet with parchment paper. Place the salmon pieces on the baking sheet and bake for 5 to 6 minutes, then broil for an additional 2 minutes for a golden finish. Watch closely to avoid burning.
5. Sprinkle with parsley and serve with lemon wedges, if desired.

**STORAGE:** Store leftover salmon bites in an airtight container in the fridge for up to 3 days. Reheat in the air fryer at 350°F for 3 to 4 minutes or in the oven at 350°F for about 6 to 8 minutes, until warmed through. Avoid microwaving to help maintain texture.

**PER SERVING**
Protein: 37g
Carbohydrates: 2g
Fat: 19g

No Added Sugar
**IF MODIFIED:**
Gluten-Free
Grain-Free

# Oven-Baked Beefy Burritos

**SERVES 4 • PREP TIME: 5 MINUTES • COOK TIME: 20 MINUTES • TOTAL TIME: 25 MINUTES**

- 1 tablespoon avocado oil
- 1 pound ground beef
- 1 teaspoon onion powder
- 1 teaspoon ground cumin
- ½ teaspoon dried oregano
- ½ teaspoon sea salt
- 1 (10-ounce) jar mild or medium salsa, plus more for serving
- 1 (15-ounce) can refried pinto beans
- 4 large (9- to 10-inch) tortillas (I prefer Siete brand for a grain-free option)
- 1 cup shredded Monterey Jack cheese (or preferred cheese)
- ¼ cup chopped fresh cilantro
- Toppings: shredded lettuce, diced tomatoes, avocado, sour cream, salsa, lime wedges

A good burrito always hits. These are baked for crispy edges and packed with juicy beef, refried beans, and melty cheese. They also happen to be the ultimate meal-prep move as they freeze beautifully. Make a batch now, and future-you will thank you—they're hearty and exactly what you want without that too-full, can't-move taqueria feeling.

1. Preheat the oven to 375°F. Line a baking sheet with parchment paper.
2. In a large sauté pan, heat the oil over medium heat. Add the ground beef, onion powder, cumin, oregano, and salt. Cook, breaking up the meat, for about 5 minutes, until it starts to brown. Add the salsa and continue to cook for 5 to 7 minutes, until most of the liquid has evaporated.
3. Meanwhile, in a small saucepan over low heat, warm the refried beans for 2 to 3 minutes, stirring until smooth and easily spreadable. Warm the tortillas in the microwave for 30 seconds to 1 minute, or in a dry pan over medium heat until just warm.
4. Lay out the tortillas and add one-fourth each of the beans, cheese, beef, and cilantro to each tortilla. Roll up the tortillas, folding in the sides as you go.
5. Place the burritos seam side down on the baking sheet. Bake for 15 minutes, until warmed through and crispy on the bottom.
6. Serve whole or cut in half, then load up with lettuce, tomatoes, avocado, and sour cream, if desired. Serve immediately, with extra salsa and lime wedges on the side.

**STORAGE:** Store leftover burritos in an airtight container in the fridge for up to 4 days, or wrap individually and freeze for up to 2 months.

---

**PER SERVING**
Protein: 40g
Carbohydrates: 27g
Fat: 30g

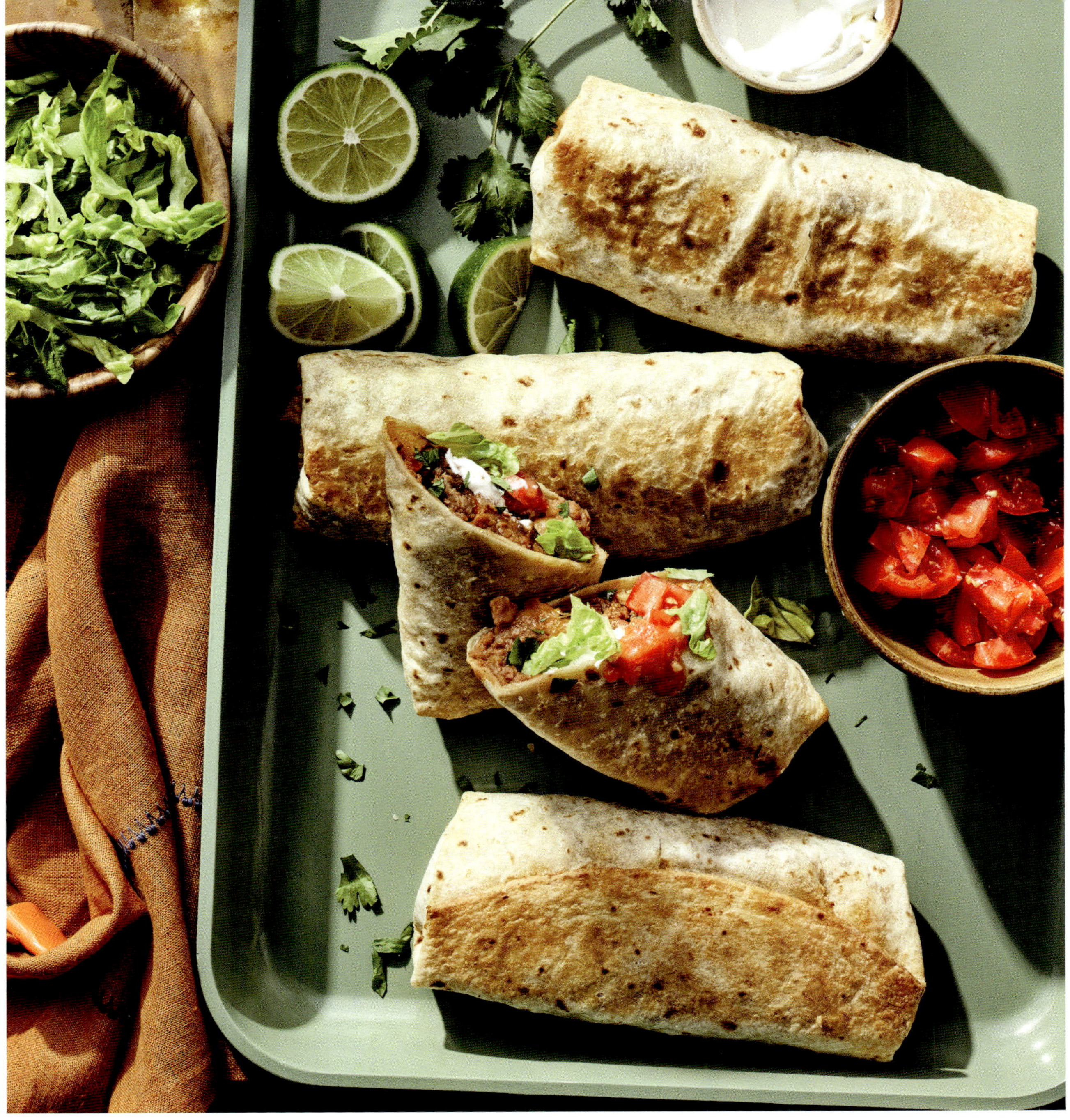

## *To reheat:*

**FROM THE FRIDGE**

- Warm in a 350°F oven for 10 to 15 minutes, or microwave until heated through.

**FROM FROZEN**

- Bake at 350°F for 25 to 30 minutes, or air-fry at 350°F for 12 to 15 minutes, flipping halfway through for even crisping. For the crispiest results, skip the microwave.

**MEAL-PREP TIP:** *Make a double batch, wrap each burrito individually in foil or parchment, and stash in the freezer. When hunger hits, just pop one in the oven or air fryer to reheat. Crispy, satisfying, and completely hands-off.*

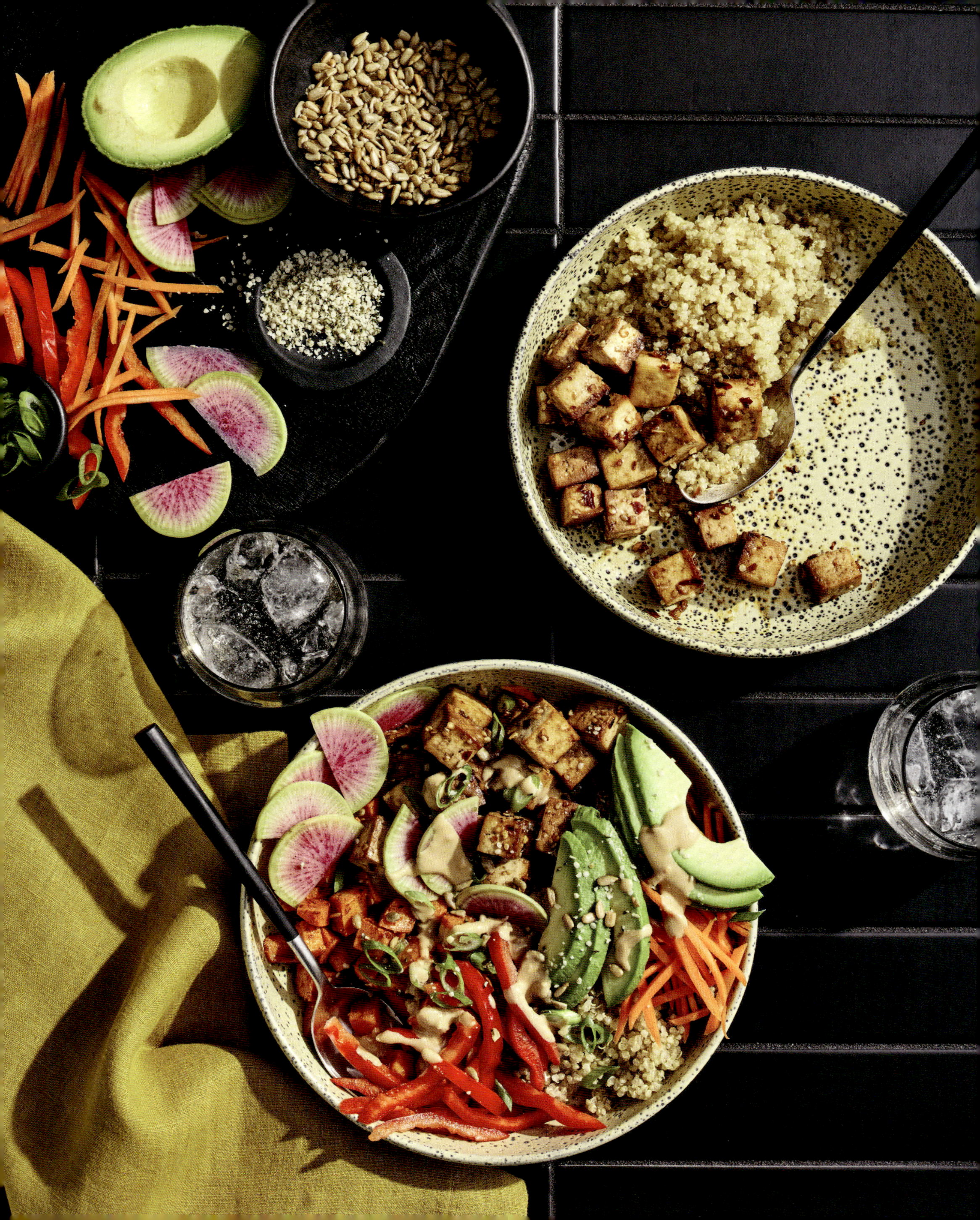

Dairy-Free
Gluten-Free

# Chili Crisp Tofu and Quinoa Power Bowls

**SERVES 2 • PREP TIME: 15 MINUTES • COOK TIME: 15 MINUTES • TOTAL TIME: 30 MINUTES**

This bowl checks all the boxes: spicy, crispy tofu, caramelized sweet potatoes, and plenty of fresh, crunchy veggies, all drizzled with creamy, zesty goodness. A vibrant 30g protein vegetarian option that's colorful, satisfying, and ready in 30 minutes.

**MARINADE AND SAUCE**

3 tablespoons coconut aminos
3 tablespoons tahini
1 tablespoon toasted sesame oil
1 tablespoon maple syrup
1 tablespoon lemon juice
2 garlic cloves, minced
1½ teaspoons chili flakes
½ teaspoon paprika
Sea salt and freshly ground black pepper

1 (12-ounce) block extra-firm tofu, pressed and cubed
1 medium sweet potato, diced
1 cup chicken bone broth or vegetable broth
½ cup white quinoa, rinsed
1 carrot, shredded
1 small bell pepper, seeded and thinly sliced
1 avocado, sliced
1 watermelon radish, thinly sliced
2 green onions, white and green parts, thinly sliced
3 tablespoons mixed seeds (hemp and sunflower)

1. **Prep the tofu and sweet potato:** Preheat the oven to 425°F. In a bowl, whisk the coconut aminos, tahini, sesame oil, maple syrup, lemon juice, garlic, chili flakes, paprika, salt, and pepper. Toss the tofu with half the sauce to coat. Drizzle 1 to 2 teaspoons of the remaining sauce over the sweet potato, season with salt and pepper, and toss to lightly coat. Reserve the rest for drizzling.
2. **Roast:** Spread the tofu and sweet potato on a parchment-lined baking sheet. Roast for 20 minutes, flipping once, until the tofu is golden and the sweet potato is tender.
3. **Cook the quinoa:** Meanwhile, bring the broth to a boil in a medium saucepan. Add the quinoa, reduce the heat to low, cover, and simmer for 15 minutes, until the water is absorbed. Fluff with a fork and set aside.
4. **Assemble:** Divide the quinoa into bowls. Top with the tofu, sweet potato, carrot, bell pepper, avocado, radish, and green onion. Drizzle with the reserved sauce and sprinkle with seeds.

**STORAGE:** Store components separately in airtight containers in the fridge for up to 4 days. For best texture, reheat tofu and sweet potatoes in a skillet or air fryer. Add fresh toppings and dressing just before serving.

**PER SERVING**
Protein: 30g
Carbohydrates: 61g
Fat: 41g

**MAKE-AHEAD TIP:** *To save some time in the moment, cook the quinoa, roast the sweet potatoes, and mix the tahini dressing up to 3 days ahead of time. You can also press and cube the tofu in advance to speed things up. Store all components separately, then just marinate, roast the tofu, and assemble when you're ready to eat.*

Dairy-Free
Gluten-Free
Grain-Free

# Chicken and Peanut Pad Thai Bowls

FOR THE SAUCE

½ cup chicken bone broth

⅓ cup unsweetened creamy peanut butter

¼ cup coconut aminos

1½ tablespoons rice vinegar

1 tablespoon maple syrup

1 tablespoon fish sauce (optional)

2 teaspoons grated fresh ginger

1 clove garlic, minced

½ teaspoon red pepper flakes (adjust to spice preference)

FOR THE NOODLES AND CHICKEN

7 ounces sweet potato glass noodles (or pad Thai noodles)

2 tablespoons avocado oil

1½ pounds chicken breasts, cut into 2-inch-long, ½-inch-thick strips

½ teaspoon sea salt

1 cup matchstick carrots (about 2 medium)

2 baby bok choy, chopped

2 large eggs, whisked

2 green onions, white and green parts, sliced

⅓ cup chopped fresh cilantro

¼ cup dry-roasted peanuts, chopped

Sea salt

1 lime, cut into wedges

**PER SERVING (FOR 5 SERVINGS)**
Protein: 39g
Carbohydrates: 49g
Fat: 22g

SERVES 4 TO 5 • PREP TIME: 15 MINUTES • COOK TIME: 15 MINUTES • TOTAL TIME: 30 MINUTES

Call me sentimental, but my travel memories are basically built around food. This dish lives rent-free in my brain from our babymoon in the Maldives—I ordered their chicken pad Thai almost daily from the hotel where we stayed, Gili Lankanfushi—it was that good. As soon as we got home, I had to re-create it. This is my spin, and it's earned a permanent spot in the book. I think you're going to be obsessed.

1. **Make the sauce:** In a medium bowl, whisk together the broth, peanut butter, coconut aminos, vinegar, maple syrup, fish sauce (if using), ginger, garlic, and red pepper flakes until smooth. Set aside.
2. **Cook the noodles:** Cook the noodles according to package instructions. Drain and set aside.
3. **Cook the chicken:** Heat 1 tablespoon of the oil in a large skillet or wok over medium-high heat. Add the chicken strips, season with salt, and cook for 6 to 7 minutes, flipping occasionally, until they are golden brown and cooked through. Drain excess liquid, then transfer the chicken to a plate and set aside.
4. In the same skillet, heat the remaining 1 tablespoon oil over medium heat. Add the carrots and bok choy, cover, and sauté for 3 to 4 minutes, until the bok choy softens and the carrots are just tender. Push the vegetables to the side and pour in the eggs. Scramble until just cooked. Return the chicken to the skillet and add the noodles. Pour the sauce over everything and toss well to coat evenly.
5. Remove from the heat and stir in the green onions and cilantro. Top with peanuts and a sprinkle of salt and serve with lime wedges.

**STORAGE:** Store leftovers in an airtight container in the fridge for up to 4 days. Reheat in a skillet over medium heat or in the microwave, adding a splash of water to loosen the sauce if needed. For the best texture, store the garnishes (peanuts or herbs) separately and add just before serving.

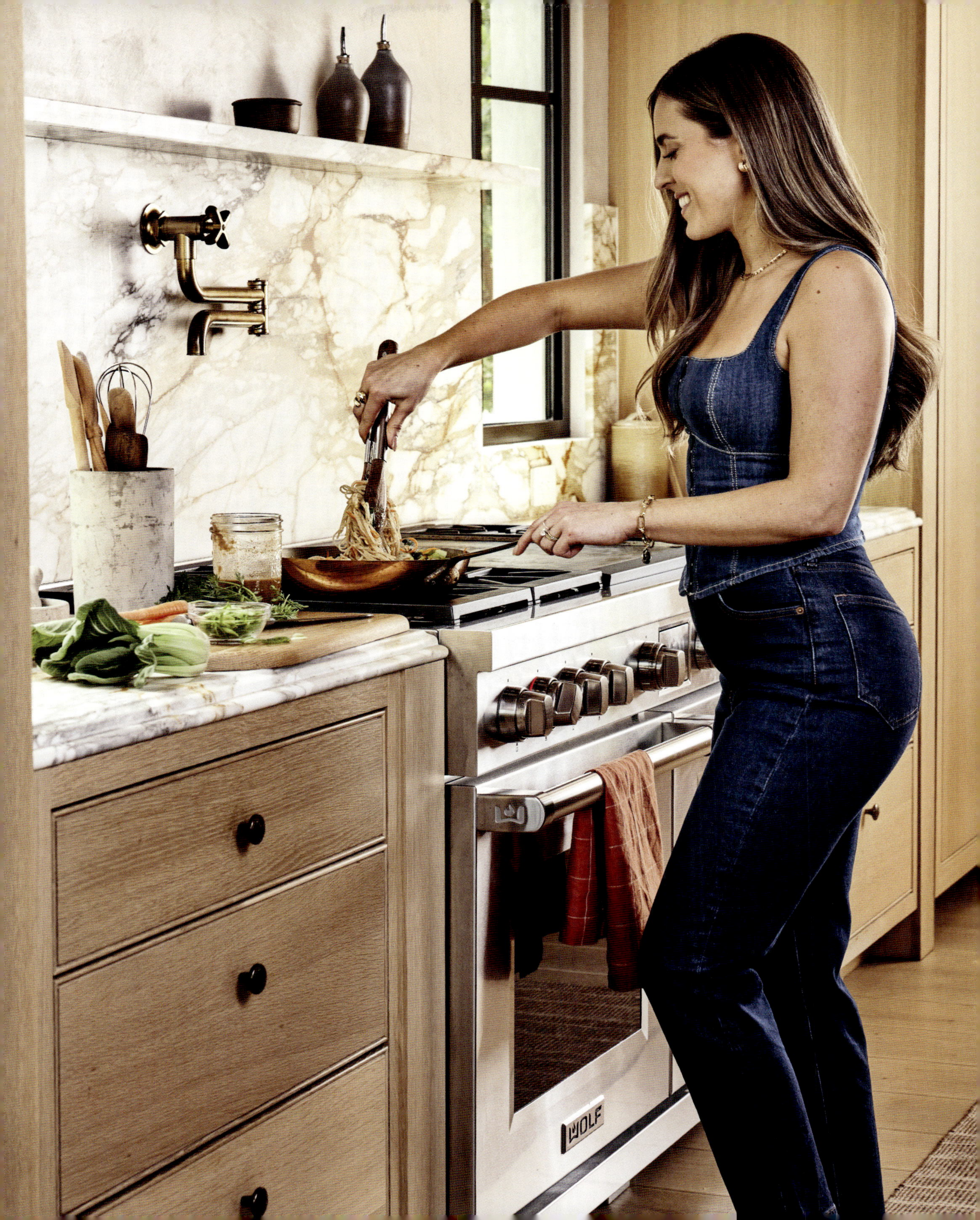
WOLF

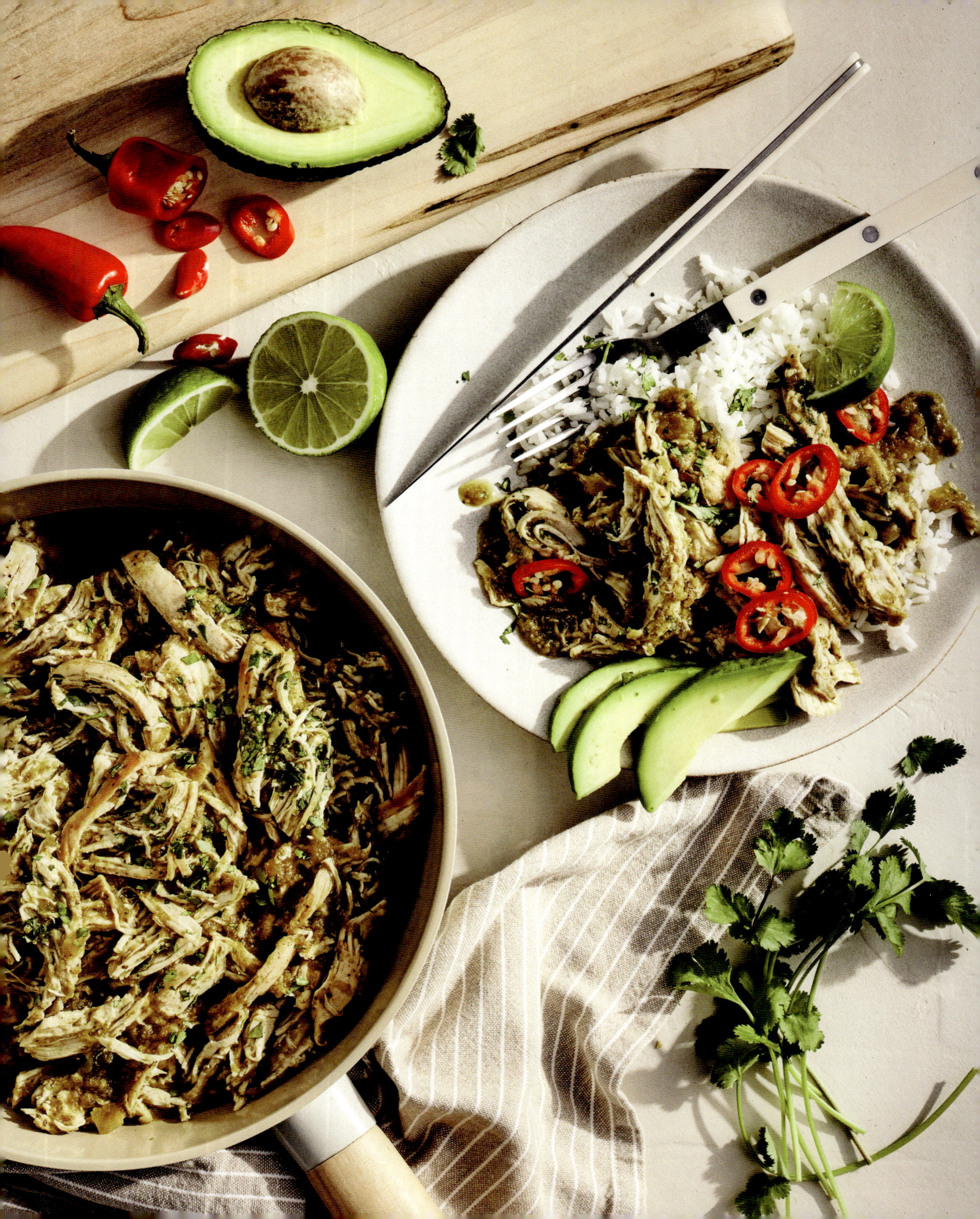

Dairy-Free
Gluten-Free
Grain-Free
No Added Sugar
Paleo

# 20-Minute Shredded Chicken Verde

SERVES 6 • PREP TIME: 5 MINUTES • COOK TIME: 15 MINUTES • TOTAL TIME: 20 MINUTES

I've been making chicken verde for as long as I can remember, and it never lets me down. Whether I have no idea what to make for dinner or I need something quick to feed my family or a small crowd, this recipe always delivers. It comes together insanely fast and is so versatile—eat it plain over greens or rice, stuff it into tacos or enchiladas, or add some bone broth to turn it into a cozy soup.

**1½ pounds boneless, skinless chicken breasts, trimmed**

**Sea salt and freshly ground black pepper**

**1 tablespoon extra-virgin olive oil**

**2 (15.5-ounce) jars salsa verde (or preferred salsa)**

**Juice of ½ lime (1 tablespoon lime juice)**

**⅓ cup finely chopped fresh cilantro**

**Red chili flakes (optional)**

**Flaky salt (optional)**

1. Season the chicken breasts with salt and black pepper on both sides.
2. In a large pot, heat the oil over medium-high heat. Add the chicken breasts and sear for 2 to 3 minutes per side, until lightly golden. Pour in the salsa verde and flip each piece of chicken to fully coat. Reduce the heat to medium-low, cover with a lid, and cook for 10 to 12 minutes, until the chicken is cooked through. Transfer the chicken to a cutting board and use two forks to shred it into thin pieces.
3. Return the chicken to the pot and stir in the lime juice and cilantro. Top with chili flakes and flaky salt, if using. Serve as is, over greens or rice, in tacos or enchiladas, or add 2 to 3 cups of broth to transform it into a protein-forward soup.

**STORAGE:** Store in an airtight container in the fridge for up to 4 days. Reheat gently on the stovetop or in the microwave with a splash of broth or salsa to keep it juicy.

**PER SERVING**
Protein: 34g
Carbohydrates: 3g
Fat: 5g

**NOTE:** *This is a great dish to prep at the start of the week for anytime meals!*

Dairy-Free
Gluten-Free
Grain-Free
No Added Sugar

# Grilled Mahi Mahi with Mango Salsa

SERVES 4 • PREP TIME: 10 MINUTES, PLUS 15 MINUTES MARINATING • COOK TIME: 5 MINUTES • TOTAL TIME: 30 MINUTES

If you need a quick, high-protein meal that tastes like a tropical escape, this is it. Mahi mahi is light and flaky and it cooks in minutes, making it perfect for busy nights. The sweet and tangy mango salsa adds the freshest pop of flavor and pairs perfectly with the smoky, spiced fish. Plus, mahi mahi is full of protein and omega-3s, so you're fueling up with every bite. Serve it over Bone Broth Jasmine Rice (page 198) with a squeeze of lime and I promise—this one will quickly make it to the top of your list!

FOR THE MAHI MAHI

1 teaspoon paprika

½ teaspoon ground cumin

½ teaspoon garlic powder

½ teaspoon onion powder

1 teaspoon sea salt

½ teaspoon freshly ground black pepper

4 (6-ounce) mahi mahi fillets (halibut works great here, too, if you can't find mahi mahi)

1 tablespoon extra-virgin olive oil

FOR THE MANGO SALSA

1 large ripe mango, cut into ½-inch dice

1 small red bell pepper, seeded and cut into ¼-inch dice

½ small red onion, finely diced

1 small jalapeño, seeded and minced

¼ cup chopped fresh cilantro

2 tablespoons freshly squeezed lime juice (1 lime), plus lime wedges for serving

½ teaspoon sea salt

1. **Season the mahi mahi:** In a small bowl, mix the paprika, cumin, garlic powder, onion powder, salt, and black pepper. Pat the mahi mahi fillets dry with a paper towel and place in a shallow dish or rimmed baking sheet. Drizzle with the oil, then coat evenly with the spice mixture. Let sit for 15 to 20 minutes.
2. **Make the mango salsa:** Meanwhile, in a medium bowl, stir together the mango, bell pepper, onion, jalapeño, cilantro, lime juice, and salt until well combined. Set aside.
3. **Grill the mahi mahi:** Preheat a grill or grill pan over medium-high heat. Once hot, add the fillets and cook for 2 to 3 minutes per side, or until opaque and just cooked through.
4. Serve the mahi mahi topped with mango salsa, with extra lime wedges on the side for squeezing.

---

**PER SERVING**
Protein: 35g
Carbohydrates: 17g
Fat: 5g

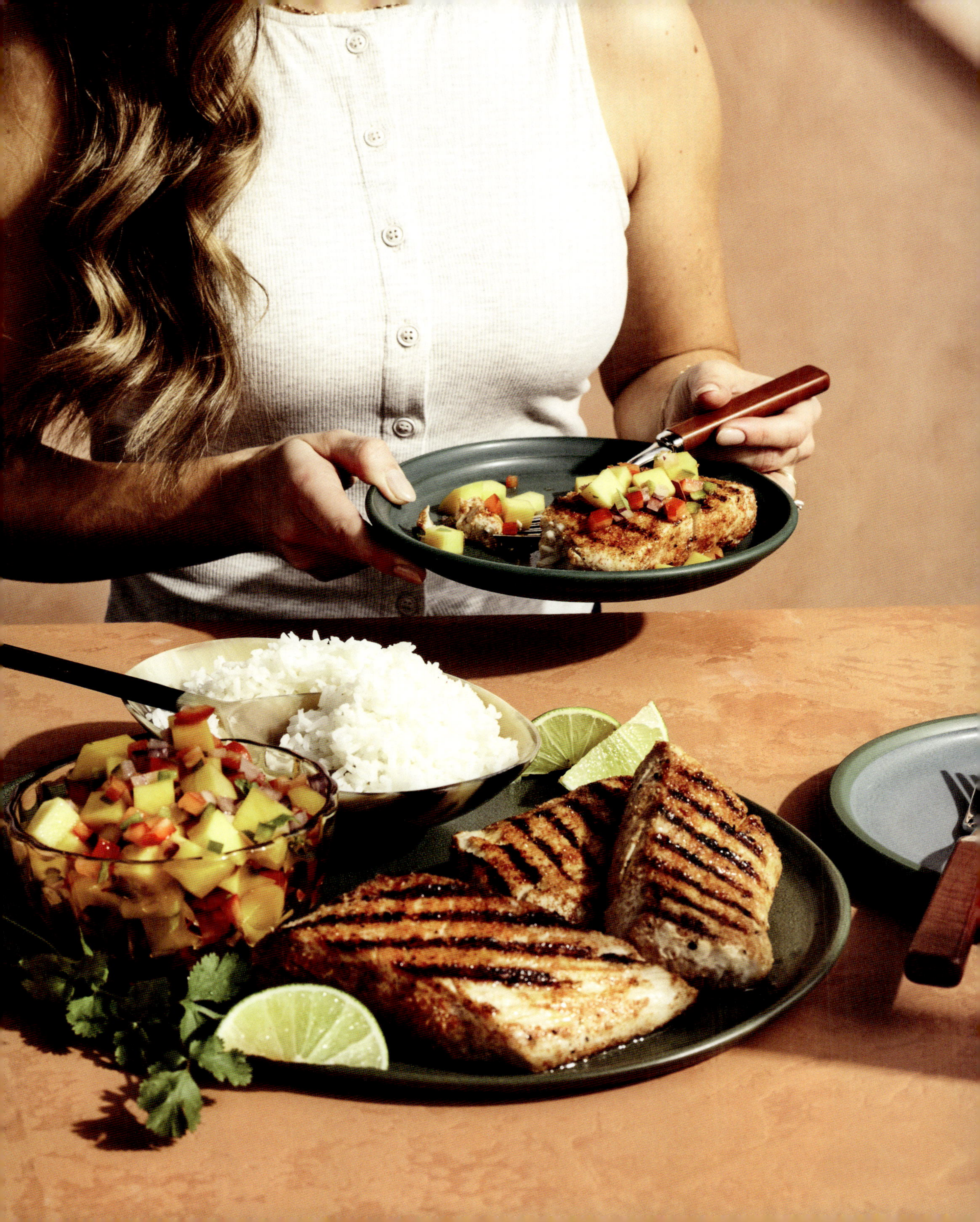

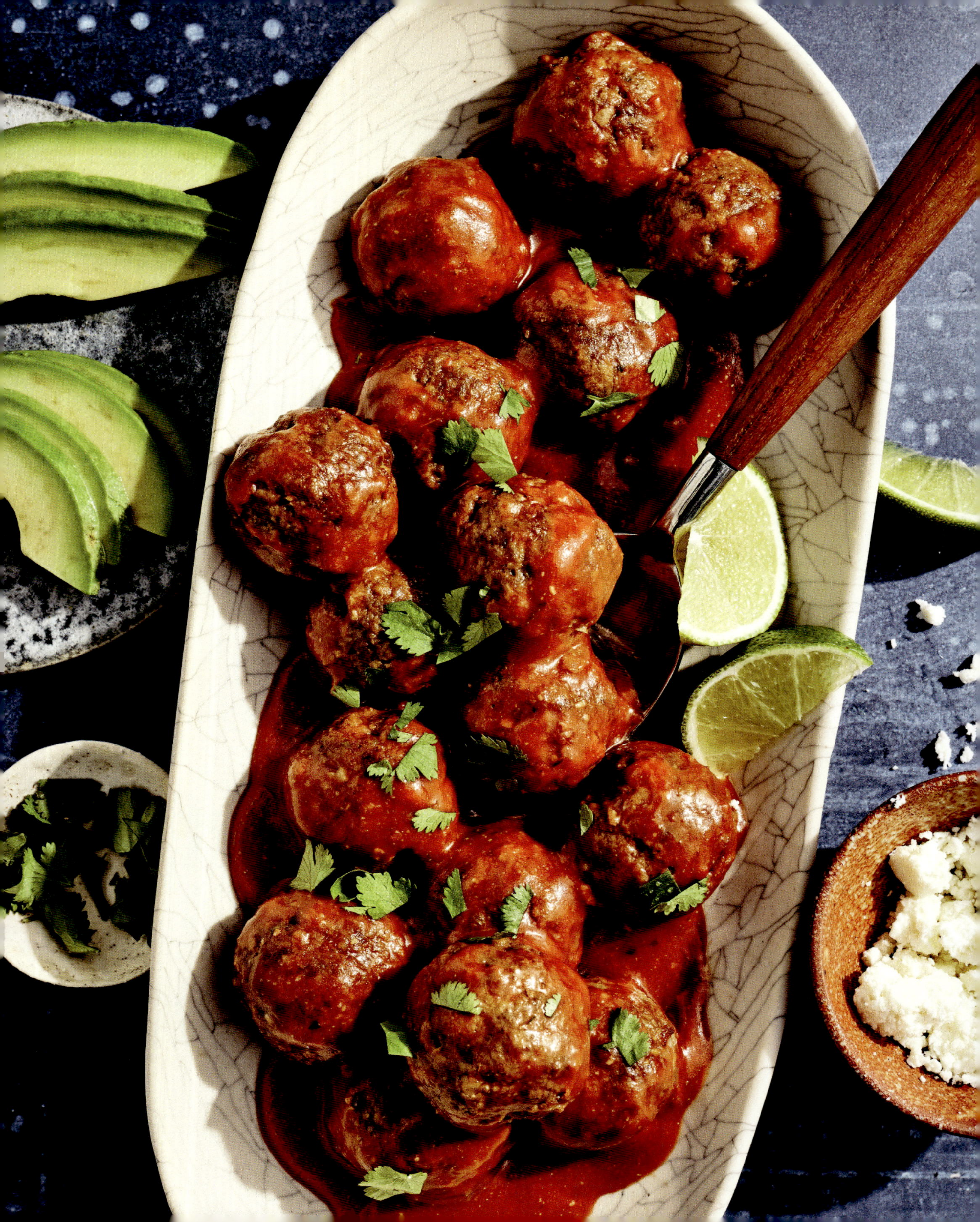

Gluten-Free
Grain-Free
No Added Sugar
**IF MODIFIED:**
Dairy-Free

# Mexican Meatballs in Creamy Enchilada Sauce

**SERVES 2 TO 4 • PREP TIME: 10 MINUTES • COOK TIME: 15 MINUTES • TOTAL TIME: 25 MINUTES**

Two of the best worlds collide when meatballs meet Mexican flavors. These juicy baked meatballs are simmered in the most velvety homemade enchilada sauce—one I'll happily eat by the spoonful. The sauce is creamy, spiced just right, and full of depth thanks to a quick roux and warm spices. Feel free to use a combo of ground beef and ground turkey or chicken, depending on what you have on hand. Serve over rice, tucked into tortillas, or on their own as a flavorful party app.

**FOR THE MEATBALLS**

Avocado oil spray
1 pound ground beef
1 large egg
½ cup almond flour
1 small onion, minced or grated on a box grater
2 cloves garlic, minced
1 (1.31-ounce) packet organic taco seasoning (I prefer Siete)

**FOR THE SAUCE**

3 tablespoons ghee (or vegan butter for dairy-free)
3 tablespoons arrowroot powder
1 teaspoon chili powder
1 teaspoon oregano
½ teaspoon ground cumin
½ teaspoon onion powder
½ teaspoon garlic powder
½ teaspoon sea salt
1 (6-ounce) can tomato paste
2 cups chicken bone broth
For serving (optional): white or brown rice, minced cilantro, cotija cheese, sliced avocado

1. Preheat the oven to 400°F. Spray a baking sheet liberally with avocado oil.
2. **Make the meatballs:** In a medium bowl, mix the ground beef, egg, almond flour, onion, garlic, and taco seasoning until well combined. Scoop heaping tablespoons of the mixture and roll into about 24 meatballs. Place the meatballs on the baking sheet and bake for 15 minutes, until browned and the internal temperature reaches 160°F.
3. **Make the sauce:** While the meatballs bake, melt the ghee in a large skillet over medium heat. Whisk in the arrowroot powder and cook for 1 to 2 minutes, until smooth and bubbling. Stir in the chili powder, oregano, cumin, onion powder, garlic powder, and salt. Cook for 1 minute, until the spices are toasted and fragrant. Add the tomato paste and broth, whisking until smooth. Bring to a simmer and cook for 3 to 5 minutes, until thickened.
4. Transfer the meatballs to the skillet and simmer in the sauce over low heat for 5 minutes to let the flavors meld.
5. Serve over rice if you like, and top with cilantro, cotija cheese, and avocado.

**STORAGE:** Store meatballs and sauce together in an airtight container in the fridge for up to 4 days, or freeze for up to 2 months. Reheat gently on the stovetop or in the microwave, adding a splash of broth if needed to loosen the sauce.

---

**PER SERVING (FOR 4 SERVINGS)**
Protein: 34g
Carbohydrates: 21g
Fat: 38g

No Added Sugar
**IF MODIFIED:**
Gluten-Free
Grain-Free

# Shredded Chicken Quesadillas

**SERVES 3 • PREP TIME: 10 MINUTES • COOK TIME: 20 MINUTES • TOTAL TIME: 30 MINUTES**

I swear, eating quesadillas makes me feel like a kid—probably because they were my go-to after-school snack growing up. But with all the protein and fiber packed into these, I can at least pretend like I'm adulting. The combo of shredded chicken, creamy refried beans, and melty cheese tucked inside a crispy tortilla is quick and easy and hits the spot every time. Perfect for lunch, dinner, or whenever that crispy-cheesy craving hits.

**1½ cups shredded rotisserie chicken (skin and bones removed), or sub 1 large chicken breast (see Tip below)**

**1 tablespoon ghee, melted**

**1 tablespoon avocado or extra-virgin olive oil (optional), if using chicken breast**

**½ teaspoon garlic powder**

**½ teaspoon sea salt, plus more to season the chicken breast (if using)**

**¼ teaspoon freshly ground black pepper**

**¼ cup sliced green onions, white and green parts**

**Avocado oil spray**

**6 large (10-inch) tortillas (I prefer Siete brand for a grain-free option)**

**¾ cup refried beans**

**1½ cups shredded goat cheddar cheese (or preferred cheese)**

**Optional toppings: guacamole, pico de gallo, Homemade BBQ Sauce (page 118) Southwest Sauce (page 188)**

1. In a medium bowl, mix the chicken, ghee, garlic powder, salt, pepper, and green onions until well combined.
2. Heat a large cast-iron skillet over medium heat and spray with avocado oil. Add a tortilla to the skillet and spread 3 tablespoons refried beans over it. Top with ¼ cup of the chicken mixture and ½ cup cheese. Place another tortilla on top. Cook for about 3 to 4 minutes per side, until golden brown and the cheese has melted. Repeat with the remaining ingredients to make three quesadillas.
3. Slice and serve with guacamole, pico de gallo, BBQ sauce, or Southwest sauce.

**TIP:** *To use one large chicken breast instead of the rotisserie chicken, slice the breast in half horizontally (to make 2 thinner pieces) and season both sides with salt and pepper. Heat 1 tablespoon oil in a medium skillet over medium-high heat. Add the breast and cook for 3 to 4 minutes per side, until golden and cooked through. Transfer to a cutting board and shred with two forks.*

**PER SERVING**
Protein: 34g
Carbohydrates: 27g
Fat: 35g

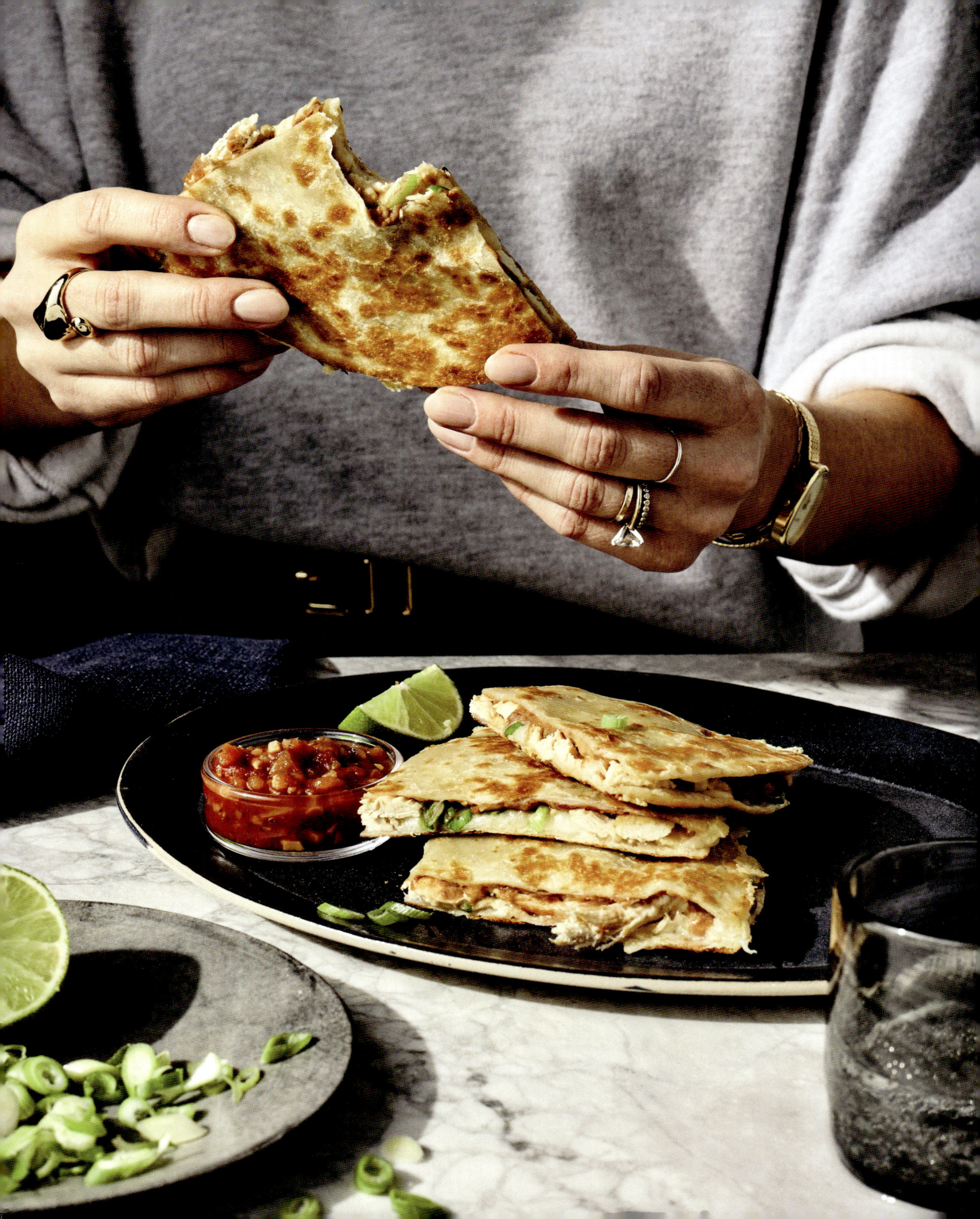

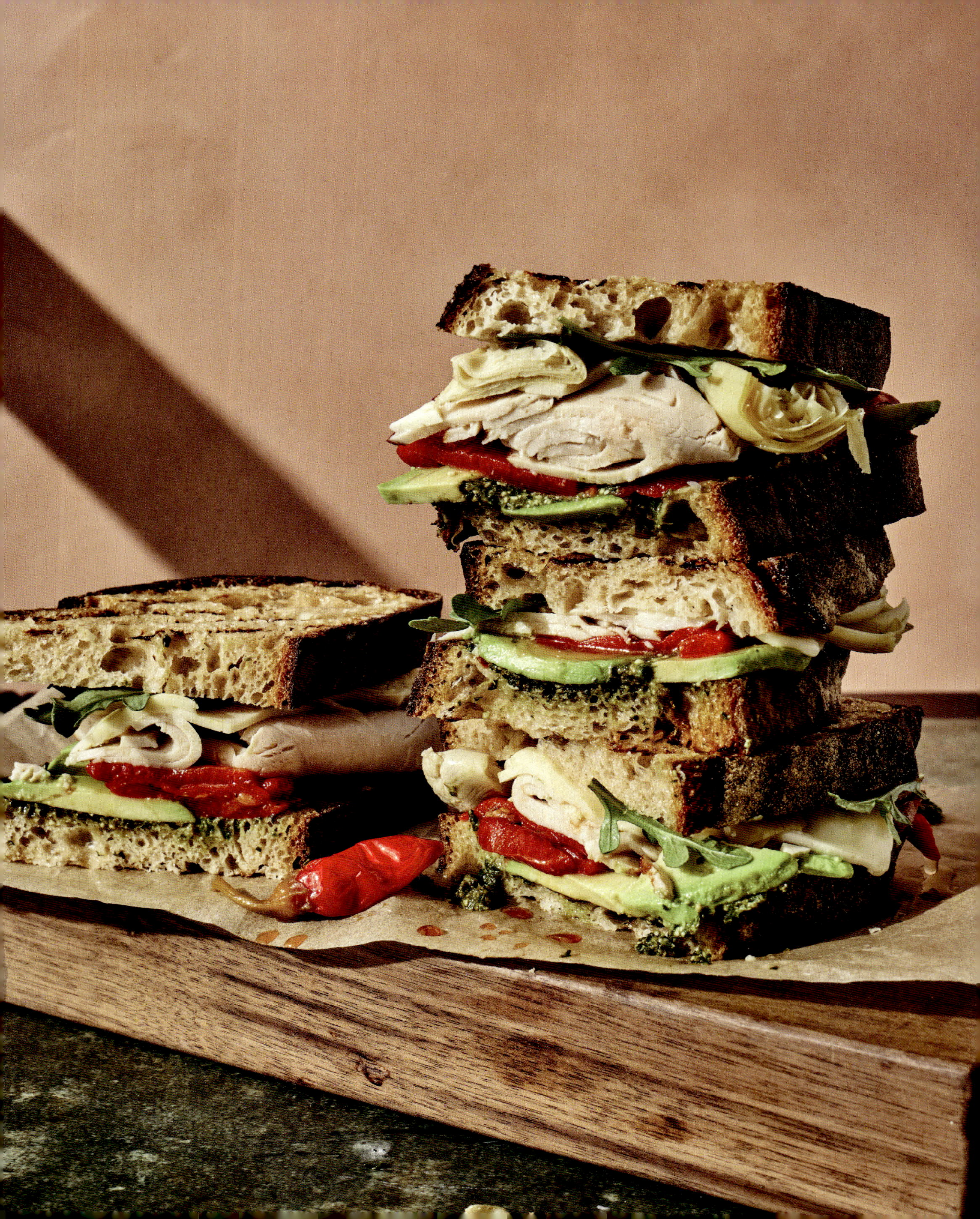

No Added Sugar
**IF MODIFIED:**
Dairy-Free
Gluten-Free
Grain-Free

# Loaded Chicken Pesto Panini

**SERVES 1 TO 2 • PREP TIME: 10 MINUTES • COOK TIME: 5 MINUTES • TOTAL TIME: 15 MINUTES**

If there's one sandwich that never gets old, it's this loaded-up panini. Melty cheese, roasted red peppers, creamy avocado, and tender chicken all stacked between two crispy slices of sourdough? Absolute perfection. And don't even get me started on the homemade basil pesto—fresh, herby, and the best way to take any sandwich to the next level. If you don't have a panini press, don't worry, I've got you covered with a simple stovetop method. Get ready to level up your sandwich game.

**FOR THE BASIL PESTO**

¼ cup extra-virgin olive oil

⅓ cup raw pine nuts

Juice of 1 lemon (about 2 tablespoons)

2 cups fresh basil leaves

1 tablespoon nutritional yeast

½ teaspoon minced garlic

½ teaspoon sea salt

¼ teaspoon freshly ground black pepper

**FOR THE PANINI**

1 tablespoon ghee (or vegan butter for dairy-free)

2 slices bread of choice (I prefer rustic sourdough)

Calabrian peppers (omit if spice is not preferred)

½ avocado, thinly sliced

3 roasted sweet red peppers

6 slices deli chicken or turkey

1 cup arugula

Sea salt and freshly ground black pepper

2 slices cheddar cheese

4 canned artichoke hearts, drained and quartered

1. **Make the basil pesto:** In a food processor, combine the oil, pine nuts, lemon juice, basil, nutritional yeast, garlic, salt, black pepper, and 2 tablespoons water and pulse until smooth.
2. **Make the panini:** Spread the ghee on one side of each bread slice. Spread about 2 tablespoons of pesto on the other side of one slice and lay Calabrian peppers, if using, on the other side of the second slice. Layer the avocado, red peppers, chicken, arugula, salt, black pepper, cheese, and artichokes on the pesto side, and top with the other bread slice, ghee side up.
3. Heat a panini press (or a large skillet over medium heat). Place the sandwich on the panini grill, press down, and cook for 3 to 5 minutes, until golden brown and the cheese has melted. (If using a skillet, place the sandwich in the hot skillet and press down firmly with a spatula or a second heavy skillet and cook for 2 to 3 minutes.) Flip the sandwich, press down again, and cook for another 2 to 3 minutes, until the bread is crisp and the cheese has melted. Serve immediately and enjoy.

---

**PER SERVING (FOR 2 SERVINGS)**
Protein: 37g
Carbohydrates: 40g
Fat: 35g

**NOTE:** *This recipe makes extra pesto. Store it in an airtight container in the fridge for up to 5 days, or freeze in a silicone ice cube tray for up to 3 months.*

Dairy-Free
Gluten-Free
Grain-Free
No Added Sugar
Paleo

# My Weeknight Hero: Ginger-Garlic Turkey Skillet

**SERVES 2 TO 4 • PREP TIME: 5 MINUTES • COOK TIME: 15 MINUTES • TOTAL TIME: 20 MINUTES**

My weeknight hero is savory, tangy, and just the right amount of garlicky—perfect for when you want something fresh and flavorful, fast. Ground turkey and veggies cook up in one pan, and if you prep the recipe and wash your lettuce at the start of the week, you've got a solid work-from-home lunch ready to go too.

- 1 tablespoon avocado oil
- 1 tablespoon sesame oil
- 1 pound ground turkey
- 1 small yellow onion, cut into ¼-inch dice
- 1 medium red bell pepper, seeded and cut into ¼-inch dice (or sub diced zucchini, shredded carrots, or chopped snap peas)
- 3 cloves garlic, minced
- 2 teaspoons minced fresh ginger
- ¼ cup coconut aminos
- 1 tablespoon rice wine vinegar
- 1 tablespoon chili garlic sauce
- 1 teaspoon arrowroot powder
- ½ teaspoon sea salt

**FOR SERVING**

- 1 head butter lettuce, leaves separated, washed, and gently patted dry
- 2 green onions, white and green parts, sliced (optional)
- ¼ cup dry-roasted salted cashews, chopped (optional)
- Flaky salt (optional)

1. In a large skillet, heat the avocado oil and sesame oil over medium heat. Add the ground turkey, breaking it into crumbles with a spatula. Cook for 5 to 7 minutes, stirring occasionally, until no longer pink. Stir in the onion, bell pepper, garlic, and ginger and sauté for 3 to 5 minutes, until the onions are translucent and the peppers are slightly tender. Add the coconut aminos, vinegar, chili garlic sauce, arrowroot powder, and salt. Stir well and simmer for 2 minutes, until the sauce thickens and coats the turkey mixture.
2. Spoon the turkey mixture into the lettuce cups. If you like, top with green onions, cashews, and flaky salt, if using.

**STORAGE:** Store the filling in an airtight container in the fridge for up to 4 days and reheat in a skillet or microwave until warmed through. Keep the lettuce leaves separate and assemble just before serving to maintain freshness and crunch.

**PER SERVING (FOR 2 SERVINGS)**
Protein: 48g
Carbohydrates: 18g
Fat: 22g

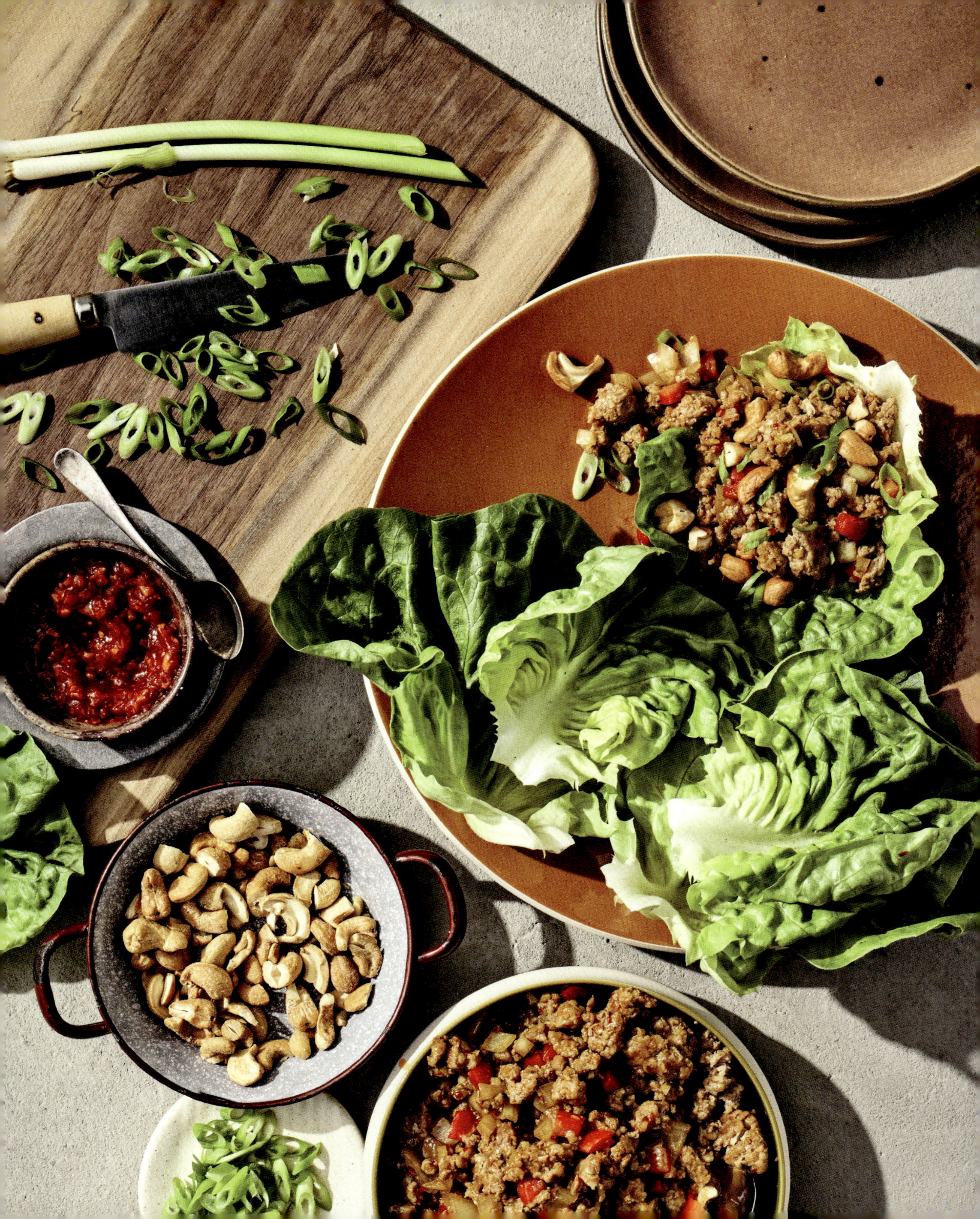

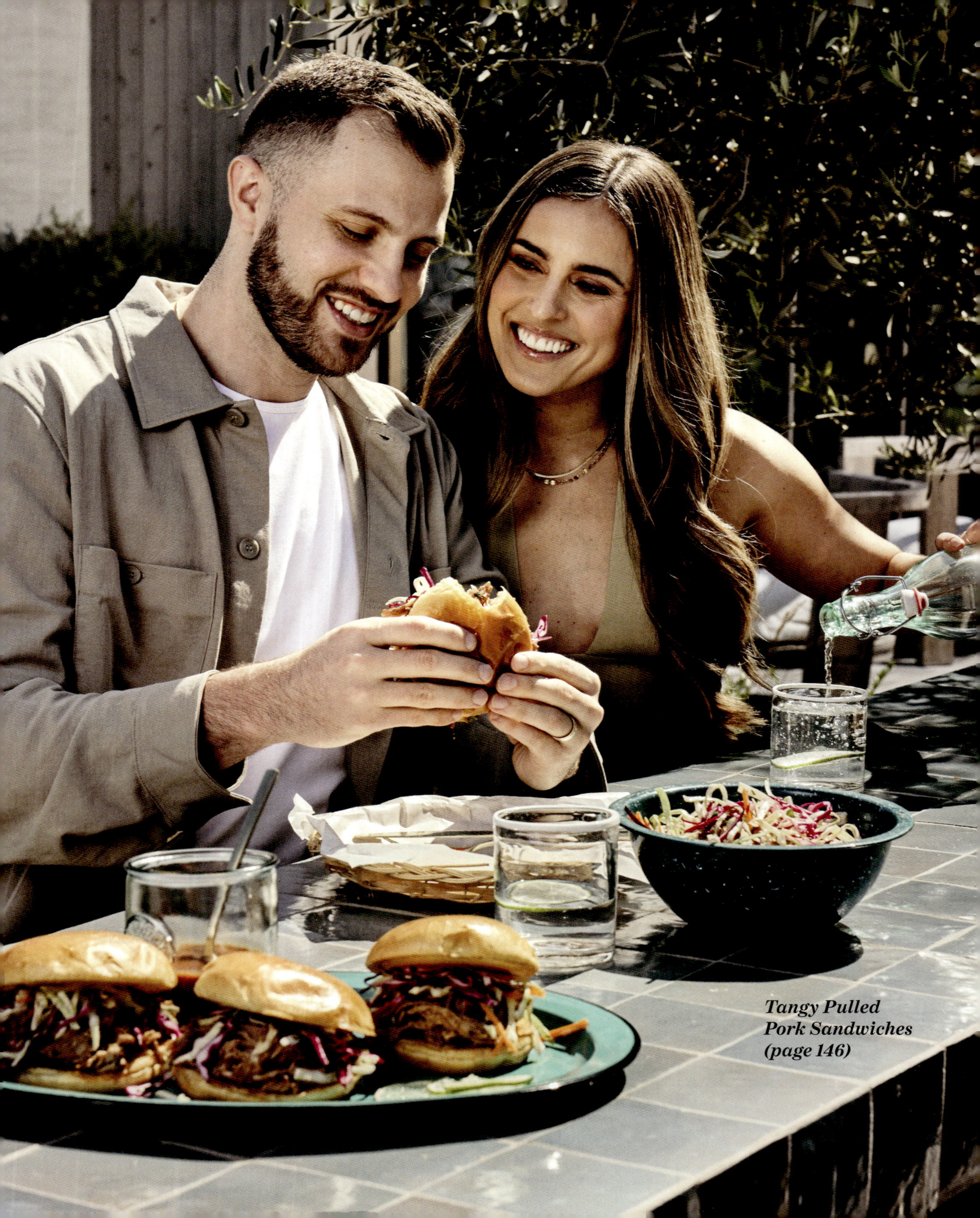

*Tangy Pulled Pork Sandwiches* *(page 146)*

*All of these slow cooker recipes can also be made in a Dutch oven. Just follow the stovetop instructions included within each recipe.*


146 **Tangy Pulled Pork Sandwiches**

148 **Buffalo Chicken Baked Tacos**

151 **Sesame-Ginger Pot Roast**

152 **Short Ribs with Bone Broth Polenta**

155 **Slow Cooker Picadillo**

156 **Brothy Beans with Zesty Chimichurri**


# Slow Cooker Mains

Dairy-Free

**IF MODIFIED:**

Gluten-Free

Grain-Free

# Tangy Pulled Pork Sandwiches

SERVES 6 • PREP TIME: 20 MINUTES • COOK TIME: 3½ TO 4 HOURS (DUTCH OVEN) OR 4 TO 10 HOURS (SLOW COOKER) • TOTAL TIME: 3 HOURS 50 MINUTES TO 4 HOURS 20 MINUTES (DUTCH OVEN) OR 4 HOURS 20 MINUTES TO 10 HOURS 20 MINUTES (SLOW COOKER)

This is the kind of meal that makes you look like a pro with almost zero effort. A pork shoulder, a handful of simple ingredients, and a slow cooker do all the heavy lifting, leaving you with melt-in-your-mouth pulled pork coated in a smoky, tangy sauce. The crisp coleslaw in the sandwich balances every bite with just the right amount of crunch and acidity. However you serve it—on a bun, over rice, or straight from the pot—it's always something everyone loves.

FOR THE PORK

- 3 to 4 pounds pork shoulder
- 2½ teaspoons sea salt
- 1½ teaspoons freshly ground black pepper
- 1 large onion, sliced
- 1 cup Homemade BBQ Sauce (page 118) or store-bought unsweetened BBQ sauce (such as Primal Kitchen, one 8.5-ounce jar)
- ½ cup chicken bone broth
- ½ cup apple cider vinegar
- ¼ cup coconut sugar
- 1 teaspoon smoked paprika
- 1 teaspoon chili powder
- ½ teaspoon ground cumin
- 3 garlic cloves, minced

FOR THE COLESLAW

- 2 cups shredded green cabbage
- 2 cups shredded red cabbage
- 1 large carrot, shredded
- ½ cup chopped fresh cilantro
- 3 tablespoons extra-virgin olive oil
- 2 tablespoons apple cider vinegar
- 1 tablespoon honey
- 1 teaspoon sea salt
- For serving: 6 brioche-style buns, Homemade BBQ Sauce (page 118), optional

1. **Prepare the pork:** Pat the pork shoulder dry with paper towels and season generously with the salt and pepper on all sides. Spread the onions across the bottom of the slow cooker. Place the seasoned pork shoulder on top.
2. In a medium bowl, whisk together the sauce, broth, vinegar, coconut sugar, paprika, chili powder, and cumin until smooth. Pour the sauce evenly over the pork, then scatter the garlic on top.
3. Cover and cook on low for 8 to 10 hours or high for 4 to 5 hours, until the pork is fork-tender and easily shredded. If the meat isn't shredding easily, let it cook for another 30 to 60 minutes until the collagen fully breaks down.
4. **To cook in a Dutch oven:** After seasoning the pork, layer the onions in a large Dutch oven and place the pork on top. Pour the sauce mixture over the meat and add the garlic. Bring to a gentle simmer over medium heat, then reduce the heat to low, cover, and cook for 3½ to 4 hours, turning the pork once or twice, until it's tender enough to shred easily with a fork.
5. Transfer the pork to a large cutting board. Use two forks to shred the meat, discarding excess fat, if desired. Return the pork to the pot and stir it into the juices for maximum flavor. Let it sit on low heat for an additional 15 to 30 minutes to soak up the sauce.
6. **Make the coleslaw:** In a large bowl, mix the green cabbage, red cabbage, carrot, cilantro, oil, vinegar, honey, and salt until well combined.

---

**PER SERVING**

Protein: 45g

Carbohydrates: 55g

Fat: 32g

7. **Assemble the sandwiches:** In a large skillet over medium heat, toast the buns cut side down until golden and crisp. Alternatively, you can toast them in a toaster oven or regular toaster if they fit—whatever's easiest.
8. Spoon the pork and onions onto the bottom buns, drizzle with some sauce, and top with coleslaw. If using, add a dollop of homemade BBQ sauce, then top with the bun tops.

**STORAGE:** The pulled pork will keep in an airtight container in the fridge for up to 4 days. Reheat gently in a saucepan over low heat or in the microwave. Store the slaw separately and assemble the sandwiches just before serving. The pork also freezes well in an airtight container for up to 3 months. To thaw, place it in the refrigerator overnight, then reheat in a skillet over low heat or in the microwave until warmed through.

The slaw will keep in an airtight container in the fridge for up to 3 days. Stir before serving to redistribute the dressing.

No Added Sugar
**IF MODIFIED:**
Gluten-Free
Grain-Free

# Buffalo Chicken Baked Tacos

**SERVES 6 • PREP TIME: 25 MINUTES • COOK TIME: 1 TO 1½ HOURS (DUTCH OVEN) OR 3 TO 8 HOURS (SLOW COOKER) • TOTAL TIME: 1 HOUR 25 MINUTES TO 2 HOURS (DUTCH OVEN) OR 3 HOURS 25 MINUTES TO 8 HOURS 25 MINUTES (SLOW COOKER)**

This one started as a "what else can I do with chicken?" moment—and turned into a top-tier dinner. Buffalo chicken gets slow-cooked and shredded, then stuffed into tortillas and baked until crispy. Load them up with avocado, green onion, jalapeño, and cilantro for that perfect creamy-fresh-spicy balance, then dig in. They're just as good for a crowd as they are for a family weeknight win. **Pro tip:** Skip the baking and serve the tacos fresh if you're short on time—they're just as irresistible.

**FOR THE CHICKEN**

1 cup sour cream (any kind)
¼ cup hot sauce (such as Frank's RedHot)
¼ cup unsweetened ketchup (like Primal Kitchen)
2 tablespoons extra-virgin olive oil
3 cloves garlic, minced
1 teaspoon ground cumin
1 teaspoon Himalayan pink salt
½ teaspoon onion powder
¼ teaspoon paprika
1½ to 2 pounds boneless, skinless chicken breasts, trimmed

**FOR THE TACOS**

8 to 10 tortillas (I prefer Siete brand for a grain-free option)
1 cup shredded cheddar cheese
2 avocados, diced
⅓ cup chopped fresh cilantro
1 jalapeño, seeded and thinly sliced
2 green onions, white and green parts, thinly sliced
Juice of 1 lime (about 2 tablespoons)
¼ teaspoon sea salt

1. **Make the chicken:** In a medium bowl, stir together the sour cream, hot sauce, ketchup, oil, garlic, cumin, pink salt, onion powder, and paprika until smooth.
2. Add the mixture to the slow cooker along with the chicken breasts, and flip until evenly coated in the sauce. Cover and cook on high for 3 to 4 hours or on low for 6 to 8 hours, until the chicken is tender and cooked through.
3. **To cook in a Dutch oven:** Combine the sauce and chicken in a large Dutch oven. Bring to a gentle simmer over medium heat, then reduce the heat to low. Cover and cook for 1 to 1½ hours, flipping the chicken once, until fall-apart tender.
4. Shred the chicken right in the pot using two forks and toss to coat in the sauce.
5. **Bake the tacos:** Preheat the oven to 410°F. Line a baking sheet with parchment paper.
6. In a dry skillet over medium heat, warm each tortilla for 30 seconds to 1 minute, until slightly charred.
7. Fill each tortilla with a few tablespoons of cheese, followed by about ½ cup (or more) of the chicken. Fold each taco and press shut. Transfer the tacos to the baking sheet and bake for 10 to 12 minutes, until crisp.
8. Serve immediately, topping each taco with avocado, cilantro, jalapeño, and green onions. Finish with a squeeze of lime juice and a sprinkle of salt.

**STORAGE:** The shredded Buffalo chicken will keep in an airtight container in the fridge for up to 4 days. Reheat gently on the stovetop or in the microwave. Assemble the tacos when you're ready to eat them, so they are fresh and don't get soggy.

---

**PER SERVING**
Protein: 35g
Carbohydrates: 20g
Fat: 28g

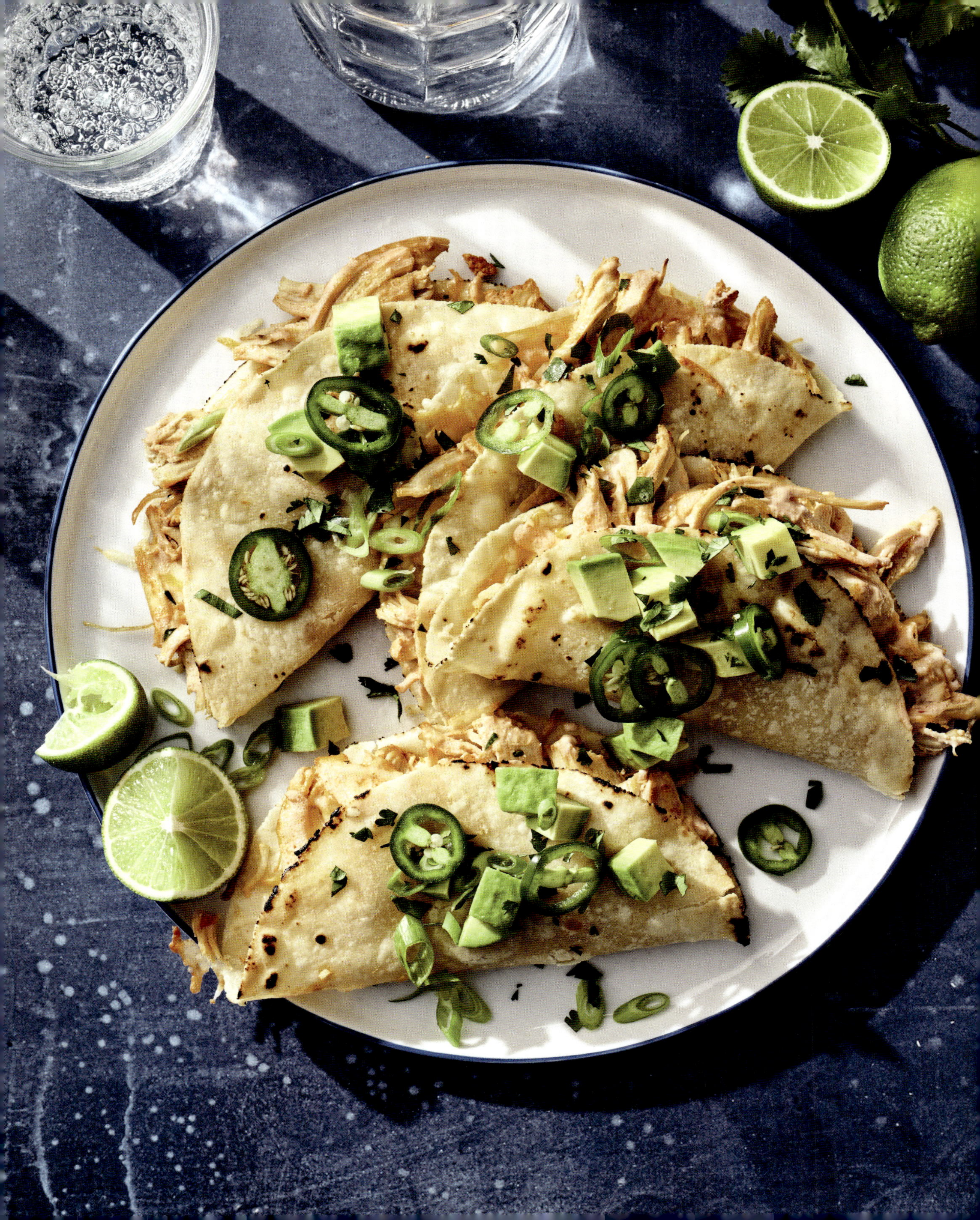

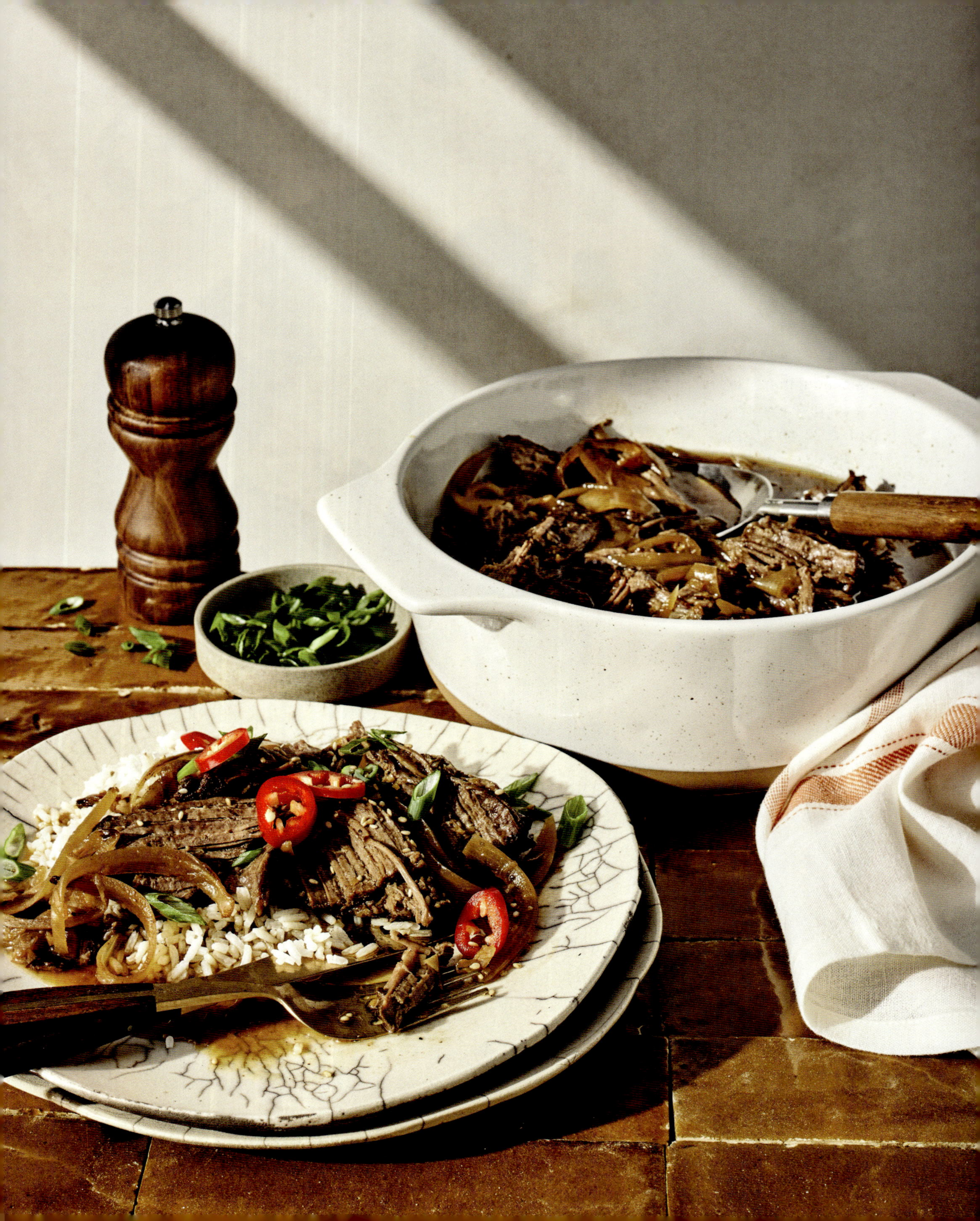

Dairy-Free
Gluten-Free
Grain-Free

# Sesame-Ginger Pot Roast

SERVES 6 • PREP TIME: 20 MINUTES • COOK TIME: 2½ TO 3 HOURS (DUTCH OVEN) OR 6 TO 8 HOURS (SLOW COOKER) • TOTAL TIME: 2 HOURS 50 MINUTES TO 3 HOURS 20 MINUTES (DUTCH OVEN) OR 6 HOURS 20 MINUTES TO 8 HOURS 20 MINUTES (SLOW COOKER)

- 3 pounds beef chuck roast
- 1 teaspoon sea salt
- 1 teaspoon freshly ground black pepper
- 1 tablespoon avocado oil
- 1 yellow onion, thinly sliced
- 3 garlic cloves, minced
- 1-inch piece fresh ginger, minced
- 1½ cups beef bone broth
- ⅓ cup coconut aminos
- 2 tablespoons toasted sesame oil
- 1 tablespoon unseasoned rice vinegar
- 1 tablespoon honey
- Optional toppings: sliced green onion, fresh cilantro, thinly sliced red chili pepper, toasted sesame seeds, sea salt

Leaving a chuck roast to slow cook in the morning so it's perfectly tender by dinnertime? That's the kind of life hack we all need, especially when chasing little ones around the house. It makes the house smell incredible, takes zero effort once it gets going, and pairs well with just about any side. This recipe has even earned a permanent spot on our Thanksgiving menu because it's that good.

1. Season the chuck roast with the salt and pepper. In a large skillet, heat the avocado oil over medium-high heat. Add the roast and sear for about 5 minutes per side, or until deeply browned. (Alternatively, if your slow cooker has a sauté or browning function, you can do this step directly in the insert to save time and cleanup.)
2. Transfer the roast to the slow cooker and add the onion, garlic, ginger, broth, coconut aminos, sesame oil, vinegar, and honey. Cover and cook on low for 6 to 8 hours or high for 4 hours, until the meat is tender and falling apart. If the roast isn't shredding easily, it likely needs more time for the collagen to break down. Continue cooking in 30-minute increments until the meat is fall-apart tender.
3. **To cook in a Dutch oven:** Sear the roast directly in a large Dutch oven over medium-high heat until browned on all sides. Add the onion, garlic, ginger, broth, coconut aminos, sesame oil, vinegar, and honey. Bring to a simmer over medium heat, then reduce the heat to low, cover, and cook for 2½ to 3 hours, flipping the roast once halfway through. Check for doneness—if the meat isn't tender enough to shred, continue simmering in 20- to 30-minute increments until it easily falls apart.
4. Shred the meat with two forks or tongs directly in the pot, tossing to coat it in the sauce.
5. Serve topped with some of the braising sauce from the pot and garnish with green onion, cilantro, red chili, toasted sesame seeds, and salt, if desired.

**PER SERVING**
Protein: 34g
Carbohydrates: 7g
Fat: 22g

**STORAGE:** This pot roast will keep in an airtight container in the fridge for up to 4 days. The flavors get even better the next day. Reheat on the stovetop over low heat until warmed through.

Gluten-Free
No Added Sugar

# Short Ribs with Bone Broth Polenta

**SERVES 4 TO 6 • PREP TIME: 30 MINUTES • COOK TIME: 3 TO 3½ HOURS (DUTCH OVEN) OR 8 TO 10 HOURS (SLOW COOKER) • TOTAL TIME: 3 HOURS 30 MINUTES TO 4 HOURS (DUTCH OVEN) OR 8 HOURS 30 MINUTES TO 10 HOURS 30 MINUTES (SLOW COOKER)**

This one's got Sunday dinner energy—but it's easy enough to pull off any day of the week. The short ribs go low and slow until they're fall-apart tender, then get spooned over creamy, cheesy bone broth polenta.

**FOR THE SHORT RIBS**

- 3 pounds boneless beef short ribs, cut into 2- to 3-inch pieces
- 1 teaspoon sea salt
- 1 teaspoon freshly ground black pepper, plus more for garnish
- 1 tablespoon avocado oil
- 3 medium carrots, cut into 1-inch pieces
- 6 ounces cremini mushrooms, halved
- 3 cups beef bone broth
- 4 sprigs fresh thyme, plus more for garnish
- 1 large yellow onion, sliced ½ inch thick
- 6 garlic cloves, minced
- 2 tablespoons tomato paste

**FOR THE POLENTA**

- 4 cups beef bone broth
- 1 cup polenta
- 1 teaspoon sea salt
- 1 tablespoon ghee
- ½ cup grated pecorino romano cheese

1. **Sear the short ribs:** Season the short ribs all over with the salt and pepper. Heat the oil in a large cast-iron skillet over medium heat. Brown the short ribs for 3 to 4 minutes per side. Transfer to the slow cooker and add the carrots, mushrooms, 1 cup of the broth, and the thyme sprigs.
2. In the same skillet, sauté the onions for 5 to 6 minutes, until they begin to caramelize. Stir in the garlic and tomato paste and cook for 1 to 2 minutes more. Pour in the remaining 2 cups broth and use a wooden spoon to scrape up the browned bits from the bottom—this is called deglazing and adds rich flavor. Simmer for 7 to 8 minutes, until reduced by half. Transfer to the slow cooker.
3. **Cook the ribs:** Set the slow cooker to low for 8 to 10 hours or high for 4 to 6 hours, until the short ribs are tender and falling apart. Shred the meat into bite-size pieces and return to the pot.
4. **To cook in a Dutch oven:** After searing the ribs and sautéing the vegetables, transfer all to a Dutch oven. Deglaze the skillet as directed above, then pour the reduced broth into the pot. Bring everything to a simmer, cover, and cook on low heat for 3 to 3½ hours, turning the ribs once or twice. Shred and return to the pot.
5. **Make the polenta:** In a medium saucepan, bring the broth to a boil over high heat. Slowly whisk in the polenta and salt, stirring constantly to prevent lumps. Reduce the heat to low, cover, and cook for 30 minutes, stirring every 10 minutes. If it becomes too thick, stir in a bit of broth or water, 1 tablespoon at a time. Stir in the ghee and pecorino until smooth and creamy.
6. Serve the polenta topped with the short ribs and a spoonful of sauce from the pot. Finish with pepper and thyme.

**STORAGE:** The short ribs will keep in an airtight container in the fridge for up to 4 days. Reheat gently with a splash of broth or water to loosen the sauce. Store polenta separately in an airtight container for up to 3 days, and stir while reheating to maintain its creaminess.

**PER SERVING (FOR 6 SERVINGS)**
Protein: 51g
Carbohydrates: 29g
Fat: 48g

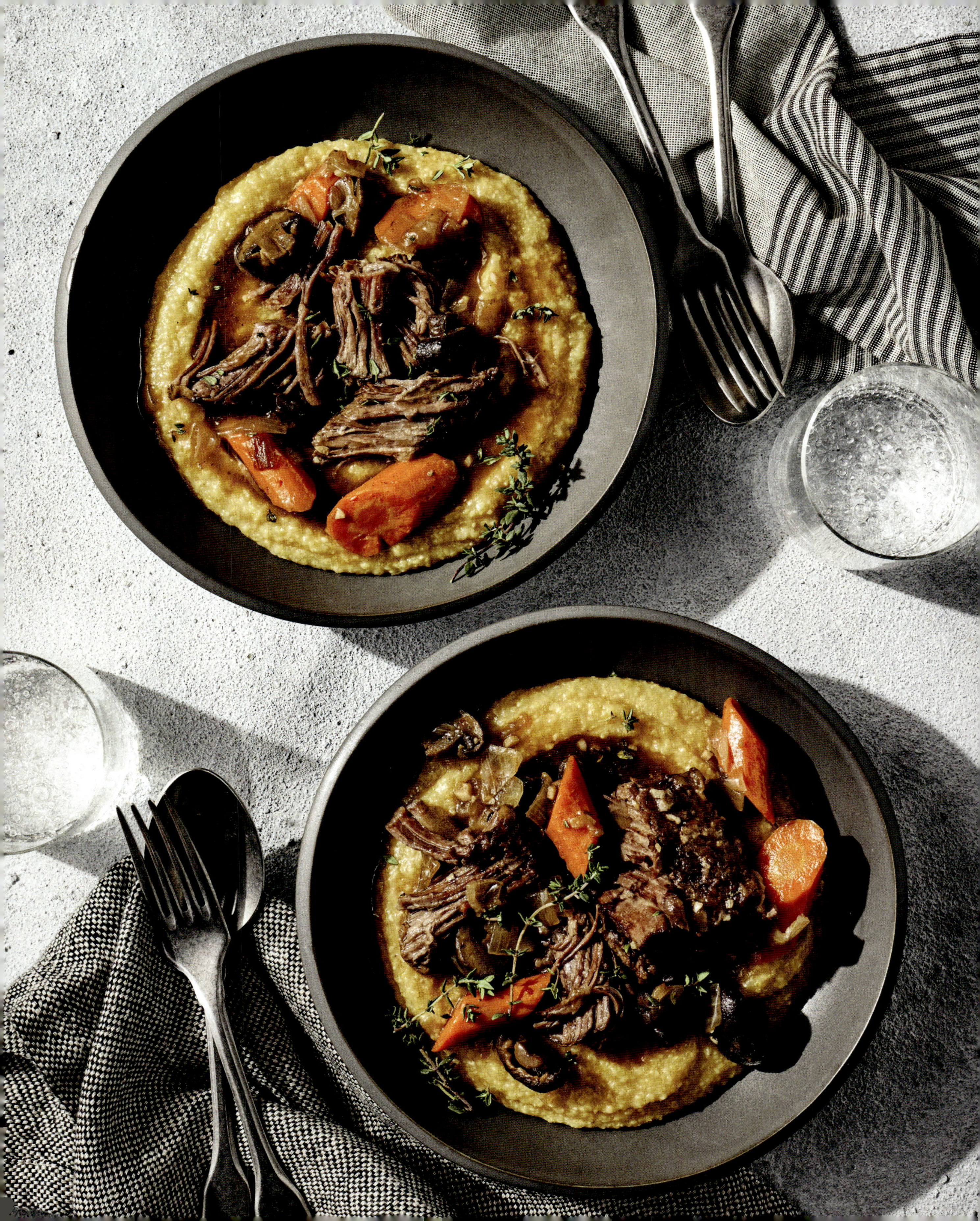

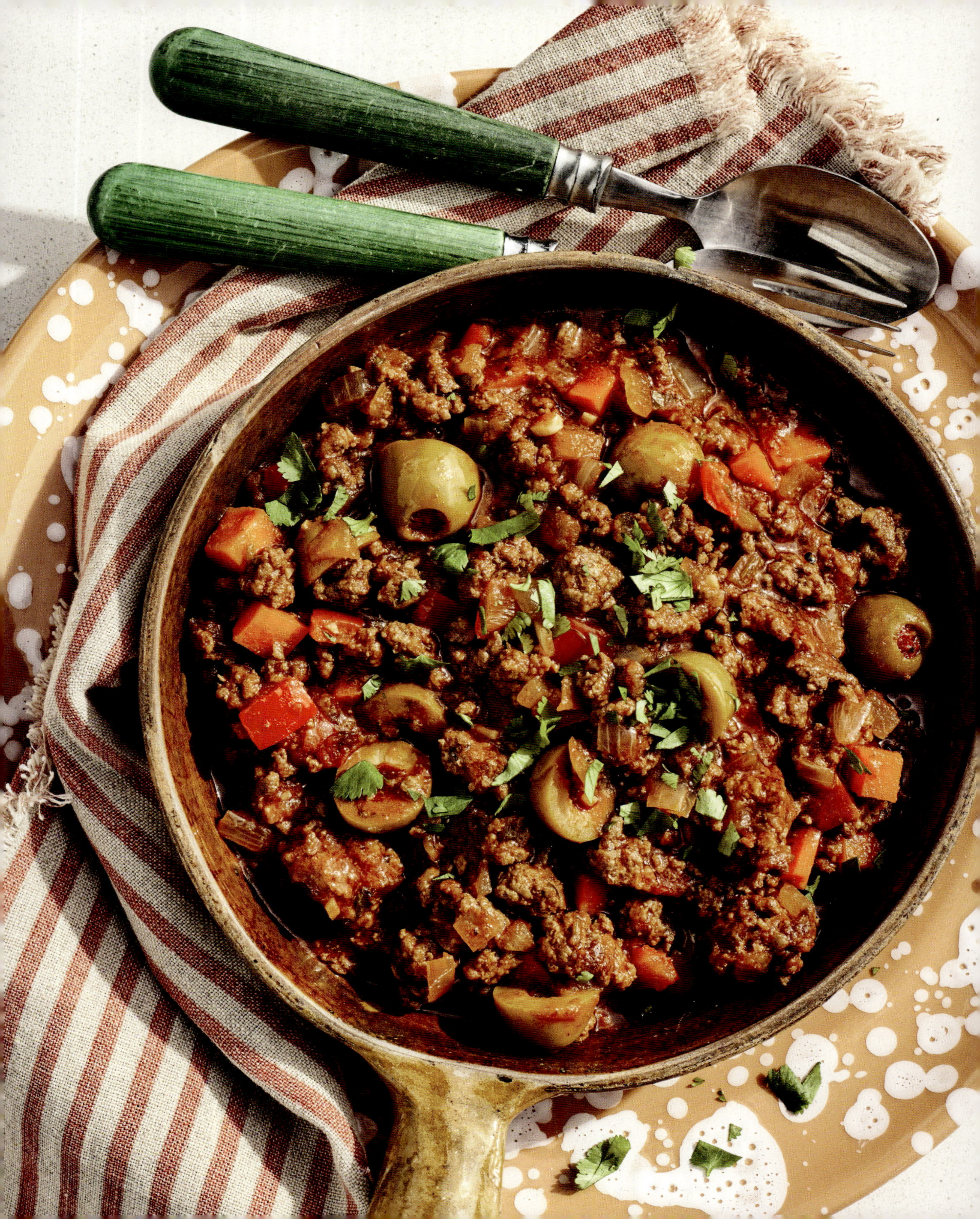

Dairy-Free
Gluten-Free
Grain-Free
No Added Sugar

# Slow Cooker Picadillo

SERVES 4 TO 6 • PREP TIME: 20 MINUTES • COOK TIME: 45 MINUTES TO 1 HOUR (DUTCH OVEN) OR 6 TO 8 HOURS (SLOW COOKER) • TOTAL TIME: 1 HOUR 5 MINUTES TO 1 HOUR 20 MINUTES (DUTCH OVEN) OR 6 HOURS 20 MINUTES TO 8 HOURS 20 MINUTES (SLOW COOKER)

If you've never had picadillo, get ready—this one's a flavor bomb. Ground beef simmers low and slow in a mix of tomato, spices, briny olives, and aromatics until it's rich and savory, then hits you with flavor at first bite. Every bite has that salty-sweet thing going on, with tender carrots and pops of fresh cilantro to round it out. I love it over rice with black beans, but it's bold enough to stand on its own.

- 2 tablespoons extra-virgin olive oil
- 2 pounds ground beef
- 1 teaspoon sea salt
- 1 teaspoon freshly ground black pepper
- 1 yellow onion, diced
- 1 red bell pepper, seeded and diced (or sub diced zucchini, carrots, or mushrooms—whatever you've got on hand)
- 5 cloves garlic, minced
- 2 tablespoons tomato paste
- 2 teaspoons ground cumin
- 1 teaspoon dried oregano
- ½ teaspoon ground cinnamon
- 1 (14-ounce) can tomato sauce
- 2 large carrots, chopped
- ¼ cup chopped fresh cilantro
- 2 bay leaves
- 1 cup pimento-stuffed olives, drained and halved (save ¼ cup olive brine to add to the picadillo)
- For serving (optional): Bone Broth Jasmine Rice (page 198), black beans, Farro (page 182), Garlicky Roasted Broccolini (page 183)

1. In a large skillet, heat 1 tablespoon of the oil over medium heat. Add the ground beef and season with the salt and black pepper. Cook, breaking up the meat, for 7 to 8 minutes, until it starts to brown. Using a slotted spoon, transfer the beef to the slow cooker.
2. If needed, pour off excess fat from the skillet, then return the skillet to the heat. Add the remaining 1 tablespoon oil, then the onion, bell pepper, and garlic and cook until softened, about 5 minutes. Stir in the tomato paste, cumin, oregano, and cinnamon and cook for 1 to 2 minutes, until the tomato paste turns brick red and the spices are toasted. Pour in the tomato sauce and stir to scrape up any browned bits from the pan.
3. Transfer the mixture to the slow cooker. Add the carrots, cilantro, bay leaves, olives, and reserved olive brine. Cover and cook on high for 3 to 4 hours or low for 6 to 8 hours, until the flavors meld and the carrots are tender.
4. **To cook in a Dutch oven:** Brown the ground beef directly in a large Dutch oven over medium heat. Add the onion, bell pepper, and garlic, and cook until softened, about 5 minutes. Add the tomato sauce, carrots, cilantro, bay leaves, olives, and olive brine. Bring to a simmer, then cover and cook over low heat for 45 minutes to 1 hour, stirring occasionally, until the carrots are tender and the flavors are fully developed. Discard the bay leaves and adjust seasoning with additional salt if needed.

**STORAGE:** Picadillo will keep in an airtight container in the fridge for up to 4 days. Reheat in a skillet over medium heat or in the microwave.

---

**PER SERVING (FOR 4 SERVINGS)**
Protein: 41g
Carbohydrates: 18g
Fat: 40g

Gluten-Free
Grain-Free
No Added Sugar

# Brothy Beans with Zesty Chimichurri

**SERVES 4 TO 6 • PREP TIME: 20 MINUTES • COOK TIME: 1½ TO 2 HOURS (DUTCH OVEN) OR 6 TO 8 HOURS (SLOW COOKER) • TOTAL TIME: 1 HOUR 50 MINUTES TO 2 HOURS 20 MINUTES (DUTCH OVEN) OR 6 HOURS 20 MINUTES TO 8 HOURS 20 MINUTES (SLOW COOKER)**

Some days we just need a big bowl of comfort food (with benefits!), ya know? These brothy beans are simmered in collagen-rich bone broth and loaded with fiber, iron, and B vitamins for steady energy and gut support. Crispy bacon and a zesty chimichurri take it from simple to next-level. Serve with crusty sourdough and, if you're feeling fancy, throw a poached egg on top. This was my go-to for batch cooking in those early postpartum days.

**FOR THE BEANS**

1 tablespoon extra-virgin olive oil

1 yellow onion, halved

1 head garlic, halved, as much papery peel removed as possible

1 lemon, halved

1 pound dried cannellini beans, rinsed

10 cups bone broth or water

2 sprigs fresh rosemary

6 fresh sage leaves

1 Parmesan rind (any size works)

1 teaspoon sea salt

½ teaspoon freshly ground black pepper

1 (8-ounce) package bacon (or ½ pound pancetta), diced

**FOR THE CHIMICHURRI**

½ cup chopped fresh parsley

1 garlic clove, grated

½ teaspoon dried oregano

½ teaspoon chili flakes

Grated zest of 1 lemon

2 tablespoons freshly squeezed lemon juice (1 lemon)

¼ cup extra-virgin olive oil

½ teaspoon sea salt

Crusty sourdough, for serving (optional)

---

**PER SERVING (FOR 6 SERVINGS)**
Protein: 38g
Carbohydrates: 29g
Fat: 22g

1. **Make the beans:** In a large skillet, heat the oil over medium heat. Add the onion, garlic, and lemon cut side down. Sear for about 5 minutes, until deeply golden and caramelized. Transfer the aromatics to the slow cooker. Reserve the skillet to cook the bacon later.
2. Add the beans, broth, rosemary, sage, Parmesan rind, salt, and pepper to the slow cooker. Cover and cook on low for 6 to 8 hours, until the beans are tender but still hold their shape.
3. **To cook in a Dutch oven:** Sauté the onion, garlic, rosemary, sage, and lemon directly in a large Dutch oven over medium heat. Add the remaining ingredients and bring to a simmer. Cover and cook over low heat for 1½ to 2 hours, until the beans are tender but not falling apart. Stir occasionally and add more broth as needed.
4. Just before the beans are done, reheat the reserved skillet over medium-high heat. Cook the bacon until crispy and browned. Transfer to a paper towel–lined plate.
5. Once the beans are tender, remove and discard the onion, garlic, lemon, rosemary, sage, and Parmesan rind.
6. **Make the chimichurri:** In a small bowl, combine the parsley, garlic, oregano, chili flakes, lemon zest, lemon juice, oil, and salt. Stir well and set aside.
7. Ladle the beans into bowls and top with bacon and a drizzle of chimichurri. Serve with crusty sourdough, if desired.

**STORAGE:** The beans will keep in an airtight container in the fridge for up to 4 days. Reheat on the stovetop over low heat, adding more broth as needed. Store the chimichurri separately in an airtight container in the fridge for up to 5 to 7 days, and drizzle fresh when serving.

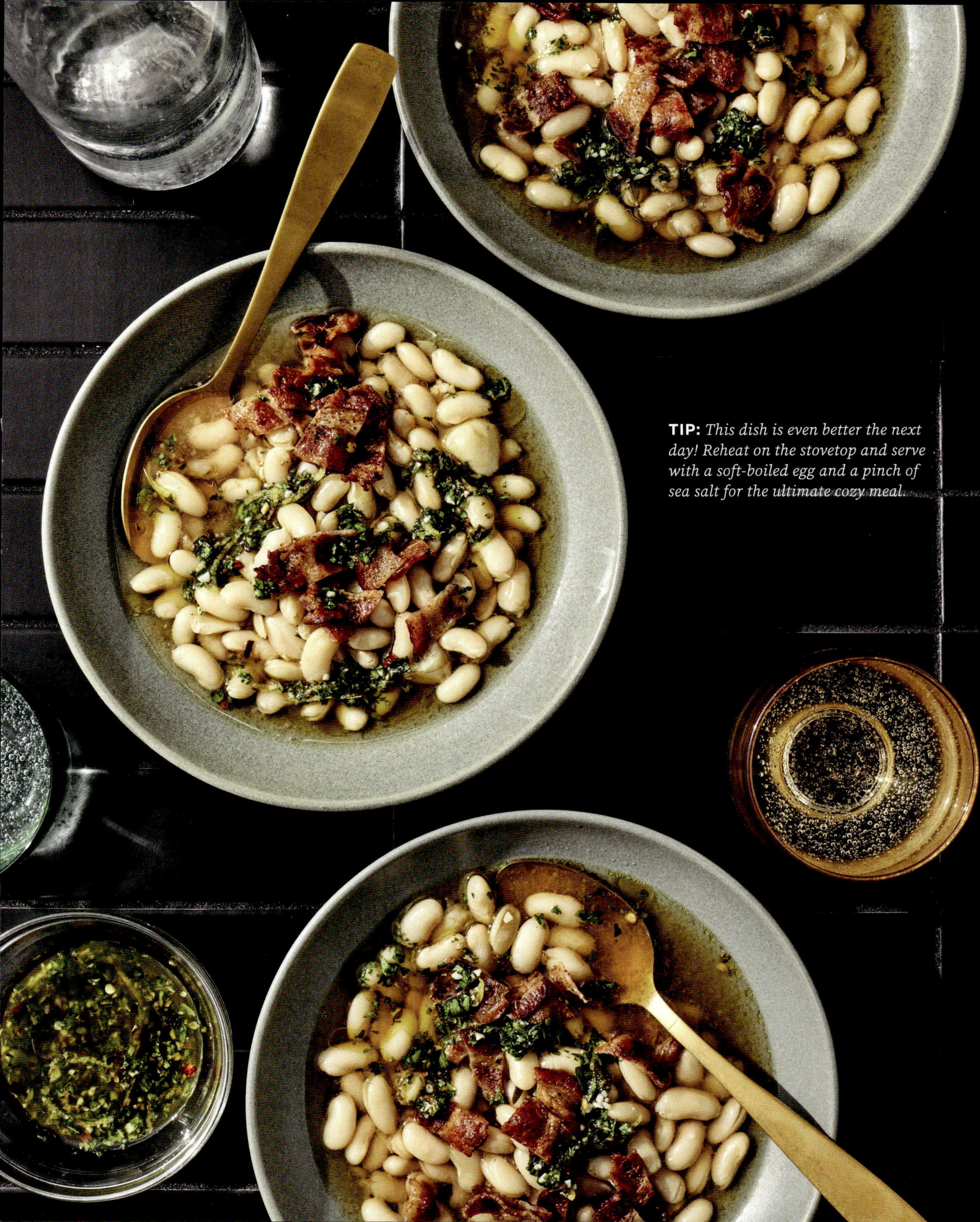

**TIP:** *This dish is even better the next day! Reheat on the stovetop and serve with a soft-boiled egg and a pinch of sea salt for the ultimate cozy meal.*

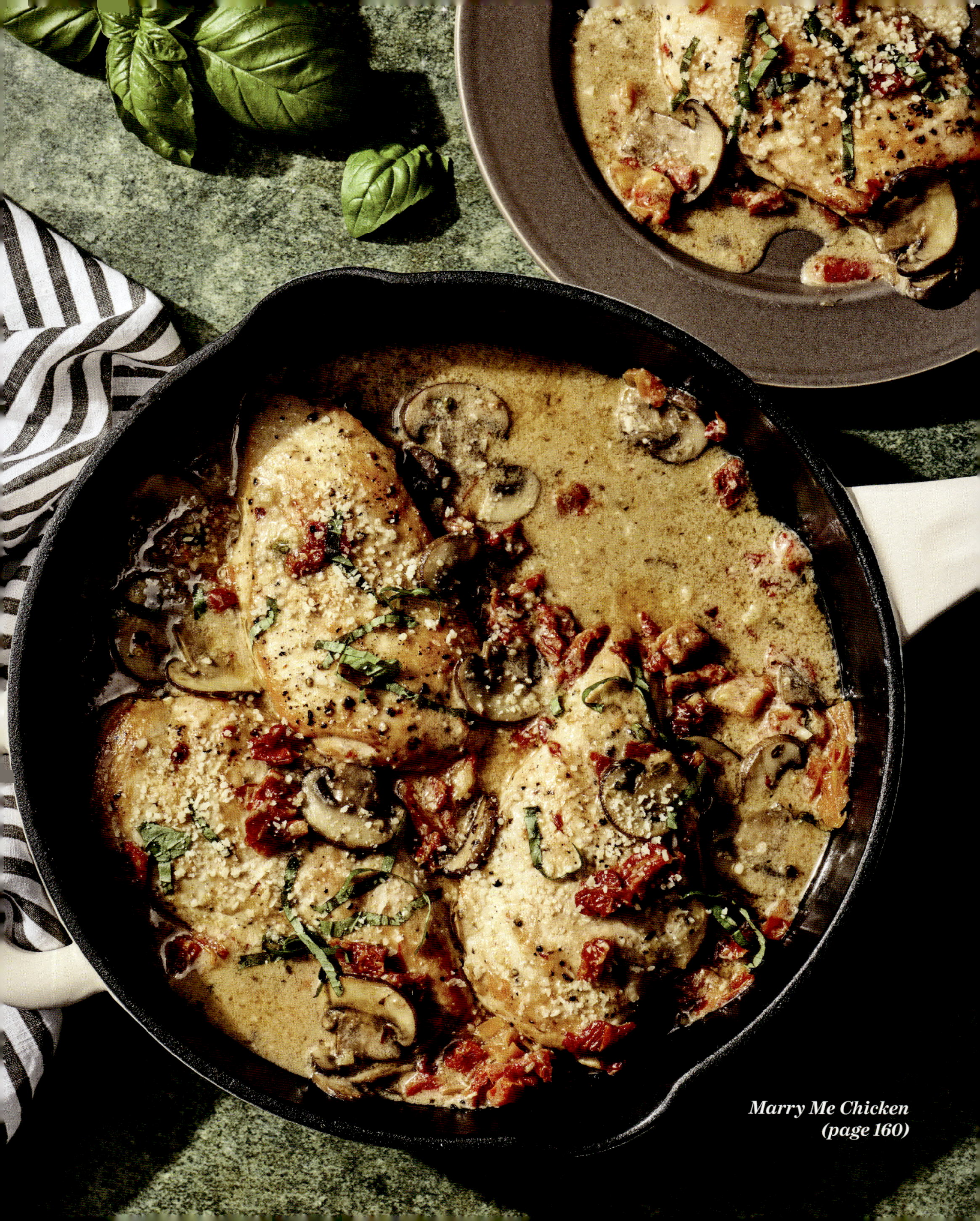

*Marry Me Chicken*
*(page 160)*

160 Marry Me Chicken

163 Beef Fried Rice

164 Sheet-Pan Brats and Potatoes

167 Crispy Lemon-Garlic Chicken Thighs

168 Pesto-Crusted Baked Cod

171 Egg Roll in a Bowl

172 One-Pan Beef and Broccoli

175 Salsa Verde Shrimp and Rice

176 Sloppy Joe Bowls

179 Double Double-Cheeseburger Bowls

180 Sheet-Pan Turmeric Chicken with Romesco

Simple One-Pan Sides

182 Sautéed Greens with Lemon and Olive Oil

182 Farro

183 Roasted Japanese Sweet Potatoes

183 Garlicky Roasted Broccolini

# One-Pan Meals

Gluten-Free
Grain-Free
No Added Sugar
Paleo
**IF MODIFIED:**
Dairy-Free

# Marry Me Chicken

**SERVES 4 • PREP TIME: 10 MINUTES • COOK TIME: 35 MINUTES • TOTAL TIME: 45 MINUTES**

- 4 (6- to 8-ounce) chicken breasts (about 1½ to 2 pounds total), trimmed
- 1 teaspoon sea salt
- ½ teaspoon freshly ground black pepper
- 2 tablespoons avocado oil or extra-virgin olive oil
- 1 tablespoon minced garlic (3 to 4 cloves)
- 1½ cups sliced mushrooms (optional)
- 1 teaspoon dried thyme
- 1 teaspoon dried oregano
- ¼ teaspoon red chili flakes
- ¾ cup chicken bone broth
- ¾ cup canned coconut cream (scoop the thick cream from the top of a 13.5-ounce can and add liquid as needed to measure ¾ cup)
- 1½ teaspoons arrowroot powder
- ½ cup olive oil–packed sun-dried tomatoes, chopped
- ⅓ cup finely grated Parmesan (or 3 tablespoons nutritional yeast for dairy-free)
- Finely chopped fresh basil, for serving

If you've spent any time online, you've probably seen Marry Me Chicken making the rounds—so this is my take on the viral classic. Legend has it the dish got its name because it's so good that someone proposed after the first bite. And honestly? I get it. I've been making this version for years, and if I could marry the sauce alone, I would. It's creamy, garlicky, a little tangy from the sun-dried tomatoes, and lightened up with coconut cream and bone broth instead of heavy cream.

1. Preheat the oven to 375°F and prepare a large oven-safe skillet.
2. Place the chicken breasts between two pieces of parchment paper or plastic wrap and use a meat mallet or rolling pin to pound them to an even ¾-inch thickness. Season both sides with the salt and pepper.
3. In the skillet, heat the oil over medium-high heat. Add the chicken and sear for about 5 minutes per side, until golden brown. Remove from the skillet and set aside on a plate.
4. Reduce the heat to low, add the garlic to the skillet, and cook for 1 minute, until fragrant. If using, add the mushrooms and cook for 3 to 4 minutes, until softened. Stir in the thyme, oregano, chili flakes, broth, and coconut cream.
5. In a small bowl, mix the arrowroot powder with 2 tablespoons water until dissolved. Stir into the skillet to thicken the sauce. Add the sun-dried tomatoes and Parmesan, stirring to combine. Return the chicken to the skillet, flipping a few times to coat in the sauce.
6. Transfer the skillet to the oven and bake for 20 minutes to cook through, or until the chicken reaches 165°F internally. Remove from the oven and spoon sauce over the chicken, top with basil, and serve with roasted broccolini, blanched asparagus, or green beans for a fresh, vibrant contrast to the rich, creamy sauce.

**STORAGE:** Store leftovers in an airtight container in the fridge for up to 4 days. Reheat gently on the stovetop or in the microwave, adding a splash of broth or water to loosen the sauce if it thickens.

**PER SERVING**
Protein: 49g
Carbohydrates: 8g
Fat: 22g

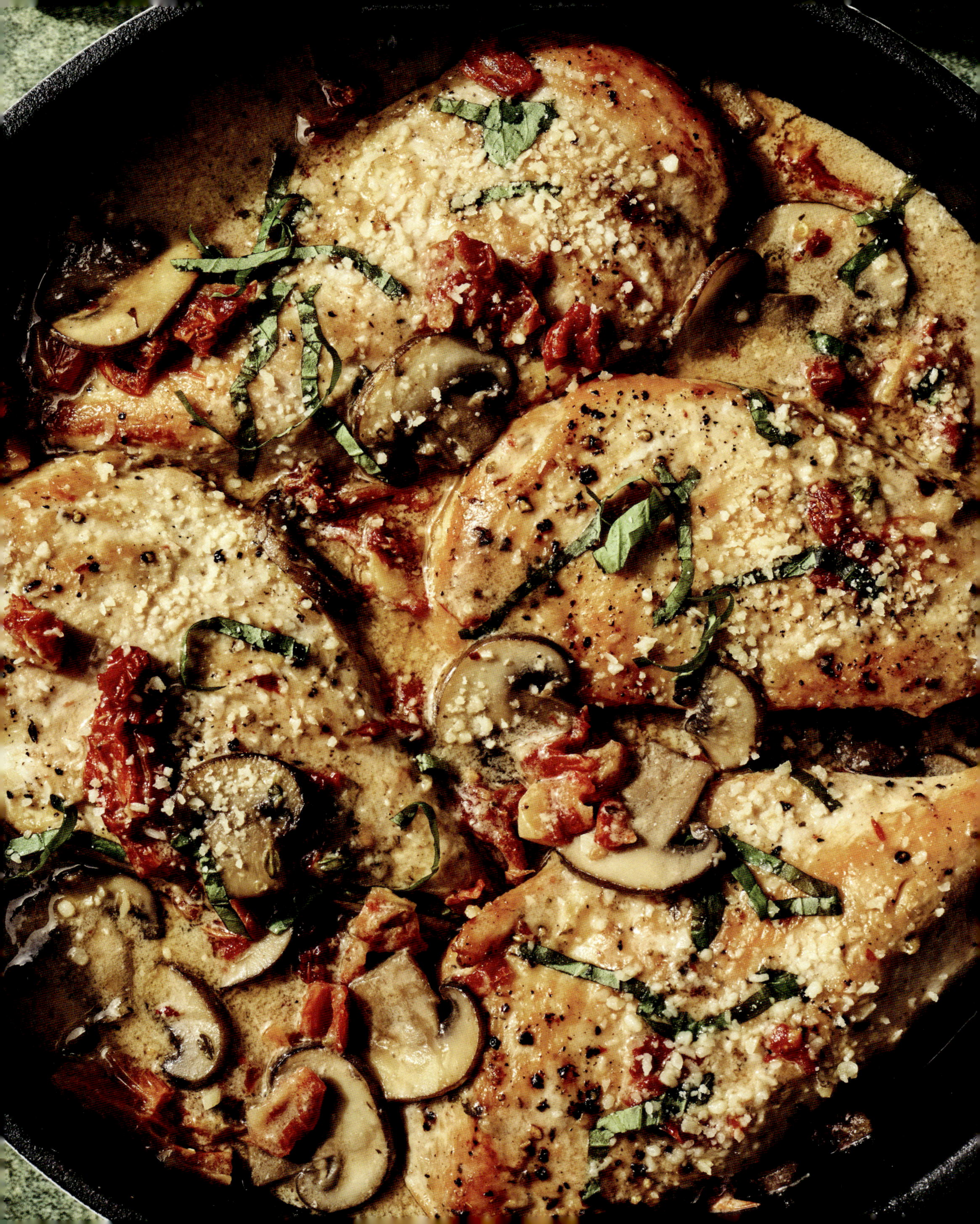

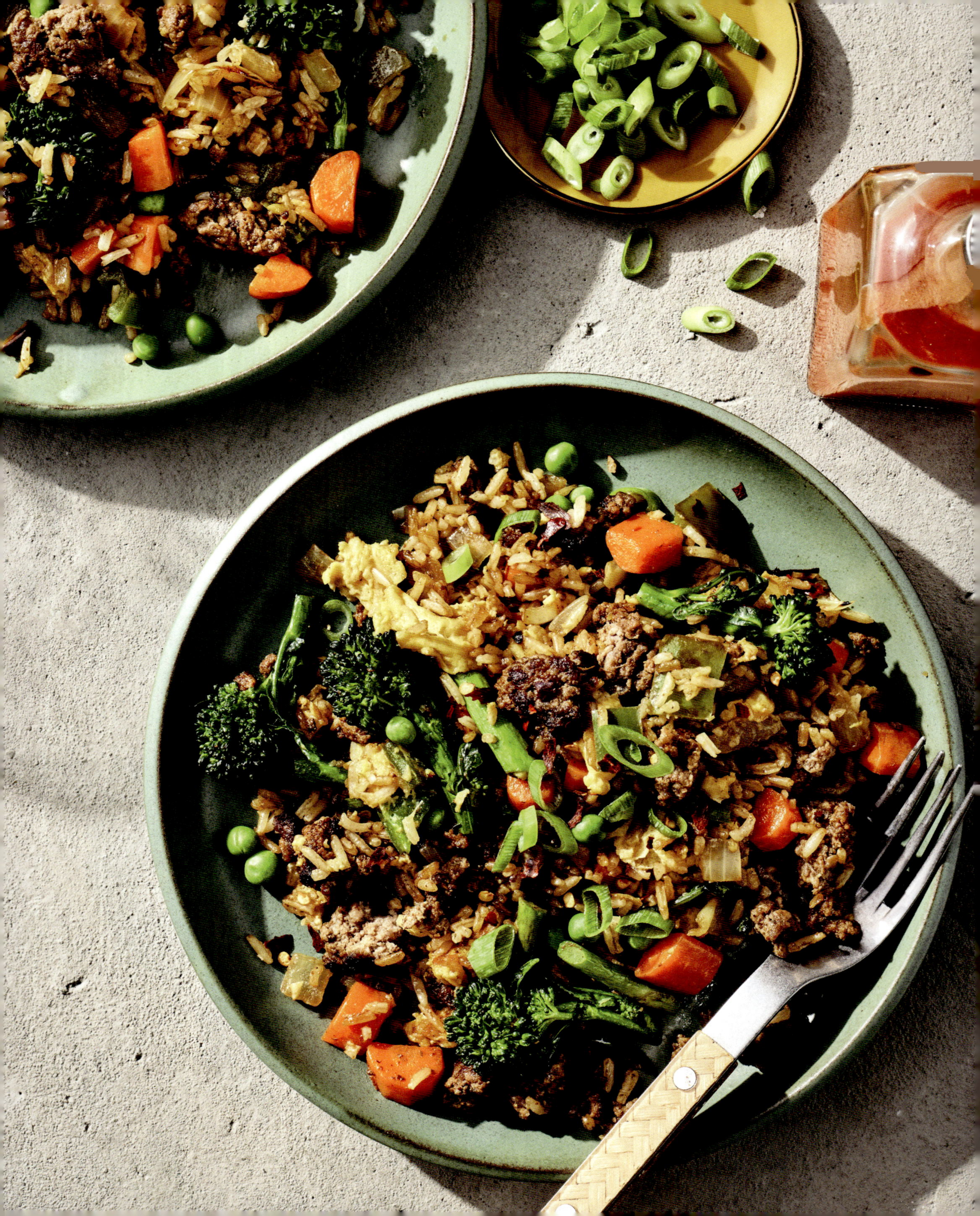

Gluten-Free
No Added Sugar
**IF MODIFIED:**
Dairy-Free

# Beef Fried Rice

**SERVES 4 • PREP TIME: 10 MINUTES • COOK TIME: 25 MINUTES • TOTAL TIME: 35 MINUTES**

I started making this beef fried rice because I always cook up a batch of taco-seasoned ground beef at the start of the week—it's my fail-safe for staying on track and getting enough protein in during busy days. One day I had leftovers—rice, veggies, and that beef—tossed them together, and just like that, it became a staple meal for Bridger and me. Honestly, I couldn't think of a better recipe to reheat when I've got 27 tabs open and no time to think.

3 tablespoons avocado oil
1 pound ground beef
1 tablespoon taco seasoning (I like Siete)
½ large onion, diced
2 large carrots, diced
1 bunch broccolini, trimmed and chopped
1 Anaheim chili, seeded and diced (or poblano or green bell pepper; or jalapeño for more heat)
1 tablespoon minced garlic
1 tablespoon minced fresh ginger
1½ cups Bone Broth Jasmine Rice (page 198), or leftover rice if you have it on hand
1 to 2 tablespoons ghee or butter (or vegan butter for dairy-free)
1 tablespoon sesame oil
3 tablespoons tamari
Avocado oil spray
2 large eggs
¾ cup frozen peas
2 teaspoons sea salt
1 teaspoon freshly ground black pepper
Chopped green onion
Red chili flakes (optional)

1. In a large skillet or wok, heat 1 tablespoon of the avocado oil over medium-high heat. Add the ground beef and cook, breaking it up, for 7 to 8 minutes, until browned. Add the taco seasoning with 2 tablespoons water and stir. Push the beef to one side of the skillet and add the onion and remaining 2 tablespoons avocado oil to the empty side. Cook for 1 minute, then stir in the carrots, broccolini, Anaheim chili, garlic, and ginger. Cook for 5 to 6 minutes, until the veggies are just tender.
2. Stir in the cooked rice and ghee, breaking up any rice clumps. Drizzle in the sesame oil and tamari and stir until the rice is evenly coated and everything is well combined.
3. Create a space in the center of the skillet and spray lightly with avocado oil. Crack the eggs directly into the center and scramble gently with a spatula, gradually folding them into the rice mixture. Stir in the peas, salt, and black pepper. Cook for another 3 to 4 minutes, until the peas are warm and everything is hot and cohesive.
4. Remove from the heat and serve hot. Top with green onion and season with salt, black pepper, and chili flakes, if desired.

**STORAGE:** Store in an airtight container in the fridge for up to 4 days. Reheat in a skillet over medium heat or in the microwave, adding a splash of water or broth if needed to refresh the texture.

**PER SERVING**
Protein: 30g
Carbohydrates: 24g
Fat: 33g

Dairy-Free
Gluten-Free
Grain-Free

# Sheet-Pan Brats and Potatoes

SERVES 2 TO 4 • PREP TIME: 10 MINUTES • COOK TIME: 30 MINUTES • TOTAL TIME: 40 MINUTES

1 pound baby potatoes, halved

2 tablespoons extra-virgin olive oil

1 teaspoon onion powder

½ teaspoon smoked paprika

Sea salt and freshly ground black pepper

1 tablespoon apple juice

1 teaspoon stone-ground mustard, plus more for serving

1 teaspoon honey

½ teaspoon sea salt

½ head purple cabbage, sliced into ¾-inch-thick wedges

4 bratwurst sausages (look for uncooked, high-quality pork, turkey, or chicken brats; you can add 1 to 2 more if you want to bump the protein—just make sure there's enough space on the pan so everything still roasts and browns properly)

2 tablespoons chopped fresh parsley

This recipe is proof that weeknight dinners don't have to be complicated to be good. Everything is roasted on one baking sheet here—juicy brats, crispy potatoes, and cabbage with a smoky mustard glaze—and it all comes out golden, flavorful, and ready to devour. Cleanup? Practically nonexistent. Want to bump the protein? Toss on an extra brat or two—just make sure they've got space to roast. If not, use a second pan or cook them in batches so everything crisps up properly.

1. Preheat the oven to 400°F. On a large rimmed baking sheet, toss the potatoes with 1 tablespoon of the oil, the onion powder, paprika, salt, and pepper. Spread out the potatoes on one-third of the baking sheet.
2. In a small bowl, whisk the remaining 1 tablespoon oil with the apple juice, mustard, honey, and salt. Arrange the cabbage wedges on the other half of the baking sheet and brush all over with the mustard sauce. Place the bratwurst in the center of the pan.
3. Roast for 30 minutes, flipping the sausages halfway through, until the brats are golden brown and cooked through, 160°F for pork, 165°F for chicken or turkey.
4. Sprinkle the parsley over the potatoes and cabbage and serve with extra mustard for dipping.

**STORAGE:** Store leftovers in an airtight container in the fridge for up to 4 days. Reheat in the oven at 375°F for 10 to 12 minutes, or in a skillet over medium heat until warmed through and crisped.

**PER SERVING (FOR 4 SERVINGS)**
Protein: 21g
Carbohydrates: 27g
Fat: 30g

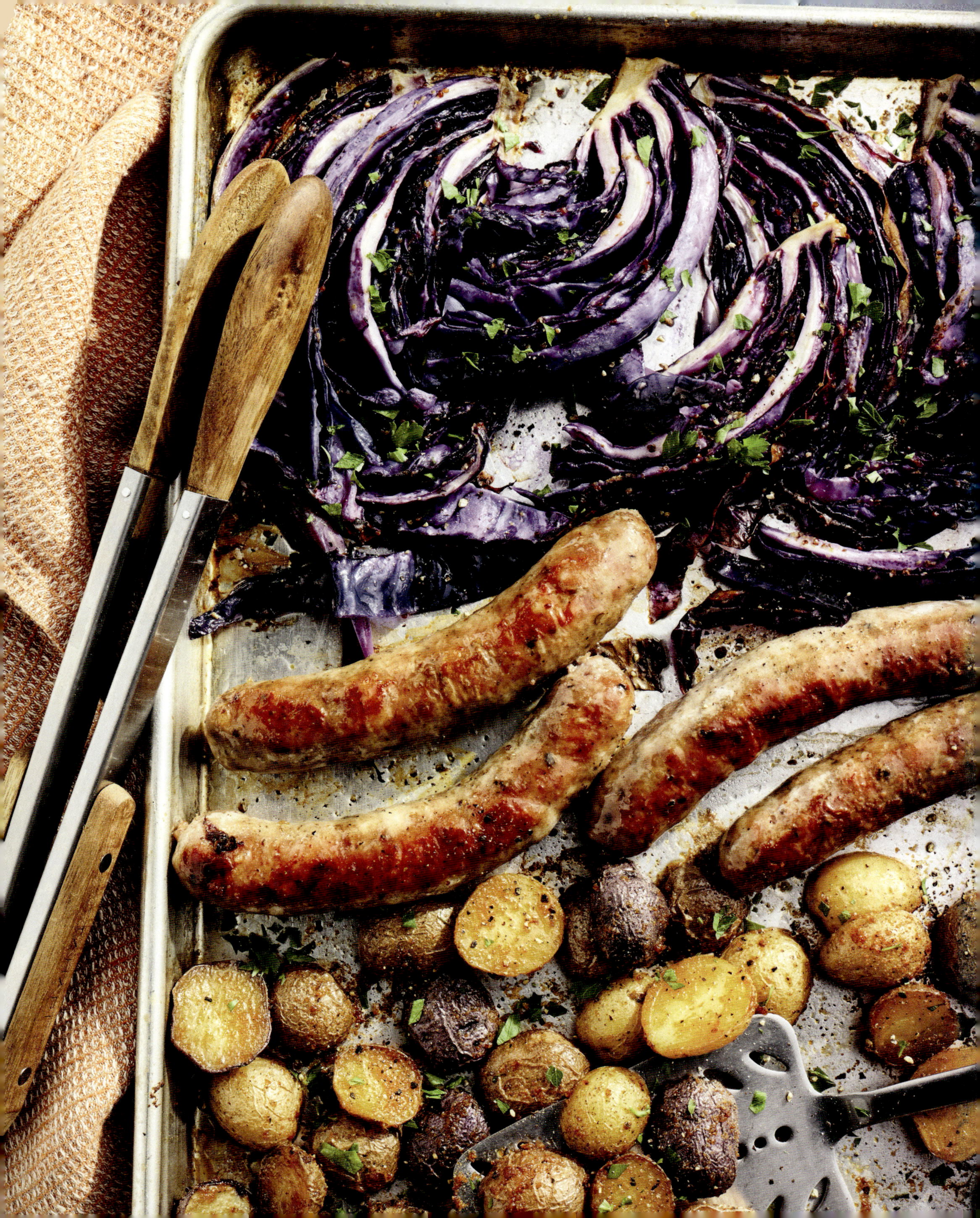

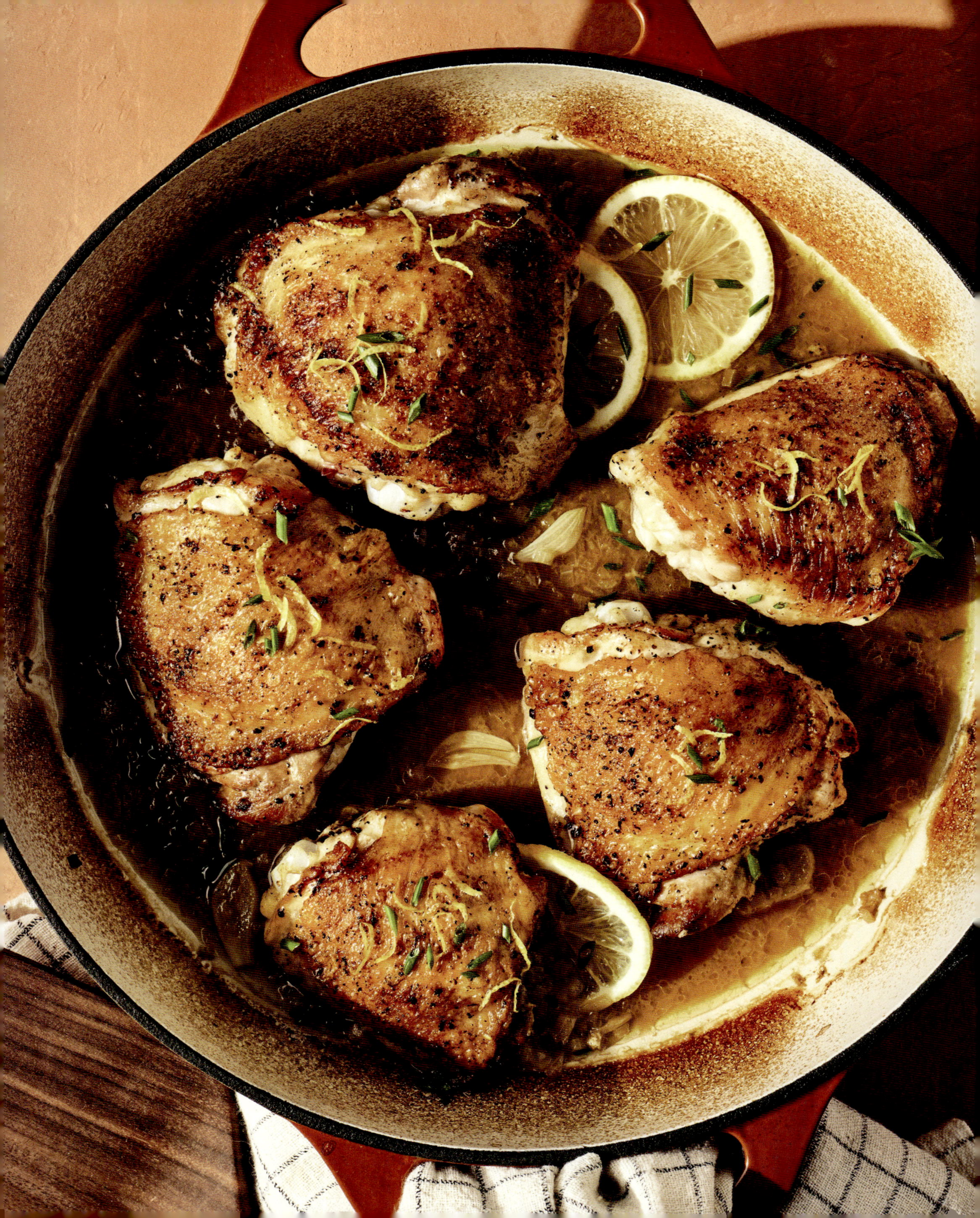

Gluten-Free
Grain-Free
No Added Sugar
Paleo
**IF MODIFIED:**
Dairy-Free

# Crispy Lemon-Garlic Chicken Thighs

**SERVES 2 TO 4 • PREP TIME: 10 MINUTES • COOK TIME: 40 MINUTES • TOTAL TIME: 50 MINUTES**

- 2 pounds bone-in skin-on chicken thighs
- 1 teaspoon sea salt
- ½ teaspoon freshly ground black pepper
- ½ teaspoon garlic powder
- Grated zest of 1 lemon, plus lemon slices and additional zest for serving
- 2 tablespoons extra-virgin olive oil
- 1 medium shallot, finely diced
- 2 cloves garlic, sliced
- 1 cup chicken bone broth or dry white wine
- 1 tablespoon Dijon mustard
- 2 tablespoons ghee (or vegan butter for dairy-free)
- Chopped fresh chives, for garnish (optional)

Chicken thighs are unmatched in flavor—they stay juicy and tender in the oven, self-basting in their own drippings while crisping up perfectly. This one-pan meal has a bright, garlicky lemon-butter sauce that delivers major payoff for minimal effort. Serve with roasted potatoes (sweet potatoes are great for extra fiber and vitamins!).

1. Preheat the oven to 425°F. Season the chicken thighs with the salt, pepper, garlic powder, and lemon zest.
2. In a large cast-iron skillet, heat the oil over medium heat. Add the chicken thighs, skin side down, and sear for about 5 minutes, until the skin is golden and crisp. Transfer the chicken to a plate and reserve the skillet, saving all those flavorful drippings!
3. In the same skillet with the drippings, add the shallot and garlic. Sauté for about 3 minutes, until the shallot is softened and translucent. Pour in the broth and mustard, stir to combine and scrape up any browned bits from the bottom of the skillet.
4. Nestle the chicken back in the skillet, skin side up. Transfer the skillet to the oven and roast for 25 to 30 minutes, until the internal temperature of the chicken reaches 165°F. Remove the skillet from the oven and transfer the chicken to the plate again.
5. Place the skillet back on the stove and simmer the sauce over medium heat for about 5 minutes, until slightly thickened. Stir in the ghee until melted and fully incorporated. Return the chicken to the skillet for a final warm-through. Garnish with chives, lemon zest, and lemon slices, if desired. Serve over Cheesy Bone Broth Mashed Potatoes (page 210), Roasted Japanese Sweet Potatoes (page 183), or your favorite veggie side.

**STORAGE:** Store in an airtight container in the fridge for up to 4 days. Reheat in a skillet over medium heat or in a 375°F oven until warmed through and the skin is crisp again. Avoid microwaving if you want to keep the skin crispy.

---

**PER SERVING (FOR 4 SERVINGS)**
Protein: 41g
Carbohydrates: 3g
Fat: 39g

Dairy-Free
Gluten-Free
Grain-Free
No Added Sugar

# Pesto-Crusted Baked Cod

**SERVES 4 • PREP TIME: 20 MINUTES • COOK TIME: 20 MINUTES • TOTAL TIME: 40 MINUTES**

**FOR THE PESTO**

- ½ cup slivered almonds, toasted (or try pine nuts, walnuts, or pumpkin seeds)
- 1 garlic clove
- Juice of 1 lemon
- 2 cups basil leaves
- ¼ cup extra-virgin olive oil
- Sea salt and freshly ground black pepper

**FOR THE COD**

- ¾ cup gluten-free panko breadcrumbs
- ½ teaspoon Italian seasoning
- ½ teaspoon sea salt
- 1 tablespoon extra-virgin olive oil
- 4 (6-ounce) boneless, skinless wild cod fillets

**FOR THE TOMATOES**

- 2 tablespoons extra-virgin olive oil
- 8 ounces cherry tomatoes, halved (about 1½ cups)
- 2 garlic cloves, sliced
- 1 tablespoon balsamic vinegar
- ½ teaspoon sea salt
- ½ teaspoon freshly ground black pepper
- 2 tablespoons fresh basil, sliced, for garnish

Cod is one of those proteins that doesn't ask for much but offers up everything—it's mild, flaky, and super quick to cook. This version gets an upgrade with a crispy panko crust and a bright basil-almond pesto that makes it feel way fancier than the effort it takes. It's light yet filling, and loaded with selenium from the cod, which supports your immune system and thyroid health. Paired with juicy sautéed cherry tomatoes and a splash of balsamic? It's the kind of dinner that's secretly simple but still impresses.

1. Preheat the oven to 400°F.
2. **Make the pesto:** In a food processor, blend the almonds, garlic, lemon juice, and basil. With the motor running, slowly drizzle in the oil until the pesto is smooth and emulsified. Season with salt and pepper and set aside.
3. **Bake the cod**: In a small bowl, mix the breadcrumbs, Italian seasoning, salt, and oil. Place the cod fillets in an oven-safe skillet and spread 1 tablespoon pesto over the top of each fillet. Press the breadcrumb mixture onto the tops, gently pressing it into the fish so it adheres. Bake for 12 to 15 minutes, until the fish is flaky and just cooked through. Carefully remove the skillet from the oven and transfer the fish to a plate to rest.
4. **Make the tomatoes:** In the same skillet, heat the oil over medium heat. Add the cherry tomatoes and garlic and cook, stirring occasionally, for about 5 minutes, until the tomatoes and garlic soften. Stir in the vinegar, salt, and pepper.
5. To serve, place the fillets over the tomatoes, then drizzle the cod with additional pesto and garnish with basil.

**STORAGE:** Store leftovers in an airtight container in the fridge for up to 3 days. Reheat gently in a 325°F oven until just warmed through. Avoid microwaving to help preserve the texture of the fish and crust.

---

**PER SERVING**
Protein: 40g
Carbohydrates: 16g
Fat: 21g

**NOTE:** *This goes well with Farro (page 182) and Sautéed Greens with Lemon and Olive Oil (page 182) for serving, and extra pesto for drizzling*

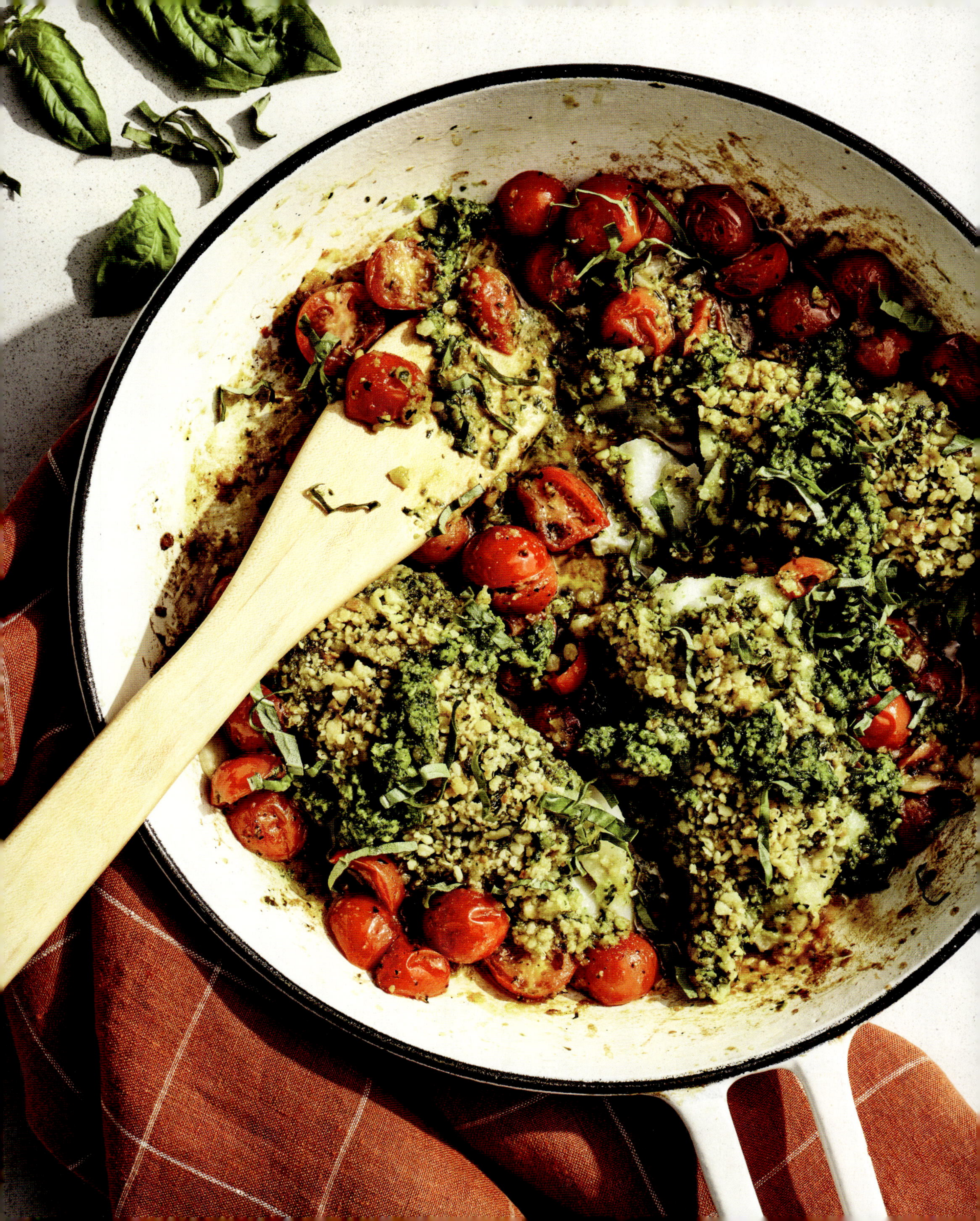

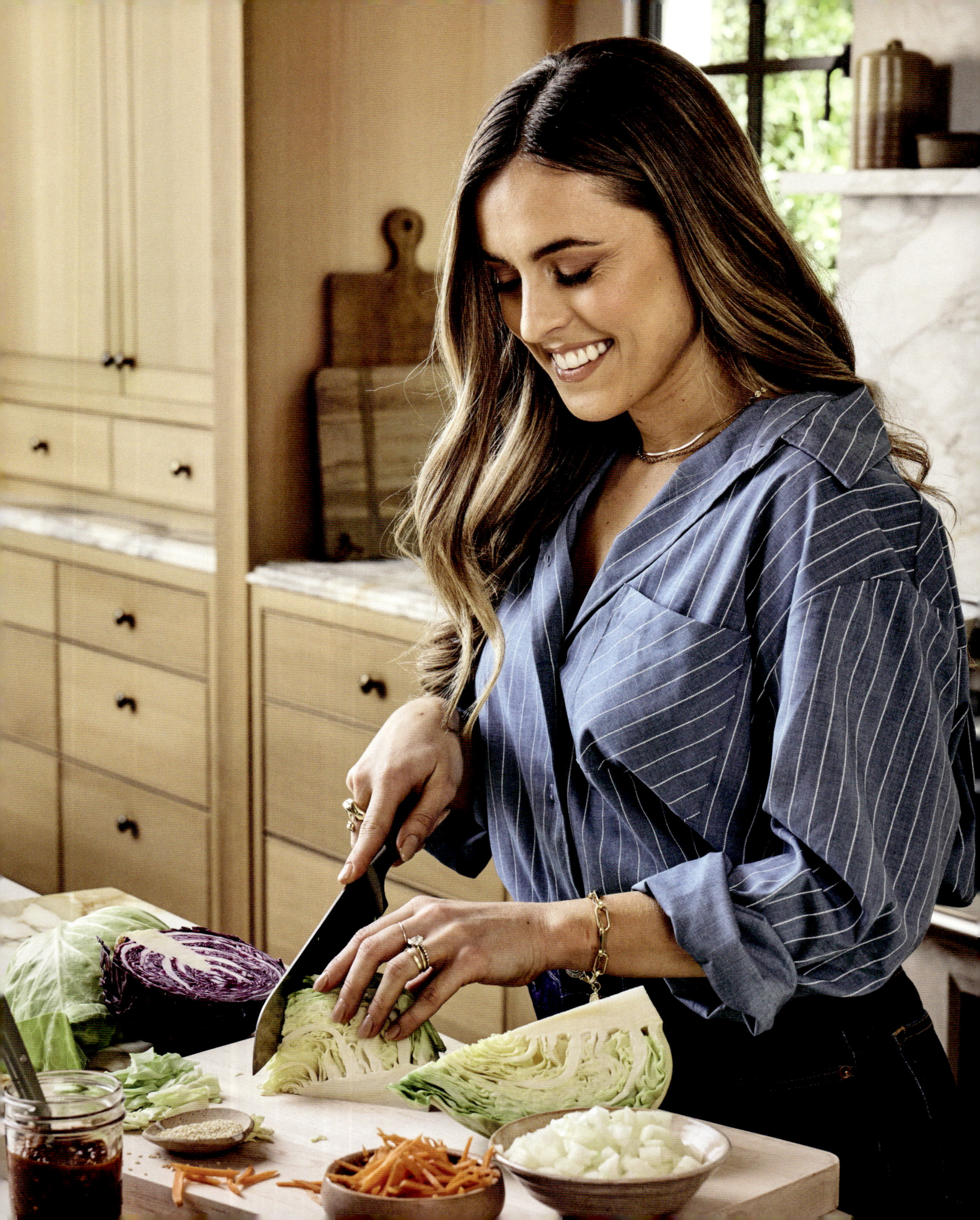

Dairy-Free
Gluten-Free
Grain-Free
No Added Sugar

# Egg Roll in a Bowl

SERVES 2 TO 4 • PREP TIME: 15 MINUTES • COOK TIME: 10 MINUTES • TOTAL TIME: 25 MINUTES

FOR THE TOPPING (OPTIONAL)

1 to 2 sheets rice paper

Avocado oil spray

FOR THE EGG ROLL BOWL

1 tablespoon avocado oil

1 pound ground pork (ground chicken or tofu also work great)

½ yellow onion, chopped

3 garlic cloves, minced

1-inch piece fresh ginger, minced

3 cups shredded green cabbage

2 cups shredded red cabbage

1 large carrot, shredded or grated

3 green onions, white and green parts, thinly sliced

¼ cup coconut aminos

1 tablespoon toasted sesame oil

1 tablespoon sambal oelek

1 teaspoon rice vinegar

½ teaspoon sea salt, plus more to taste

1 tablespoon toasted sesame seeds

3 tablespoons chopped fresh cilantro

This fast, flavorful meal has everything you love about an egg roll—savory ground pork (or your favorite protein), crispy cabbage, and a punchy sauce—minus the fuss of assembly. It's crunchy, flavorful, and comes together in one pan, perfect for weeknights when you want something good, fast. And if you're craving that extra crackly finish, you can bake crispy rice paper strips to scatter on top. Not necessary, but totally worth it if you've got 5 minutes and an extra pan.

1. **Make the crispy rice paper topping:** If making the topping, preheat the oven to 400°F. Slice the rice paper into thin strips, arrange on a parchment-lined baking sheet, and spray lightly with avocado oil. Bake for 4 to 6 minutes, until golden and crisp. Set aside to cool while you make the egg roll bowls.
2. **Make the bowls:** In a large skillet, heat the avocado oil over medium heat. Add the ground pork, breaking it up with a wooden spatula, and cook for about 5 minutes, until no longer pink. Stir in the onion, garlic, ginger, green cabbage, red cabbage, carrot, green onions, coconut aminos, sesame oil, sambal oelek, vinegar, and salt. Sauté for 5 minutes, stirring occasionally, until the cabbage is tender and everything is well combined.
3. Divide between two bowls and top with sesame seeds, cilantro, rice paper strips, if using, and salt to taste.

**STORAGE:** Store the pork mixture in an airtight container in the fridge for up to 4 days. Reheat in a skillet over medium heat or in the microwave until warmed through. Add a splash of coconut aminos or water if it needs moisture.

**PER SERVING (FOR 2 SERVINGS)**
Protein: 44g
Carbohydrates: 10g
Fat: 49g

Dairy-Free
Gluten-Free
Grain-Free
No Added Sugar

# One-Pan Beef and Broccoli

**SERVES 2 TO 4 • PREP TIME: 15 MINUTES • COOK TIME: 15 MINUTES • TOTAL TIME: 30 MINUTES**

Beef and broccoli is a classic for a reason. It hits every time. This version takes the combo to a new level thanks to a rich, savory sauce that's just the right balance of salty, garlicky, and a little sweet. It pulls everything together, and the fact that it's a one-pan meal makes it even better. Broccolini brings fiber and minerals like calcium and magnesium, while bell pepper adds natural sweetness and a pop of color. Grass-fed beef delivers protein and nutrients that help support energy and strength. Swap in sugar snap peas or cherry tomatoes if you're feeling wild—but any way, this one's a keeper.

**FOR THE SAUCE**

½ cup hot water
¾ cup coconut aminos
3 tablespoons sesame oil
1 heaping tablespoon minced garlic
4 teaspoons arrowroot powder
2 teaspoons sea salt

**FOR THE BEEF AND VEGETABLES**

2 pounds flank or flap steak
3 tablespoons avocado oil or extra-virgin olive oil
2 bunches broccolini, trimmed
2 red bell peppers, seeded and sliced
1 tablespoon sesame seeds
Extra sesame seeds, for garnish
Cooked rice, for serving (optional)

1. **Make the sauce:** In a medium bowl, whisk together the hot water, coconut aminos, sesame oil, garlic, arrowroot powder, and salt until smooth. Set aside.
2. **Prepare the beef and vegetables:** Slice the steak at an angle, cutting against the grain into very thin strips (about 2 inches long).
3. In a large skillet, heat 2 tablespoons of the avocado oil over medium-high heat. Add the broccolini and bell peppers and sauté for 4 to 5 minutes, stirring frequently, until just tender. Remove from the skillet and set aside.
4. In the same skillet, heat the remaining 1 tablespoon avocado oil over medium-high heat. Add the steak and sesame seeds and cook for 2 minutes, until the steak starts to brown. Stir in the sauce and cook for 2 minutes, until it begins to thicken.
5. Return the broccolini and bell peppers to the skillet. Cook for 5 to 7 minutes, until the steak is cooked through and coated in the sauce. Garnish with additional sesame seeds and a sprinkle of salt to taste.

**STORAGE:** Store in an airtight container in the fridge for up to 4 days. Reheat in a skillet over medium heat or in the microwave, adding a splash of water or broth if needed to loosen the sauce.

---

**PER SERVING (FOR 4 SERVINGS)**
Protein: 49g
Carbohydrates: 16g
Fat: 30g

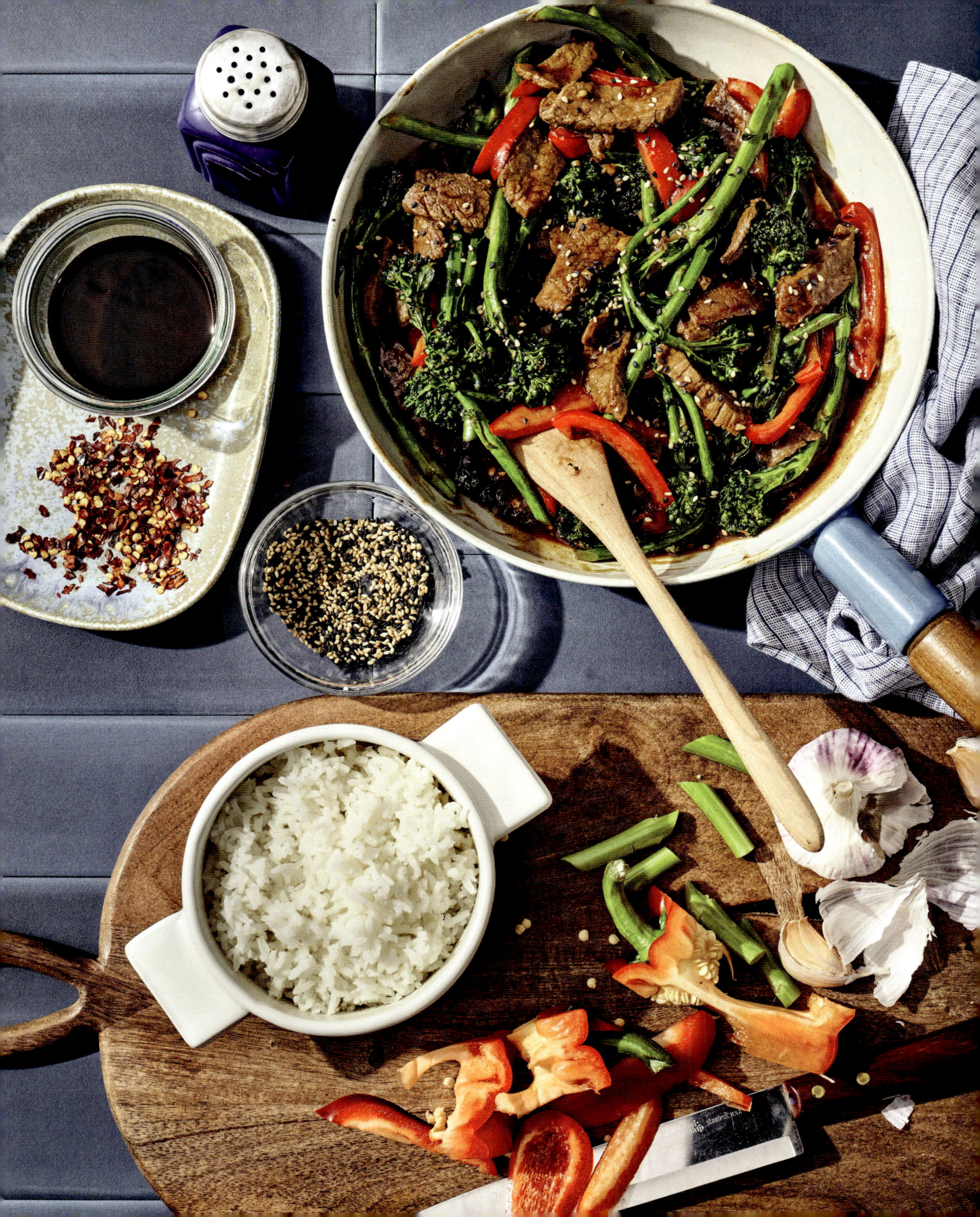

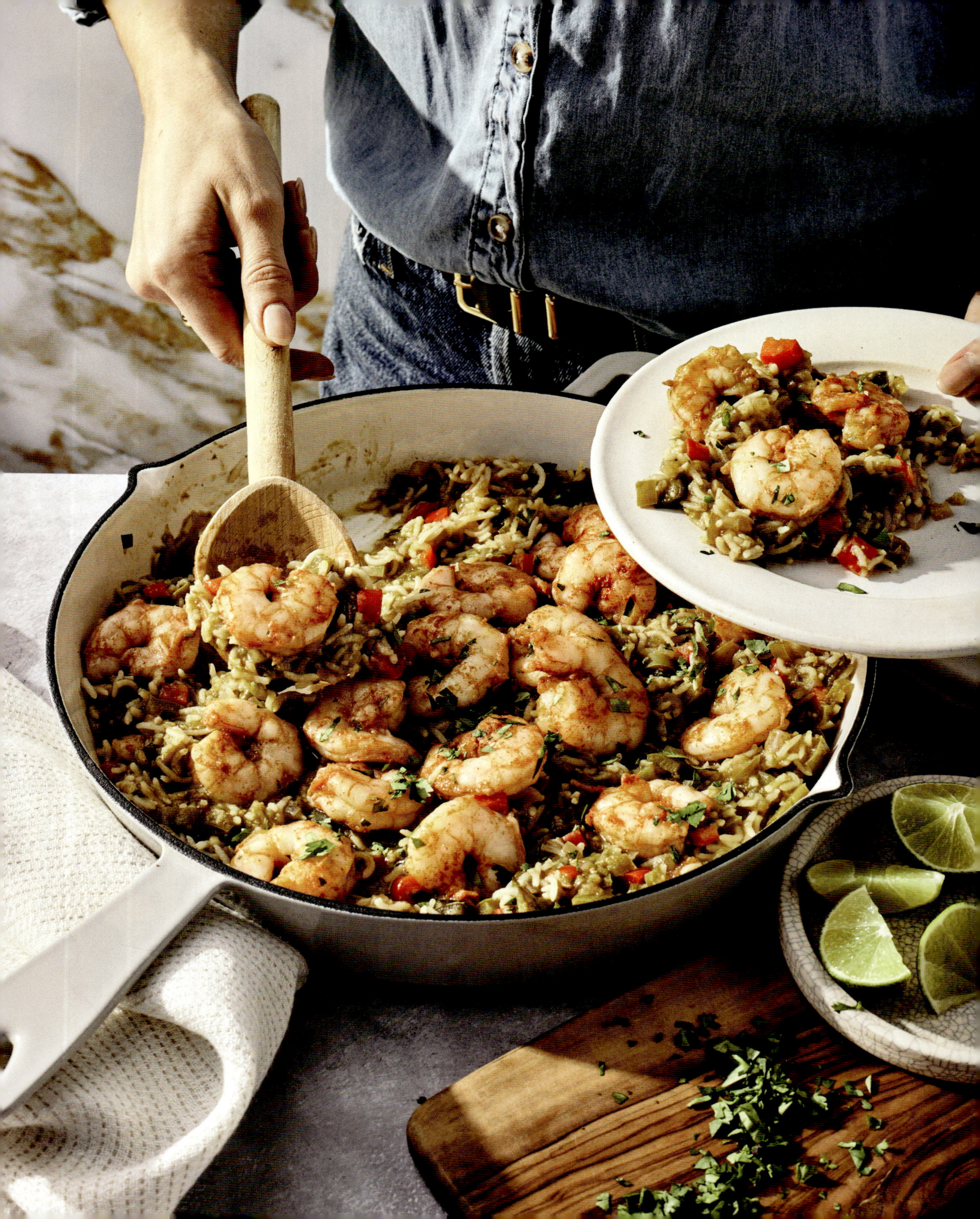

Dairy-Free
Gluten-Free
No Added Sugar

# Salsa Verde Shrimp and Rice

**SERVES 2 TO 3 • PREP TIME: 15 MINUTES • COOK TIME: 30 MINUTES • TOTAL TIME: 45 MINUTES**

- 1 tablespoon extra-virgin olive oil
- 1 cup diced red onion
- 2 Anaheim chilies, seeded and diced (or substitute green bell pepper, or jalapeño for more heat)
- 1 poblano pepper, seeded and diced
- 1 red bell pepper, seeded and diced
- 3 cloves garlic, minced
- ½ cup basmati rice
- 1 cup bone broth
- 1 (16-ounce) jar salsa verde
- 1 to 1½ pounds small or medium wild shrimp, peeled, deveined, and tails removed
- 1 teaspoon ground cumin
- ½ teaspoon smoked paprika
- 2 teaspoons Himalayan pink salt
- ½ cup chopped fresh cilantro, plus more for garnish (optional)
- Juice of 1 lime, plus (optional) wedges for garnish
- Freshly ground black pepper

When a one-pan meal delivers this much flavor, you know it's going to be a repeat recipe. Juicy well-seasoned shrimp, tender rice, and three kinds of peppers soak up the zesty salsa verde, giving this dish a bit of heat—in the best way. It's protein-forward, veggie-loaded, and has the perfect balance of everything.

1. In a large skillet, heat the oil over medium heat. Add the onion, Anaheim chilies, poblano pepper, and bell pepper. Cook for 5 to 7 minutes, stirring occasionally, until softened. Add the garlic and cook for 1 minute more. Stir in the rice and cook for 1 to 2 minutes, until lightly toasted. Pour in the broth and salsa verde. Stir to combine, then bring the mixture to a boil. Reduce the heat to low, cover, and simmer for 15 minutes, until the rice is tender.
2. Season the shrimp with the cumin, paprika, and 1 teaspoon of the salt. Arrange the shrimp in an even layer on the top of the rice. Cover and cook for 5 to 7 minutes, until the shrimp is pink and cooked through. Uncover and gently stir the shrimp into the rice mixture. Stir in the cilantro, lime juice, and remaining 1 teaspoon salt. Adjust the seasoning with black pepper to taste. Serve hot, garnished with extra cilantro and lime wedges, if desired.

**STORAGE:** Store in an airtight container in the fridge for up to 3 days. Reheat gently in a skillet over medium heat or in the microwave. Avoid overcooking to keep the shrimp tender.

---

**PER SERVING (FOR 3 SERVINGS)**
Protein: 39g
Carbohydrates: 36g
Fat: 6g

Dairy-Free
Gluten-Free
Grain-Free
No Added Sugar
Paleo

# Sloppy Joe Bowls

**SERVES 2 TO 4 • PREP TIME: 10 MINUTES • COOK TIME: 20 MINUTES • TOTAL TIME: 30 MINUTES**

- 1 tablespoon extra-virgin olive oil
- ¼ cup diced yellow onion
- 1 green bell pepper, seeded and diced
- 3 garlic cloves, minced
- 1 pound ground beef
- 1 tablespoon apple cider vinegar
- 3 tablespoons unsweetened ketchup (I prefer Primal Kitchen)
- 2 tablespoons tomato paste
- ½ cup bone broth
- 1 teaspoon chili powder
- 1 teaspoon yellow or Dijon mustard
- ½ teaspoon paprika
- ½ teaspoon sea salt, plus more for serving
- ¼ teaspoon freshly ground black pepper
- Chopped fresh chives, for garnish

If you grew up loving sloppy joes, try this grown-up version—just as saucy and satisfying as the joe you knew as a kid, but with more nutrients and less sugar. The rich, tangy, smoky sauce coats perfectly seasoned ground beef, making for a high-protein, feel-good meal. And if you're feeling nostalgic (or just extra hungry), go ahead and slap this between two toasted burger buns for the real deal—or keep it bun-free and pair with Roasted Japanese Sweet Potatoes (page 183).

1. In a large skillet, heat the oil over medium heat. Add the onion and bell pepper and cook for 4 to 5 minutes, stirring occasionally, until softened. Stir in the garlic, and cook for another 30 seconds, until fragrant.
2. Push the onion and bell peppers to one side of the skillet and add the ground beef to the empty side. Cook, breaking up the meat with a spatula, for 6 to 8 minutes, until browned and cooked through. Mix the onion, bell peppers, and beef together, then stir in the vinegar, ketchup, and tomato paste to coat everything evenly. Pour in the broth and add the chili powder, mustard, paprika, salt, and pepper. Stir to combine and bring the mixture to a simmer. Reduce the heat to low and simmer for 5 to 7 minutes, allowing the flavors to meld and the sauce to thicken.
3. Garnish with salt and chives, if you wish, and serve.

**STORAGE:** Store the meat mixture and any sides (like rice or potatoes) in separate airtight containers in the fridge for up to 4 days. Reheat in a skillet over medium heat or in the microwave until hot.

---

**PER SERVING (FOR 4 SERVINGS)**
Protein: 32g
Carbohydrates: 12g
Fat: 32g

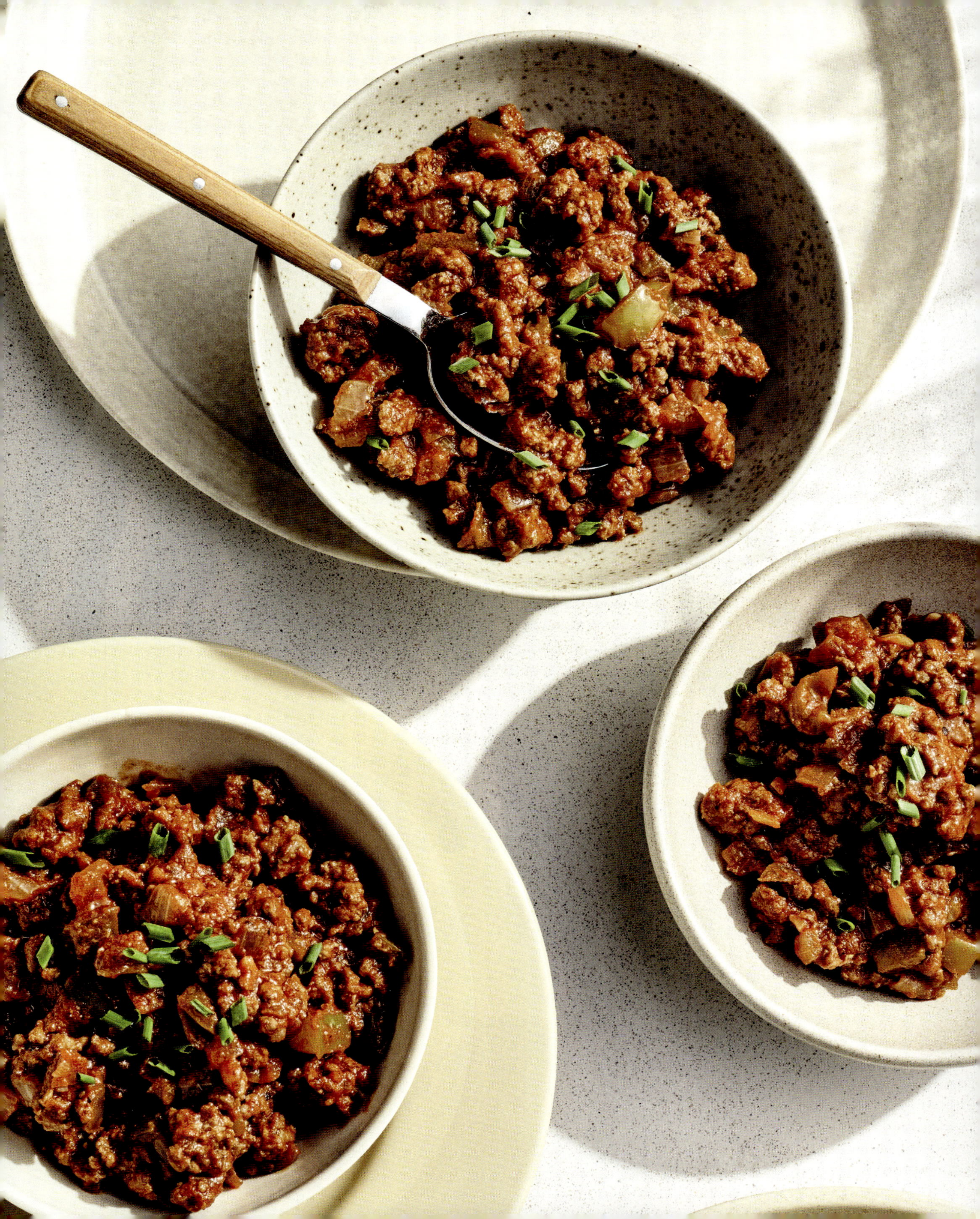

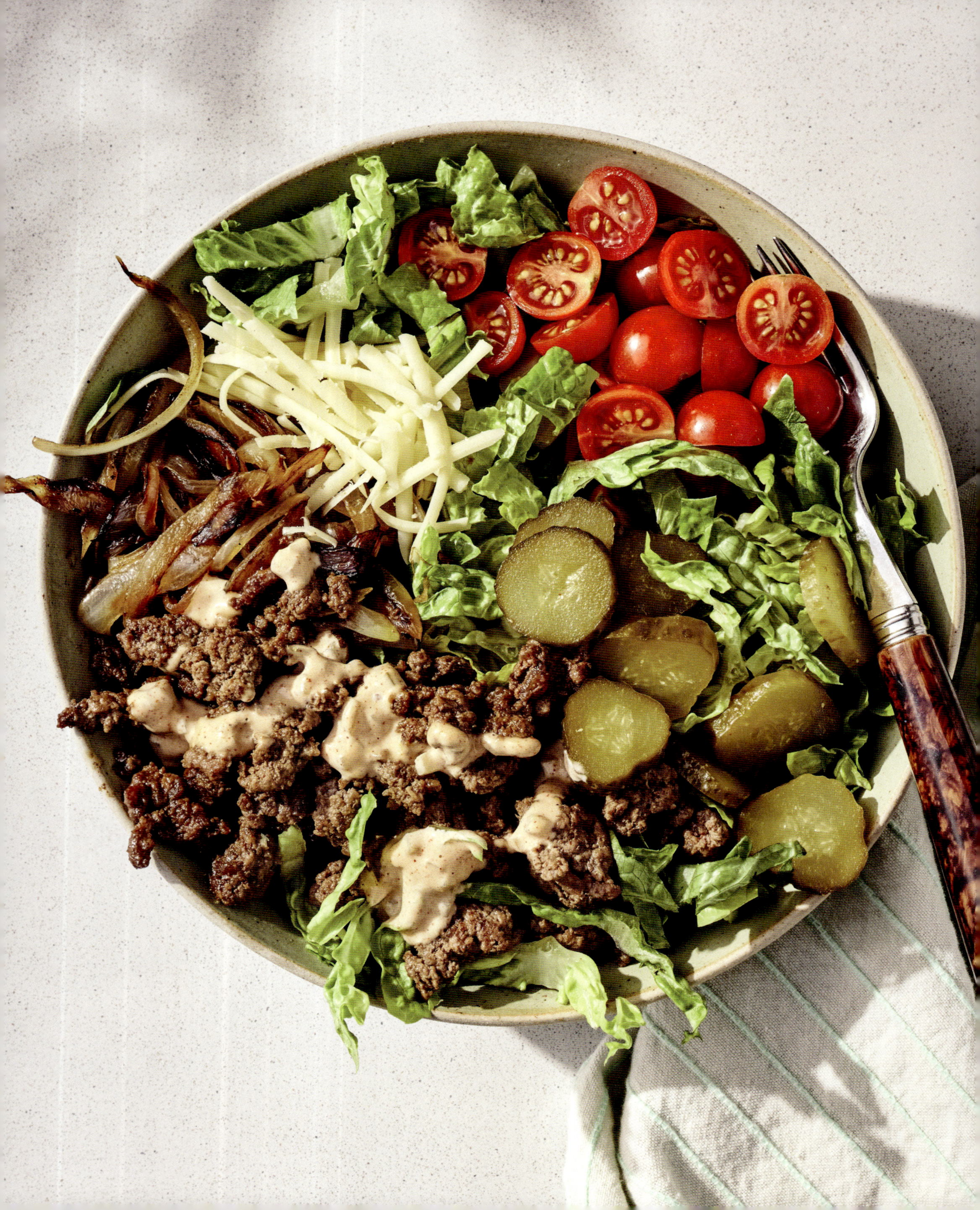

Gluten-Free
Grain-Free
No Added Sugar

# Double Double-Cheeseburger Bowls

**SERVES 4 • PREP TIME: 15 MINUTES • COOK TIME: 20 MINUTES • TOTAL TIME: 35 MINUTES**

**FOR THE BEEF**

2 tablespoons avocado oil

2 yellow onions, thinly sliced

2 teaspoons sea salt

2 pounds ground beef

1 teaspoon onion powder

1 teaspoon garlic powder

½ teaspoon paprika

½ teaspoon freshly ground black pepper

1 cup shredded cheddar cheese, plus more for topping (optional)

**FOR THE SPECIAL SAUCE**

¼ cup avocado-oil mayonnaise

2 tablespoons unsweetened ketchup (I prefer Primal Kitchen)

1 tablespoon yellow mustard

1 tablespoon finely chopped dill pickle

¼ teaspoon onion powder

¼ teaspoon paprika

**FOR THE BOWLS**

1 head romaine lettuce, finely shredded

2 cups cherry tomatoes, halved

4 dill pickles, sliced into rounds

Optional: mustard, ketchup, sliced avocado, Homemade BBQ Sauce (page 118)

**PER SERVING**
Protein: 54g
Carbohydrates: 13g
Fat: 58g

If you're a burger lover (and aren't we all?), this one's for you. This recipe delivers everything you love in a double double cheeseburger: juicy beef, melty cheese, caramelized onions, and that signature special sauce. But it's all served bowl-style so you can skip the bun and still get that full burger experience.

1. In a large skillet, heat 1 tablespoon of the oil over medium heat. Add the onions and 1 teaspoon of the salt and sauté for 10 to 15 minutes, stirring occasionally, until golden and starting to brown around the edges. If needed, add a tablespoon of water while cooking to prevent sticking or burning. Transfer the onions to a plate and set aside.
2. In the same skillet over medium heat, add the remaining 1 tablespoon oil, then the ground beef, onion powder, garlic powder, paprika, remaining 1 teaspoon salt, and the pepper. Cook, breaking up the beef as it browns, for 8 to 10 minutes, until fully cooked. If needed, drain excess grease. Sprinkle the cheese over the beef, cover the skillet with a lid, and let the cheese melt for 1 to 2 minutes. Once melted, stir to incorporate.
3. **Make the special sauce:** Meanwhile, in a small bowl, whisk together the mayonnaise, ketchup, mustard, chopped pickle, onion powder, and paprika until smooth.
4. **Assemble the bowls:** Layer the lettuce, cheesy beef, caramelized onions, cherry tomatoes, sliced pickles, and extra cheese, if desired. Drizzle with the special sauce, add any extra toppings, and enjoy!

**TIP:** *This recipe doubles easily, so you can have it for lunch the next day. Just reheat the beef mixture in a skillet and build your bowl fresh with toppings when you're ready to eat.*

Dairy-Free
Gluten-Free
Grain-Free
No Added Sugar

# Sheet-Pan Turmeric Chicken with Romesco

**SERVES 4 • PREP TIME: 15 MINUTES, PLUS 15 MINUTES MARINATING • COOK TIME: 25 MINUTES • TOTAL TIME: 55 MINUTES**

Here's another clutch sheet-pan meal to add to your weeknight rotation. Golden turmeric chicken thighs roast right over chickpeas, cauliflower, and red onion—flavoring the whole pan while delivering anti-inflammatory benefits from the turmeric and ginger (great for joints and immune support). The real kicker is a bold, smoky romesco sauce—a Spanish-inspired blend of roasted red peppers, almonds, garlic, and olive oil—that takes everything up a notch. It makes extra, so stash the leftovers in the fridge to drizzle on whatever you're eating next.

**FOR THE CHICKEN**

- 1 teaspoon turmeric
- 1 teaspoon paprika
- 1 teaspoon ground ginger
- 1 teaspoon sea salt
- 1 teaspoon freshly ground black pepper
- 2 pounds boneless, skinless chicken thighs
- 2 tablespoons extra-virgin olive oil
- 2 bunches broccolini, cut into florets, or 1 head cauliflower
- 1 (15-ounce) can chickpeas, drained and rinsed
- 1 red onion, sliced into ½-inch-thick wedges

**FOR THE ROMESCO SAUCE**

- 1 (16-ounce) jar roasted red peppers, drained
- ½ cup Marcona or raw almonds
- ¼ cup olive oil–packed sun-dried tomatoes
- 1 garlic clove
- 1 tablespoon red wine vinegar
- 1 teaspoon smoked paprika
- ½ teaspoon sea salt
- ¼ cup extra-virgin olive oil
- ¼ cup chopped fresh parsley, for garnish

1. Preheat the oven to 425°F. Line a baking sheet with parchment paper.
2. **Make the chicken:** In a small bowl, mix the turmeric, paprika, ginger, salt, and black pepper. In a large bowl, toss the chicken thighs with half of the spice mixture and 1 tablespoon of the oil. Set aside to marinate for 15 to 20 minutes.
3. If using broccolini, trim the ends. If using cauliflower, slice into ½-inch-thick slabs (some florets will fall off—that's okay).
4. On the baking sheet, toss the broccolini (or cauliflower), chickpeas, and onion with the remaining 1 tablespoon oil and the remaining spice mixture. Spread out the veggies and chickpeas and place the chicken thighs on top. Roast for 25 to 30 minutes, until the chicken is golden and the internal temperature reaches 165°F.
5. **Make the romesco sauce:** Meanwhile, in a food processor, blend the red peppers, almonds, sun-dried tomatoes, garlic, vinegar, smoked paprika, and salt until mostly smooth. With the processor running, slowly drizzle in the oil until the sauce is creamy.
6. Serve the chicken over the roasted veggies and chickpeas, drizzle with romesco sauce, and garnish with parsley.

**MAKE-AHEAD TIP:** *The romesco sauce can be made up to 5 days ahead. Store in a sealed jar in the fridge and give it a good stir before drizzling over the chicken and veggies. Bonus: It's just as good later in the week on grilled veggies or scrambled eggs, or tossed with shrimp.*

---

**PER SERVING**
Protein: 52g
Carbohydrates: 29g
Fat: 43g

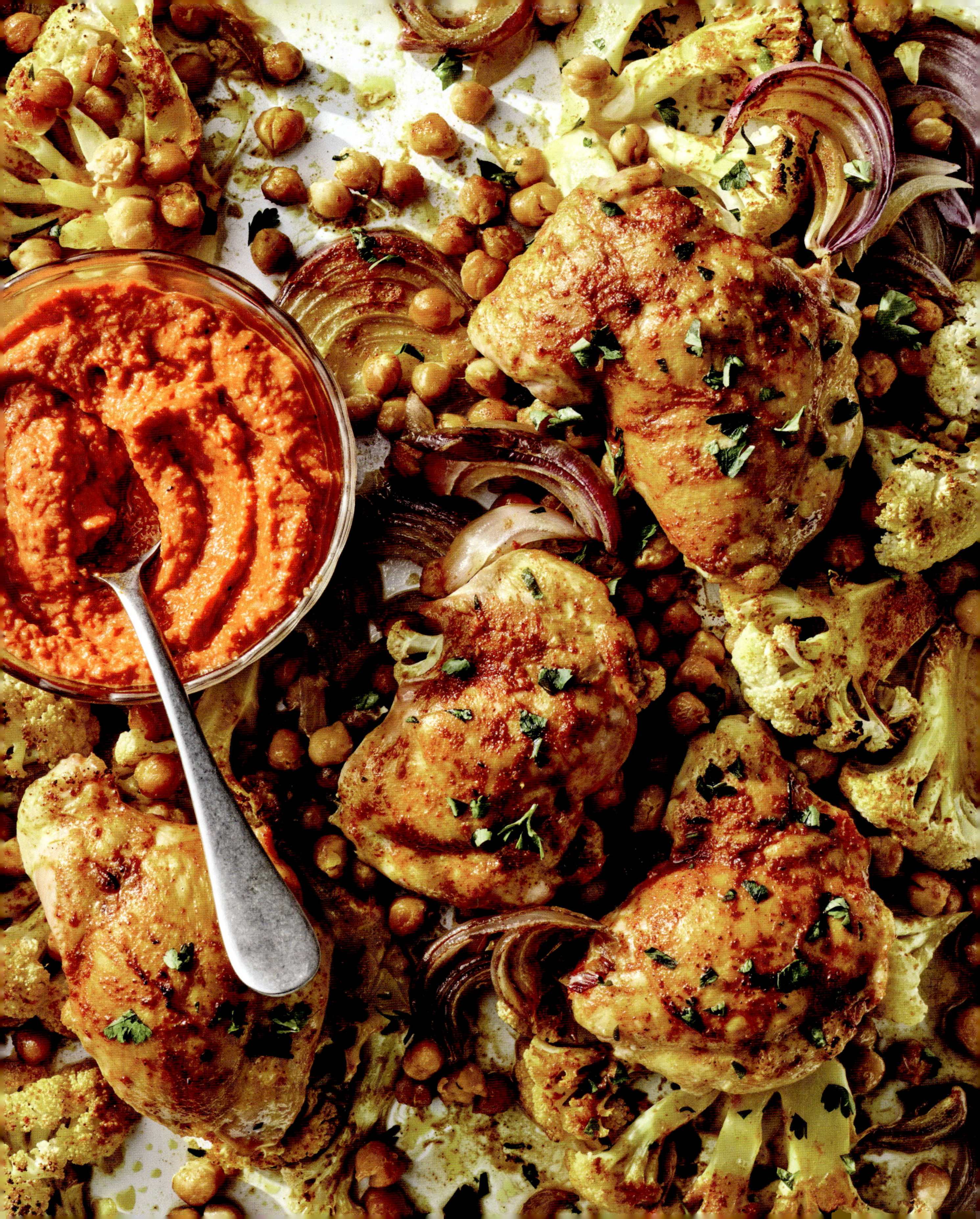

# Simple One-Pan Sides

## Sautéed Greens with Lemon and Olive Oil

Dairy-Free
Gluten-Free
Grain-Free
No Added Sugar
Paleo

SERVES 2 • PREP TIME: 5 MINUTES • COOK TIME: 5 MINUTES • TOTAL TIME: 10 MINUTES

Serve hot alongside roasted chicken, grilled steak, or baked salmon, or layer into a grain bowl.

- 1 tablespoon extra-virgin olive oil
- 1 clove garlic, minced
- 1 bunch kale, chard, or spinach, stems removed and leaves chopped
- 1 to 2 teaspoons fresh lemon juice
- Sea salt and freshly ground black pepper

Heat the oil in a medium skillet over medium heat. Add the garlic and sauté for 30 seconds. Add the greens and cook, stirring occasionally, for 3 to 5 minutes, until wilted. Finish with lemon juice, salt, and pepper. Serve immediately.

**PER SERVING**
Protein: 3g
Carbohydrates: 6g
Fat: 7g

## Farro

Dairy-Free
No Added Sugar

SERVES 4 • PREP TIME: 5 MINUTES • COOK TIME: 25 MINUTES • TOTAL TIME: 30 MINUTES

Use as a hearty base for bowls, toss into salads, or serve alongside roasted meats and veggies.

- 1 cup uncooked farro (pearled or semi-pearled)
- 3 cups water or bone broth
- ½ teaspoon sea salt
- Drizzle of extra-virgin olive oil or squeeze of lemon (optional)

Rinse the farro under cold water. Add to a medium saucepan along with the water and salt. Bring to a boil, then reduce the heat and simmer uncovered for 25 to 30 minutes, until tender but still chewy. Drain any excess liquid and fluff with a fork. Finish with oil or lemon juice, if using.

**PER SERVING**
Protein: 6g
Carbohydrates: 33g
Fat: 1g

# Roasted Japanese Sweet Potatoes

Dairy-Free
Gluten-Free
Grain-Free
No Added Sugar
Paleo

**SERVES 4 • PREP TIME: 5 MINUTES • COOK TIME: 35 MINUTES • TOTAL TIME: 40 MINUTES**

Serve hot with grilled chicken or roasted salmon, or tossed into your favorite grain bowl.

- 2 large Japanese sweet potatoes or standard yams (skin on or peeled), cubed
- 1 to 2 tablespoons avocado oil
- Sea salt and freshly ground black pepper
- Your favorite seasoning blend (garlic-herb, smoked paprika, etc.), optional

Preheat the oven to 400°F and line a baking sheet with parchment paper. Toss the sweet potatoes with the oil, salt, pepper, and seasoning blend, if using. Spread evenly on the baking sheet making sure not to crowd. Roast for 20 minutes, flip, then roast another 15 to 20 minutes, until golden and crispy at the edges.

**PER SERVING**
Protein: 2g
Carbohydrates: 24g
Fat: 5g

# Garlicky Roasted Broccolini

Dairy-Free
Gluten-Free
Grain-Free
No Added Sugar
Paleo

**SERVES 2 TO 3 • PREP TIME: 5 MINUTES • COOK TIME: 15 MINUTES • TOTAL TIME: 20 MINUTES**

Serve hot with grilled meat, fish, or something saucy.

- 1 bunch broccolini, ends trimmed
- 1 tablespoon olive oil or avocado oil
- 2 cloves garlic, minced
- Sea salt and freshly ground black pepper
- Pinch of red pepper flakes (optional)

Preheat the oven to 425°F and line a baking sheet with parchment paper. Toss the broccolini with the oil, garlic, salt, black pepper, and red pepper flakes, if using. Spread in a single layer on the baking sheet. Roast for 15 to 18 minutes, until the broccolini is tender and crisped at the edges.

**PER SERVING**
Protein: 2g
Carbohydrates: 5g
Fat: 5g

# Soups, Salads, and Satisfying Snacks

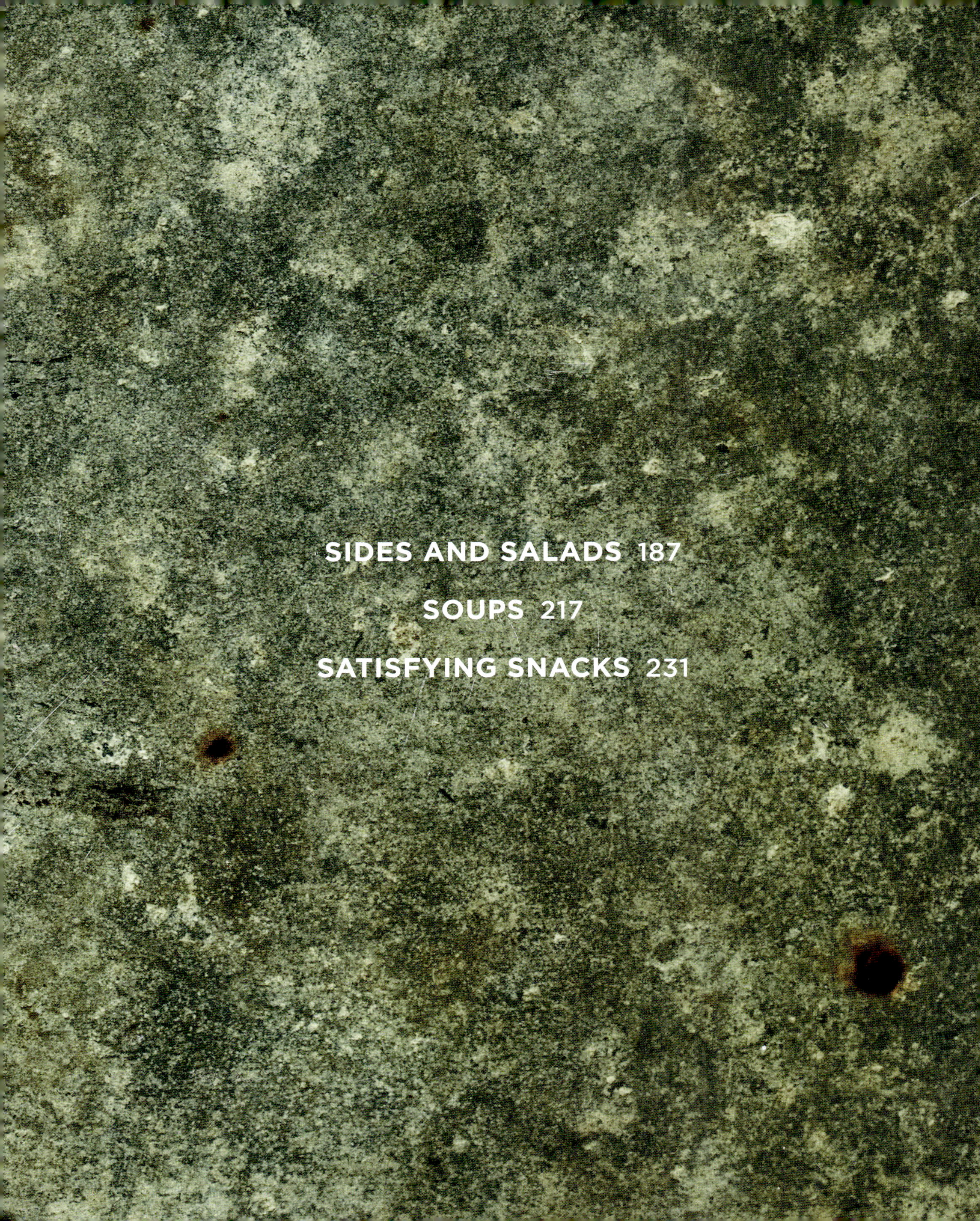

SIDES AND SALADS 187

SOUPS 217

SATISFYING SNACKS 231

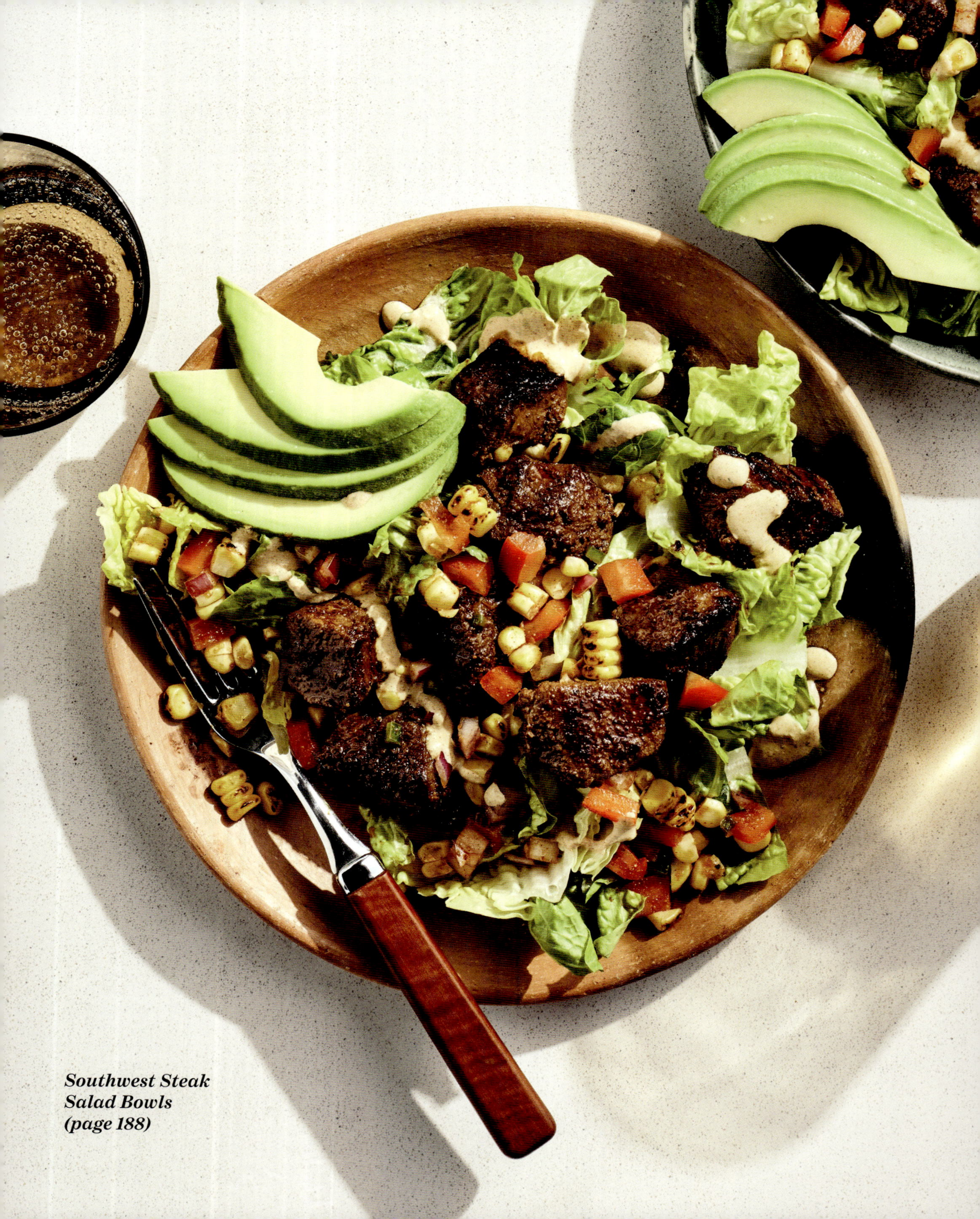

*Southwest Steak Salad Bowls* *(page 188)*

188 **Southwest Steak Salad Bowls**

190 **Italian-Style Chop Salad**

193 **Next-Level Mac and Cheese**

194 **Harvest Cobb Salad with Maple-Dijon Dressing**

197 **5-Minute Pesto Chicken Salad**

198 **Bone Broth Jasmine Rice Three Ways**

201 **Grilled Summer Pasta Salad**

202 **Roasted Sweet Potatoes with Spiced Chickpeas and Tahini Drizzle**

205 **Zucchini Fritters with Lemon-Dill Sauce**

206 **The Rachael Salad**

209 **Moroccan-Spiced Carrots with Hummus**

210 **Cheesy Bone Broth Mashed Potatoes**

212 **Sheet-Pan Greek Chicken and Chickpea Salad**

215 **Spicy Tuna Spring Rolls**

# Sides and Salads

Gluten-Free
No Added Sugar

# Southwest Steak Salad Bowls

**SERVES 4 • PREP TIME: 20 MINUTES, INCLUDING 15 MINUTES MARINATING • COOK TIME: 10 MINUTES • TOTAL TIME: 45 MINUTES**

I may be biased, but I believe this salad has it all. Perfectly seasoned steak, a zesty fire-roasted corn salad, and a creamy Southwest sauce over crisp romaine—it just hits. Bridger requests this one consistently, which says a lot. It feels restaurant-worthy but is so doable at home, and it's a solid way to hit your protein goal without overthinking it.

**FOR THE STEAK AND MARINADE**

1½ pounds top sirloin steak
¼ cup avocado oil
1 teaspoon sea salt
¾ teaspoon garlic powder
¾ teaspoon ground cumin
½ teaspoon smoked paprika
½ teaspoon onion powder
¼ teaspoon freshly ground black pepper

**FOR THE SOUTHWEST SAUCE**

½ cup full-fat cottage cheese
½ cup sour cream
Juice of 1 lime
¼ cup chopped fresh cilantro
½ teaspoon minced garlic
1 teaspoon chili powder
1 teaspoon ground cumin
1 teaspoon smoked paprika
½ teaspoon sea salt

1. **Marinate the steak:** Cut the steak into 1-inch bite-size pieces. In a large bowl, combine the steak, avocado oil, salt, garlic powder, cumin, paprika, onion powder, and black pepper. Toss until evenly coated. Let marinate at room temperature for 15 minutes.
2. **Make the Southwest sauce:** Meanwhile, in a large glass jar or container, combine the cottage cheese, sour cream, lime juice, cilantro, garlic, chili powder, cumin, paprika, and salt. Blend with an immersion blender until smooth (or use a standard blender). Set aside.
3. **Make the salad:** In a medium bowl, mix the bell pepper, corn, onion, lime juice, olive oil, jalapeño, salt, cumin, and paprika. Toss to combine and set aside.

---

**PER SERVING**
Protein: 46g
Carbohydrates: 21g
Fat: 40g

FOR THE SALAD

1 red bell pepper, seeded and diced (yellow bell pepper, cucumber, or cherry tomatoes work great too)

1 cup fire-roasted corn (I like frozen for ease)

¼ cup finely diced red onion

Juice of 1 lime

2 tablespoons extra-virgin olive oil

1½ teaspoons diced jalapeño

½ teaspoon sea salt

¼ teaspoon ground cumin

¼ teaspoon smoked paprika

3 heads romaine lettuce, chopped

2 avocados, sliced, for garnish

Chopped fresh cilantro, for garnish

Lime wedges, for garnish

4. **Cook the steak:** Heat a large skillet over medium-high heat. Place the steak in a single layer (work in batches if needed to avoid overcrowding) and sear for 2 to 3 minutes on each side, until browned and cooked to your desired doneness. Let rest for 10 minutes.

5. **Assemble the bowls:** Divide the romaine among four bowls, then top with the salad mixture and steak. Drizzle with the Southwest sauce and garnish with avocado slices, cilantro, and lime wedges. Serve immediately.

**MAKE-AHEAD TIP:** *The Southwest sauce can be made up to 4 days in advance. Store it in an airtight container in the fridge. Give it a good stir before using, and drizzle over salads, bowls, or even grilled veggies throughout the week.*

**TIP:** *The Southwest sauce also makes a delish dip or drizzle for the Shredded Chicken Quesadillas (page 138).*

Gluten-Free
Grain-Free
No Added Sugar

# Italian-Style Chop Salad

SERVES 4 • PREP TIME: 20 MINUTES • TOTAL TIME: 20 MINUTES

This recipe takes everything you love about an Italian sub and serves it up in salad form. It's layered with salami, turkey, goat cheddar, crunchy sunflower seeds, zesty pepperoncini, and a tangy oregano vinaigrette. The salad quite literally never gets old—fresh enough for lunch, hearty enough for dinner, and always dressed to impress.

**FOR THE VINAIGRETTE**

¼ cup red wine vinegar
¼ cup extra-virgin olive oil
1 garlic clove, minced
½ teaspoon dried oregano
Sea salt and freshly ground black pepper

**FOR THE SALAD**

1 small head butter lettuce, leaves washed, dried, and chopped
1 small head radicchio, thinly sliced
2 cups arugula
¼ cup diced red onion
1 cup cherry tomatoes, sliced in half
¾ cup goat cheddar cheese (or preferred cheese), diced
1 (15-ounce) can chickpeas, drained and rinsed
⅓ cup pepperoncini, sliced
12 slices Genoa salami, diced
6 ounces sliced deli turkey, chopped
½ cup toasted sunflower seeds
¼ cup hemp seeds

1. **Make the vinaigrette:** In a small bowl or jar, whisk together the vinegar, oil, garlic, oregano, salt, and pepper.
2. **Assemble the salad:** In a large bowl, combine the butter lettuce, radicchio, arugula, onion, tomatoes, cheese, chickpeas, pepperoncini, salami, turkey, sunflower seeds, and hemp seeds.
3. Pour the dressing over the salad and toss until well combined. Serve immediately.

**STORAGE:** Store all the salad components and the dressing separately in airtight containers in the fridge for up to 4 days. Toss everything together just before serving to keep the texture crisp and fresh.

**PER SERVING**
Protein: 32g
Carbohydrates: 17g
Fat: 40g

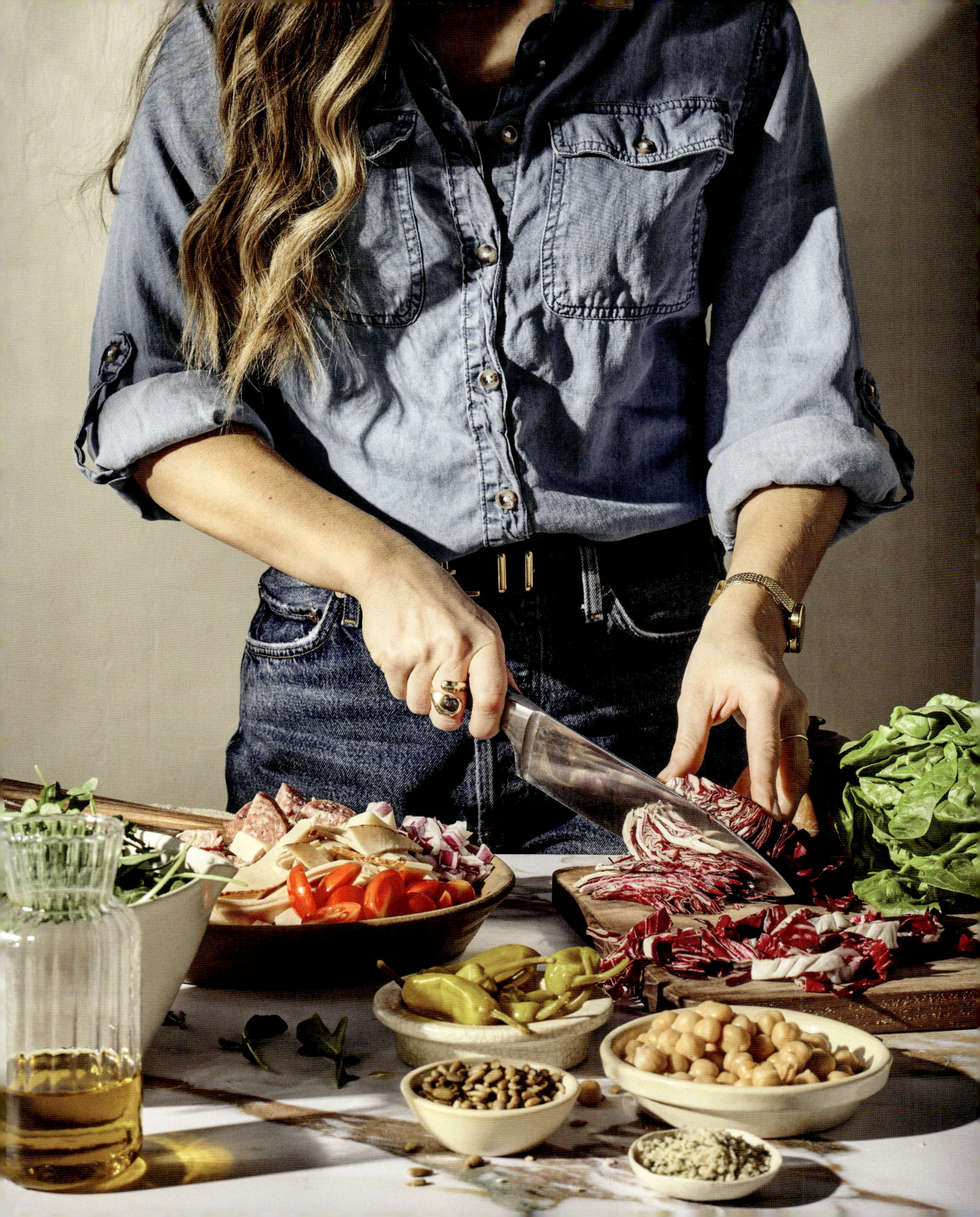

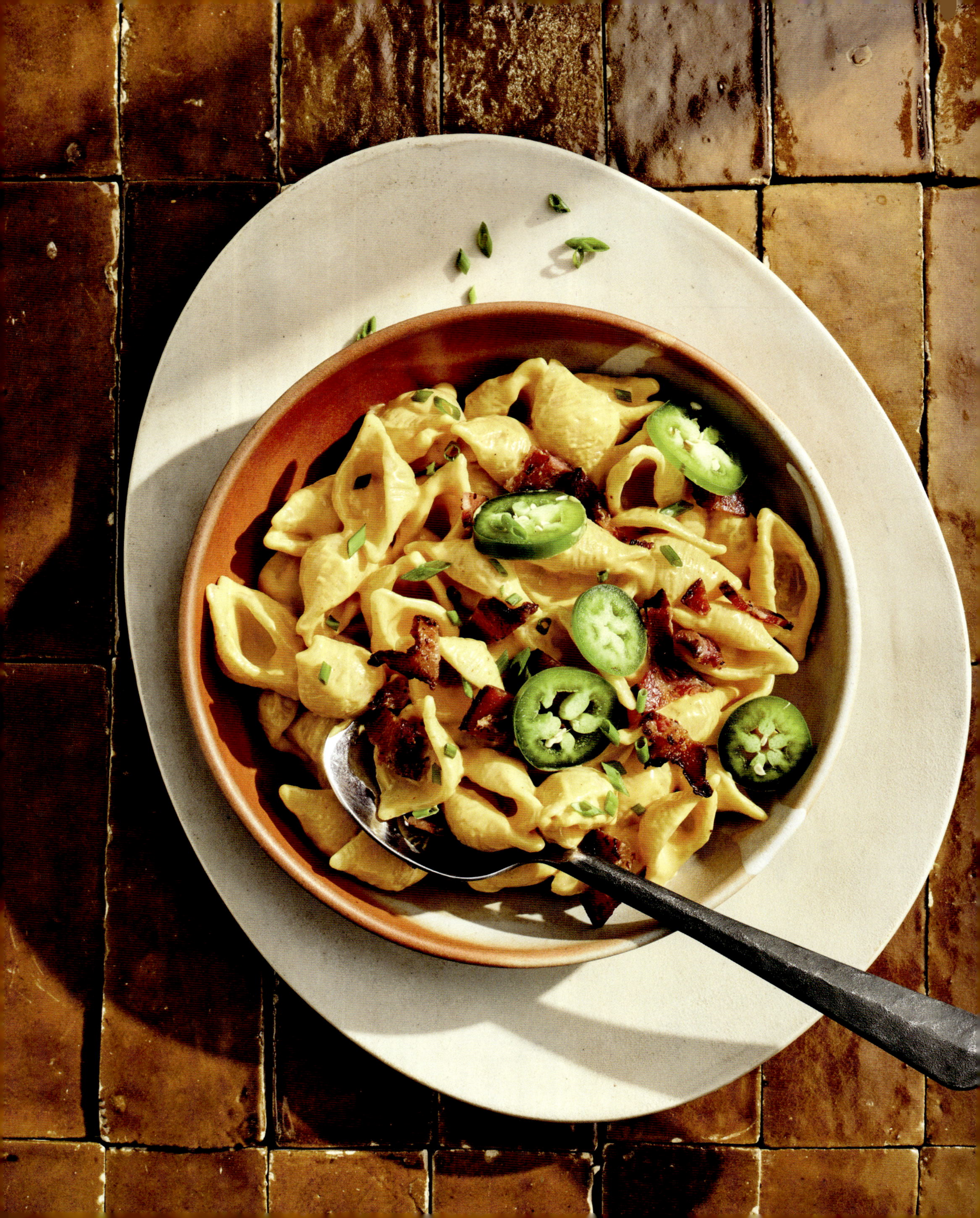

No Added Sugar
**IF MODIFIED:**
Gluten-Free

# Next-Level Mac and Cheese

**SERVES 4 TO 6 • PREP TIME: 15 MINUTES • COOK TIME: 15 MINUTES • TOTAL TIME: 30 MINUTES**

- 1 pound short pasta (such as elbows, fusilli, or shells), or gluten-free pasta of choice
- 1½ cups shredded cheddar cheese, goat cheddar, or vegan cheddar
- ½ cup full-fat cottage cheese
- ½ cup canned pumpkin puree
- ½ cup milk of choice
- ½ teaspoon paprika
- ½ teaspoon onion powder
- ½ teaspoon sea salt
- 1 tablespoon arrowroot powder
- Optional toppings: crumbled bacon, sliced jalapeño, fresh chives

This upgraded mac and cheese blends cottage cheese and pumpkin into a smooth, velvety sauce that clings to every bite of pasta. You won't taste the cottage cheese—I promise—but you'll feel good knowing this cozy bowl delivers protein, fiber, and even a little immune support thanks to the pumpkin. It hits all the nostalgic notes, just without the heaviness. I love this one for kids and parents alike—serve it as a weeknight side or load it up with toppings and call it dinner.

1. In a large pot of boiling salted water, cook the pasta according to the package instructions. Drain and return to the pot.
2. In a blender, combine the cheddar cheese, cottage cheese, pumpkin, milk, paprika, onion powder, salt, and arrowroot powder. Blend on high for 30 seconds, or until smooth.
3. Pour the blended sauce over the pasta and stir to combine. Cook over low heat for 1 to 2 minutes, until warmed through and creamy. Serve immediately, topped with crumbled bacon, jalapeño, and chives, if using.

**STORAGE:** Store in an airtight container in the fridge for up to 4 days. Reheat in a saucepan over low heat or in the microwave, adding a splash of milk or broth to bring back the creaminess.

---

**PER SERVING (FOR 6 SERVINGS)**
Protein: 20g
Carbohydrates: 55g
Fat: 11g

Gluten-Free
Grain-Free
**IF MODIFIED:**
Dairy-Free

# Harvest Cobb Salad with Maple-Dijon Dressing

**SERVES 4 • PREP TIME: 25 MINUTES • COOK TIME: 20 MINUTES • TOTAL TIME: 45 MINUTES**

Cobb salad is already a classic, but this version brings the best fall flavors to the mix. Juicy chicken, crispy bacon, and hard-boiled eggs keep it hearty and filling, while roasted butternut squash, creamy goat cheese, and pomegranate seeds add the seasonal twist. The maple-Dijon dressing ties it all together with a perfect balance of savory and sweet. For an elevated brunch or cozy dinner, this one always hits the spot!

**FOR THE DRESSING**

¼ cup apple cider vinegar
¼ cup extra-virgin olive oil
1½ teaspoons maple syrup
1 teaspoon Dijon mustard
1 garlic clove, minced
Sea salt and freshly ground black pepper
¼ cup thinly sliced red onion

**FOR THE SALAD**

½ small butternut squash, peeled and cubed (about 3 cups)
2½ tablespoons avocado oil
Sea salt and freshly ground black pepper
2 large boneless, skinless chicken breasts, halved lengthwise
4 strips bacon
6 to 8 cups baby arugula
4 hard-boiled eggs, sliced
1 avocado, sliced
½ cup roasted walnuts, chopped
¼ cup pomegranate seeds
¼ cup crumbled goat cheese (omit for dairy-free)

1. Preheat the oven to 425°F. Line a baking sheet with parchment paper.
2. **Make the dressing:** In a small bowl or jar, whisk together the vinegar, olive oil, maple syrup, mustard, garlic, salt, and pepper. Add the onion and let it marinate while you prepare the salad.
3. **Prepare the salad:** In a medium bowl, toss the butternut squash with ½ tablespoon of the avocado oil and season with salt and pepper. Spread the squash in an even layer on the baking sheet and roast for 10 to 12 minutes. Toss, then roast for 10 minutes more, or until tender and lightly golden.
4. Meanwhile, in a medium skillet, heat the remaining 2 tablespoons avocado oil over medium heat. Season the chicken with salt and pepper, then add to the skillet and cook for 7 to 8 minutes per side, until the internal temperature reaches 165°F. If the outsides are browning too quickly before the insides are fully cooked, cover the skillet for the last few minutes to help the chicken cook through evenly. Transfer the chicken to a cutting board and let rest for 5 minutes. Chop into small cubes and set aside.
5. In a large skillet over medium heat, cook the bacon for 5 to 6 minutes per side, until crisp. Transfer to a cutting board, let cool slightly, then coarsely chop.
6. In a large serving bowl, combine the butternut squash, chicken, bacon, arugula, eggs, avocado, walnuts, pomegranate, and goat cheese. Drizzle the dressing over the salad or serve it on the side.

**STORAGE:** Store the components separately in airtight containers in the fridge for up to 4 days. Keep the dressing in a small jar and toss everything together just before serving for the best texture.

---

**PER SERVING**
Protein: 40g
Carbohydrates: 20g
Fat: 40g

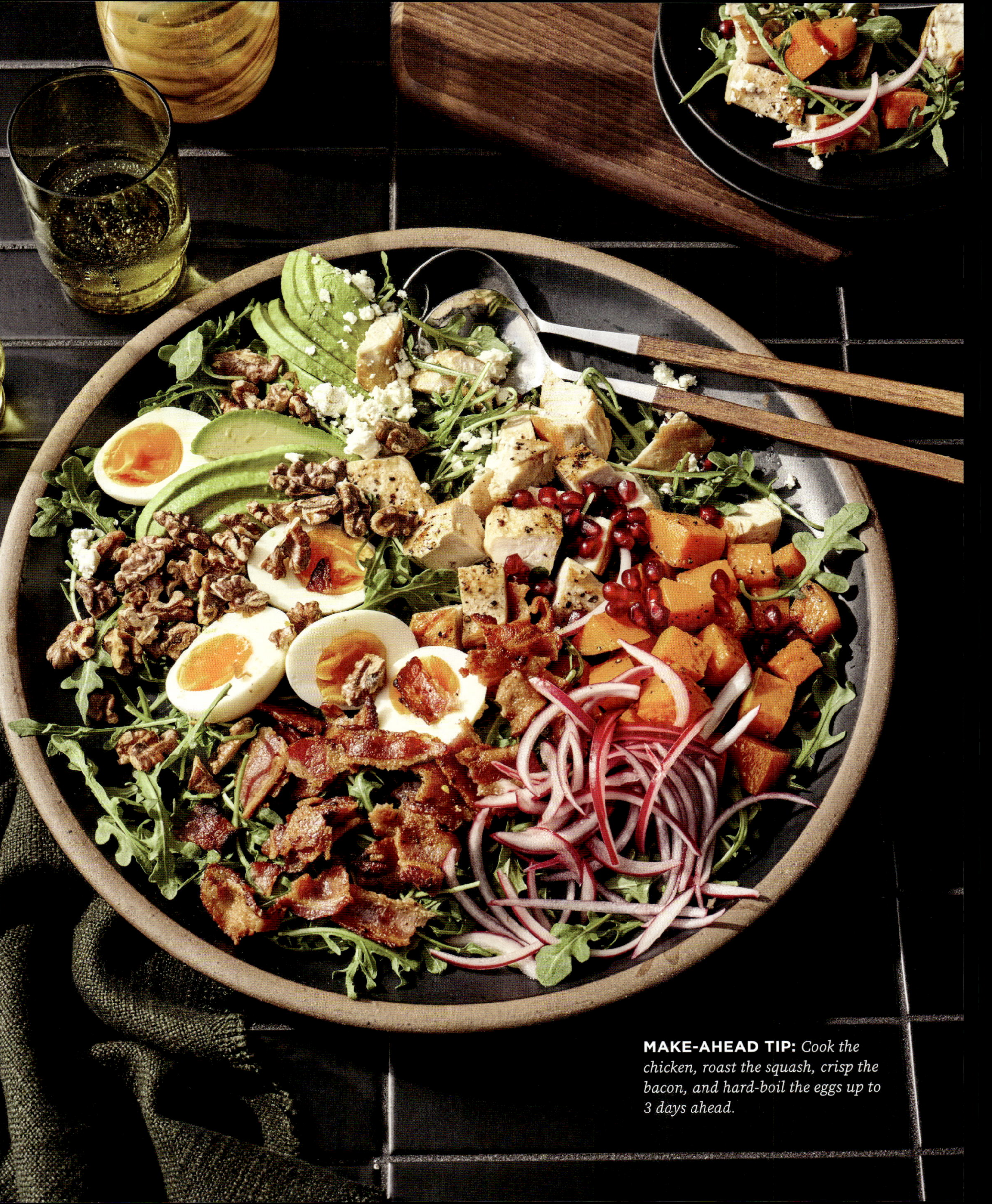

**MAKE-AHEAD TIP:** *Cook the chicken, roast the squash, crisp the bacon, and hard-boil the eggs up to 3 days ahead.*

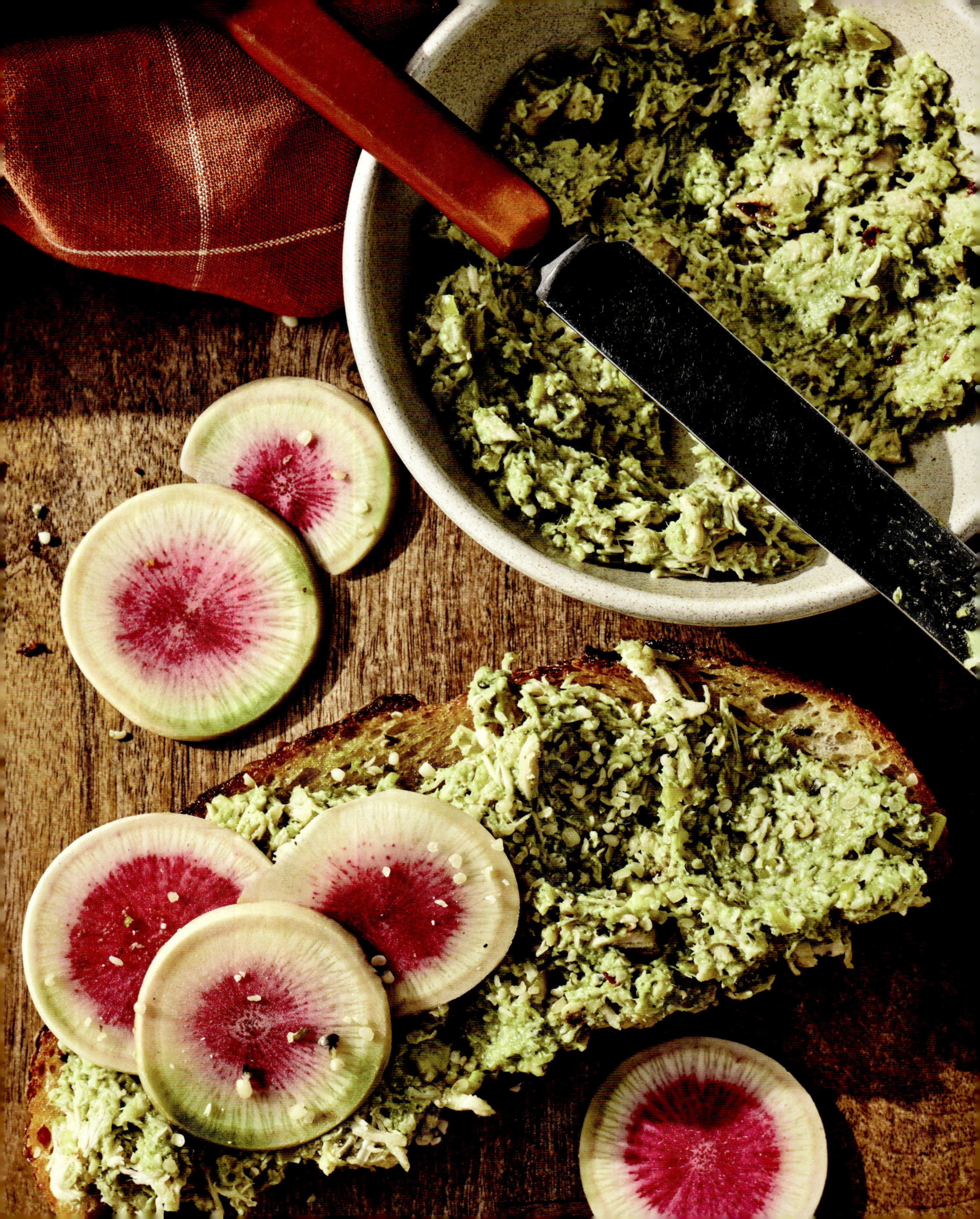

Gluten-Free
Grain-Free
No Added Sugar
Paleo
**IF MODIFIED:**
Dairy-Free

# 5-Minute Pesto Chicken Salad

**SERVES 1 • PREP TIME: 5 MINUTES • TOTAL TIME: 5 MINUTES**

- ½ medium avocado
- 2 tablespoons coarsely chopped pepperoncini
- 1 tablespoon pesto (dairy-free if preferred, or Basil Pesto, page 141)
- 1 tablespoon hemp seeds
- ½ teaspoon sea salt
- ¼ teaspoon red chili flakes
- ¼ teaspoon ground pepper
- 1 (5-ounce) can roasted chicken breast (I prefer Wild Planet), drained (or about ¾ cup shredded rotisserie or baked chicken)
- For serving: sourdough toast, crackers, veggies, or lettuce wraps

When I say this takes five minutes, I mean it. Five. Minutes. The creamy avocado, zesty pepperoncini, and herby pesto make it way more exciting than your average chicken salad. I love scooping it up with crackers, spreading it over buttery sourdough, or tossing it on greens for a no-effort meal that just hits.

In a medium bowl, mash the avocado. Add the pepperoncini, pesto, hemp seeds, salt, chili flakes, and pepper. Stir until combined. Add the chicken and mix well until fully coated. Serve immediately on toast, with crackers, with crunchy vegetables, or in lettuce wraps.

**PER SERVING**
Protein: 32g
Carbohydrates: 8g
Fat: 25g

Dairy-Free
Gluten-Free
No Added Sugar

# Bone Broth Jasmine Rice Three Ways

**SERVES 4 • PREP TIME: 5 MINUTES • COOK TIME: 15 MINUTES • TOTAL TIME: 20 MINUTES**

The easiest way to take your rice from good to very good—and actually make it work *for* you—is to swap out the water for bone broth. Just like that, you've got rich, flavorful rice full of protein, collagen, and extra nutrients. Stick with the plain version for versatility, or try the two combos I come back to again and again: a zesty cilantro-lime or a bold, tomato-infused Mexican rice. They're flavorful enough to stand on their own, but still play nice with just about anything on your plate.

**FOR BONE BROTH RICE**

1 cup jasmine rice, rinsed until the water runs clear

1¾ cups chicken bone broth

1 tablespoon ghee (optional)

**FOR MEXICAN RICE**

1 (8-ounce) can unsweetened tomato sauce

½ teaspoon chili powder

½ teaspoon ground cumin

**FOR CILANTRO-LIME RICE**

Juice of ½ lime (about 1 tablespoon)

¼ cup chopped fresh cilantro

1. In a medium saucepan with a tight-fitting lid, combine the rice, broth, and ghee, if using. If making Mexican rice, also add the tomato sauce, chili powder, and cumin, and reduce broth to 1½ cups. Bring to a boil over medium heat. Stir, reduce the heat to low, cover, and simmer for 15 minutes, until the liquid is absorbed and the rice is tender.
2. Remove from the heat and let sit, covered, for 10 minutes. Fluff with a fork. For cilantro-lime rice, stir in the lime juice and cilantro before serving.

---

**PER SERVING (BONE BROTH RICE)**
Protein: 5g
Carbohydrates: 37g
Fat: 2g (if using ghee)

---

**PER SERVING (MEXICAN RICE)**
Protein: 5g
Carbohydrates: 39g
Fat: 2g (if using ghee)

---

**PER SERVING (CILANTRO-LIME RICE)**
Protein: 5g
Carbohydrates: 37g
Fat: 2g (if using ghee)

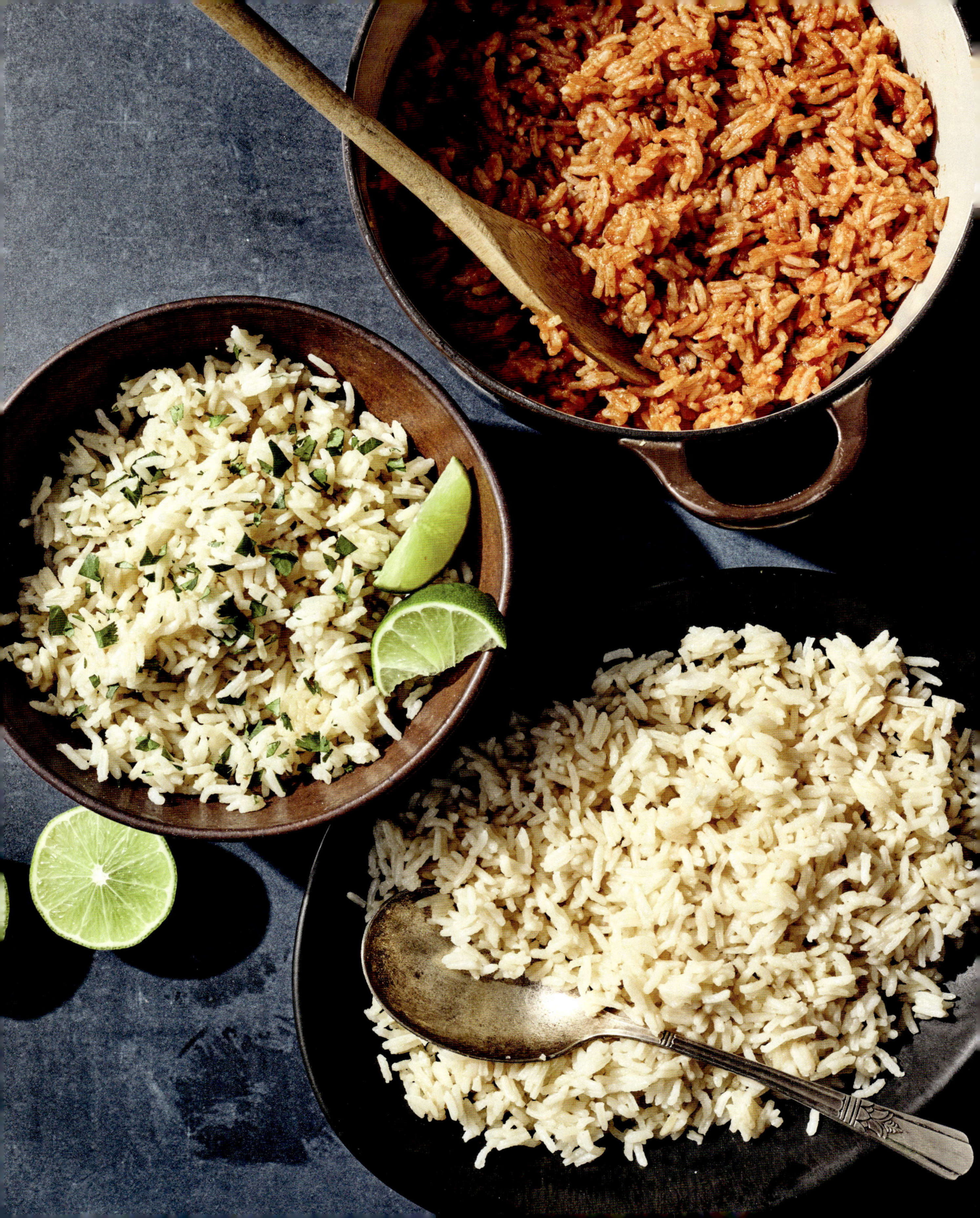

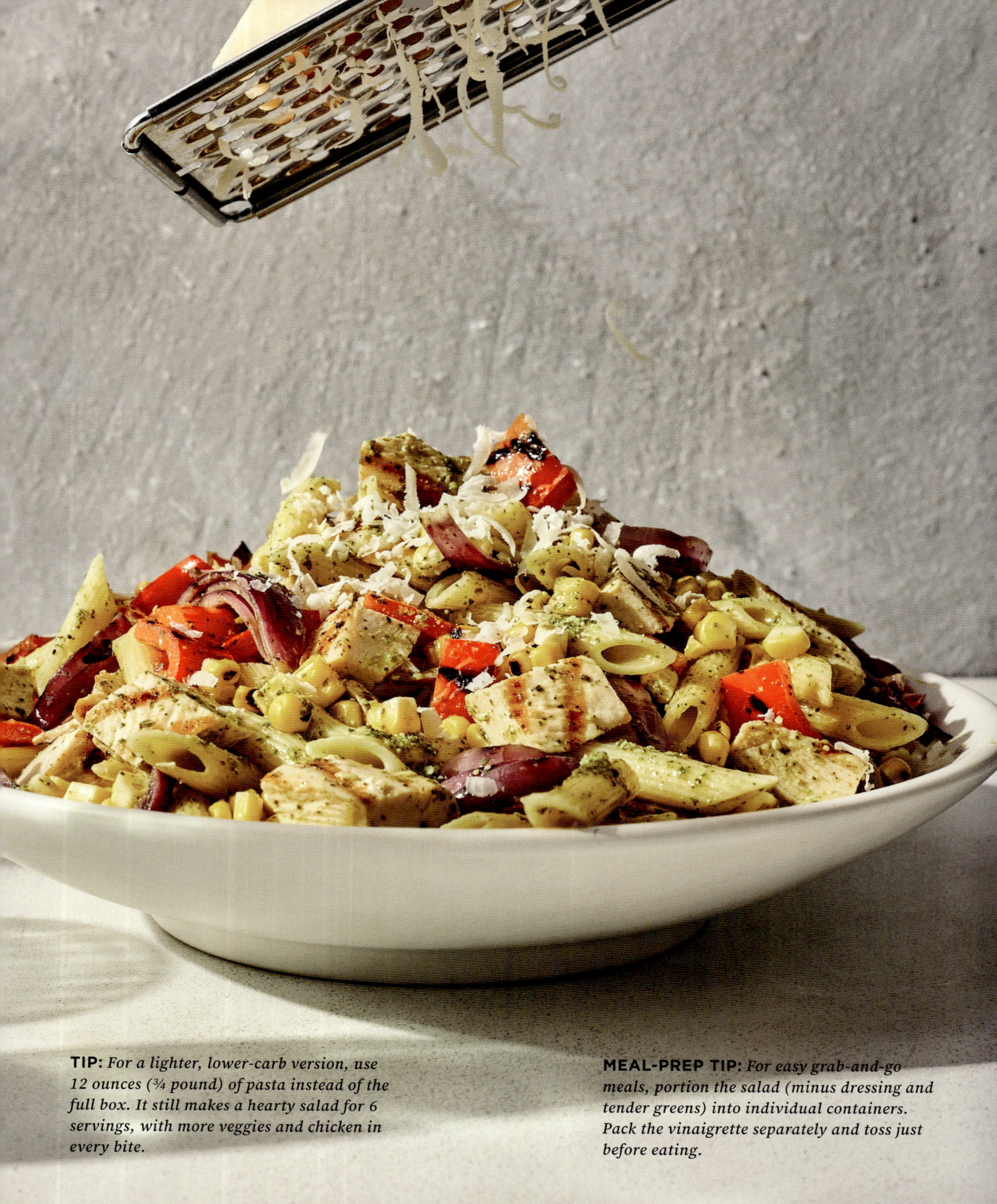

**TIP:** *For a lighter, lower-carb version, use 12 ounces (¾ pound) of pasta instead of the full box. It still makes a hearty salad for 6 servings, with more veggies and chicken in every bite.*

**MEAL-PREP TIP:** *For easy grab-and-go meals, portion the salad (minus dressing and tender greens) into individual containers. Pack the vinaigrette separately and toss just before eating.*

No Added Sugar
**IF MODIFIED:**
Dairy-Free
Gluten-Free

# Grilled Summer Pasta Salad

**SERVES 6 • PREP TIME: 30 MINUTES, PLUS 30 MINUTES MARINATING • COOK TIME: 20 MINUTES • TOTAL TIME: 1 HOUR 20 MINUTES**

- ⅓ cup pesto (see Basil Pesto, page 141)
- ¼ cup extra-virgin olive oil
- Juice of ½ lemon
- Sea salt and freshly ground black pepper
- 2 boneless chicken breasts, sliced horizontally to make 4 thinner cutlets
- 3 tablespoons chipotle ranch dressing (such as the SideDish brand)
- 2 tablespoons avocado oil
- 2 ears fresh corn, shucked
- 2 large bell peppers (red, yellow, or orange), seeded and chopped
- ½ cup thinly sliced red onion
- 1 pound short pasta (such as penne, fusilli, or shells), or gluten-free pasta of choice
- 1 tablespoon ghee (or vegan butter for dairy-free)
- 3 cups fresh spinach, chopped
- 1 cup marinated artichoke hearts, chopped
- ⅓ cup finely grated Parmesan, for garnish (omit for dairy-free)
- Flaky salt

Pesto just *tastes* like summer, and this grilled number might be the most delicious way to use it. You've got juicy chicken, smoky veggies, al dente pasta, and a bright flavorful vinaigrette all coming together in one bowl. It's perfect for BBQs, easy enough for weeknight dinners, and a total meal-prep win—serve it warm off the grill or straight from the fridge the next day. This one checks all the boxes.

1. **Make the vinaigrette:** In a medium bowl, whisk together the pesto, olive oil, lemon juice, and salt and black pepper to taste. Set aside.
2. **Marinate the chicken:** In a separate medium bowl, toss the chicken with chipotle ranch, 1 tablespoon of the avocado oil, and a generous pinch of salt and black pepper. Cover and refrigerate for 30 to 60 minutes.
3. Preheat the grill to 500°F.
4. Brush the corn with the remaining 1 tablespoon avocado oil and season with salt. Set aside on a plate.
5. Grill the marinated chicken for 4 to 5 minutes per side, or until the internal temperature reaches 165°F. Transfer to a plate and let rest for 5 minutes before slicing into 1-inch pieces.
6. **Grill the vegetables:** Grill the corn directly on the grates or in a grill basket, rotating every 2 to 3 minutes, until lightly charred. Add the bell peppers and onion directly to the grill or grill basket and cook for 7 to 8 minutes, stirring occasionally if using a basket, or flipping once or twice if grilling directly, until softened and charred. Spread the ghee over the hot corn, then slice the kernels off the cob.
7. **Cook the pasta:** Bring a large pot of salted water to a boil. Cook the pasta according to package instructions until al dente. Reserve ½ cup pasta water, then drain.
8. **Assemble the salad:** In a large bowl, combine the grilled chicken, grilled veggies, spinach, artichoke hearts, and cooked pasta. Drizzle with the vinaigrette and toss to coat. Add a splash of pasta water if needed to loosen. Serve with Parmesan and a sprinkle of flaky salt. Enjoy warm, at room temp, or chilled.

**STORAGE:** Store the salad in an airtight container in the fridge for up to 4 days. If making ahead, wait to add delicate greens or extra vinaigrette until just before serving to keep everything fresh.

---

**PER SERVING**
Protein: 28g
Carbohydrates: 72g
Fat: 35g

Dairy-Free
Gluten-Free
Grain-Free
No Added Sugar

# Roasted Sweet Potatoes with Spiced Chickpeas and Tahini Drizzle

**SERVES 4 • PREP TIME: 10 MINUTES • COOK TIME: 45 MINUTES • TOTAL TIME: 50 MINUTES**

**FOR THE SWEET POTATOES AND CHICKPEAS**

- 4 medium orange-flesh sweet potatoes
- 1 (15-ounce) can chickpeas, drained, rinsed, and patted dry
- 1 tablespoon extra-virgin olive oil
- 1 teaspoon ground cumin
- 1 teaspoon ground sumac
- 1 teaspoon smoked paprika
- ½ teaspoon garlic powder
- ½ teaspoon sea salt
- ½ teaspoon freshly ground black pepper

**FOR THE TAHINI SAUCE**

- ¼ cup tahini
- ¼ cup fresh lemon juice (1 to 2 lemons)
- 1 garlic clove, grated
- ½ teaspoon sea salt
- Optional garnishes: fresh mint, black and white sesame seeds, lemon wedges

Sweet potatoes are true superstars, and I just love 'em. They're rich in fiber, antioxidants, and nutrients like vitamin A and potassium. Roast them up with spiced chickpeas and you've got a dish that checks every box: creamy, crispy, hearty, and full of flavor. The tahini drizzle ties it all together, and while it's an incredible, totally plant-based side, you can always add shredded chicken or pulled pork if you're craving more protein.

1. **Roast the sweet potatoes and chickpeas:** Preheat the oven to 400°F. Line a baking sheet with parchment paper.
2. Scrub the sweet potatoes, prick each one a few times with a fork, and place them on one side of the baking sheet. Roast for 30 minutes.
3. Toss the chickpeas with the oil, cumin, sumac, paprika, garlic powder, salt, and pepper. Add the chickpeas to the other side of the baking sheet and roast until they are golden and crispy and the sweet potatoes are fork-tender, 15 to 20 minutes.
4. **Make the tahini sauce:** Meanwhile, in a small bowl, whisk together the tahini, lemon juice, garlic, and salt. Whisk in water, 1 tablespoon at a time, until the sauce is smooth and pourable.
5. Slice each roasted sweet potato in half lengthwise and gently fluff the flesh with a fork. Top with the chickpeas and a generous drizzle of tahini sauce, and garnish with mint, sesame seeds, and lemon wedges, if you like.

**PER SERVING**
Protein: 10g
Carbohydrates: 47g
Fat: 9g

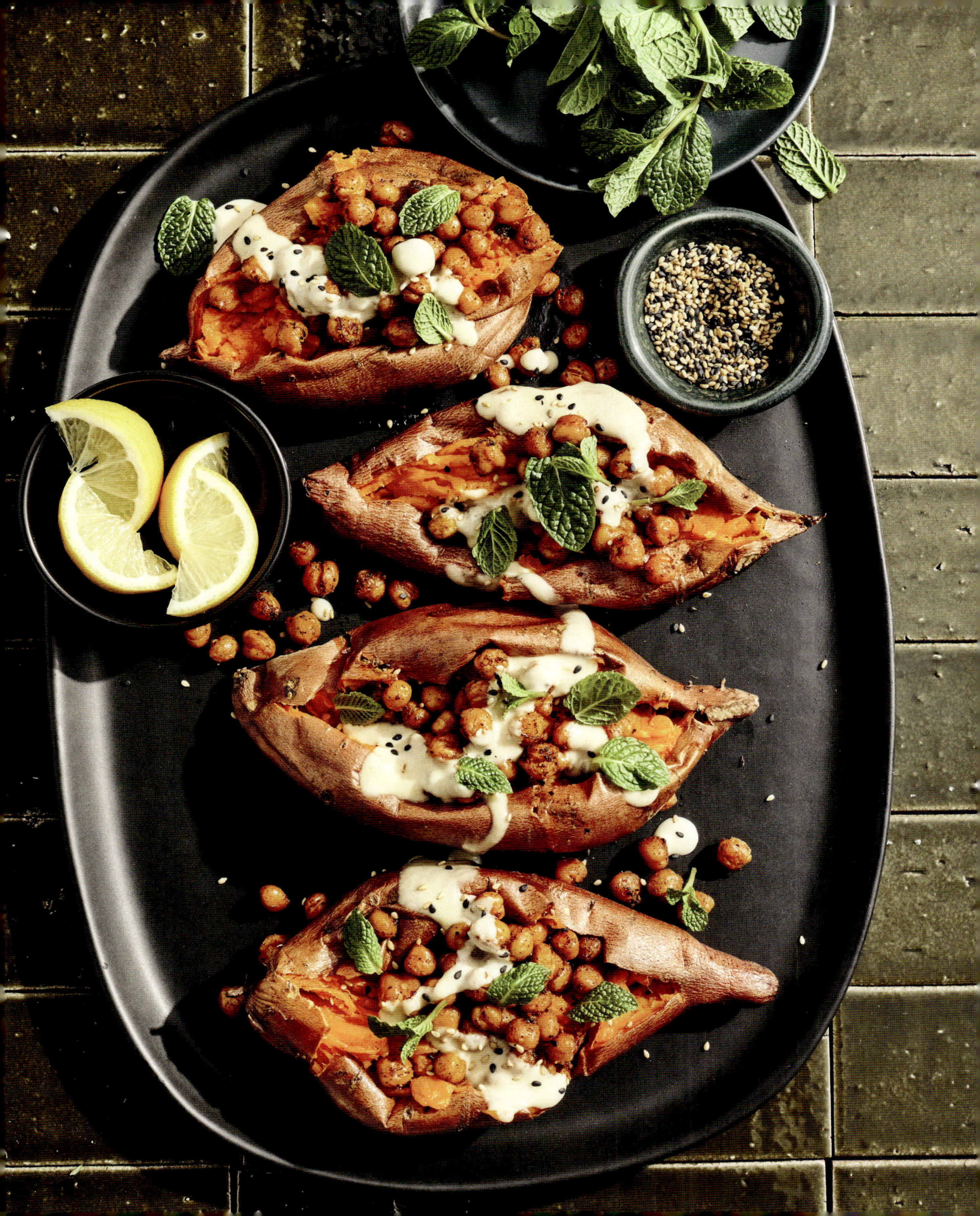

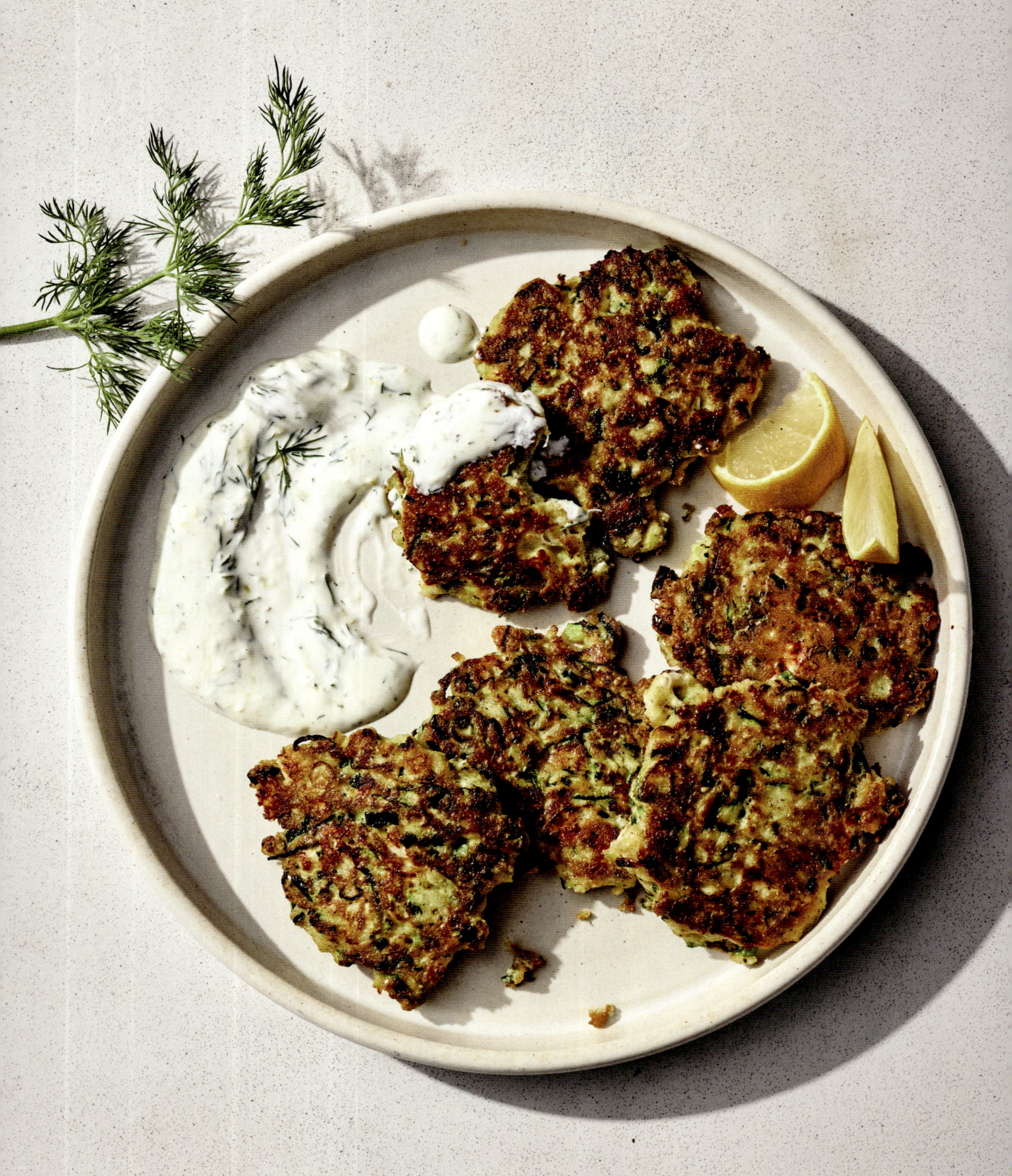

Gluten-Free
Grain-Free
No Added Sugar

# Zucchini Fritters with Lemon-Dill Sauce

MAKES 12 FRITTERS (4 SERVINGS) • PREP TIME: 15 MINUTES • COOK TIME: 15 MINUTES • TOTAL TIME: 30 MINUTES

These veggie-forward fritters are crispy on the outside and soft and cheesy on the inside. They're easy to whip up and the perfect way to turn fresh summer squash into something special. The fresh lemon-dill sauce adds a bright, herby topper to every bite. Serve them as an appetizer or side dish, and watch them disappear fast.

FOR THE SAUCE

½ cup full-fat plain Greek yogurt
1 tablespoon grated lemon zest
1 tablespoon freshly squeezed lemon juice
1 garlic clove, grated
2 tablespoons chopped fresh dill
¼ teaspoon sea salt
¼ teaspoon freshly ground black pepper

FOR THE FRITTERS

2 large zucchini
1 teaspoon sea salt
2 large eggs
3 green onions, white and green parts, finely chopped
2 garlic cloves, minced
½ cup almond flour, plus more if needed
½ cup crumbled feta
1 teaspoon za'atar
½ teaspoon freshly ground black pepper
½ teaspoon baking powder
¼ cup avocado oil
Lemon wedges, for garnish

1. **Make the sauce:** In a medium bowl, whisk together the yogurt, lemon zest, lemon juice, garlic, dill, salt, and pepper until smooth. Cover and refrigerate until ready to serve.
2. **Make the fritters:** Grate the zucchini using the large holes of a box grater. Place the shreds in a colander over the sink and give them an initial squeeze with your hands to remove as much moisture as you can. Sprinkle with the salt and let sit for 10 minutes to draw out more water. Wrap the zucchini in a clean dish towel and twist tightly over the sink until no more liquid drips out. The zucchini should feel damp but not wet and hold together when squeezed.
3. In a large bowl, mix the zucchini, eggs, green onions, garlic, almond flour, feta, za'atar, pepper, and baking powder until well combined. The batter should be thick and able to form patties. If it feels too wet, stir in 1 to 2 more tablespoons almond flour. Form into 12 loose balls (about 2 tablespoons each).
4. Heat the oil in a large sauté pan over medium heat. Line a baking sheet with a wire rack and place a few paper towels on top to absorb the oil. Add a few fritters to the pan, flattening them slightly with a spatula. Cook for 3 to 4 minutes per side, until golden brown and crisp. Transfer to the rack to drain. Repeat with remaining fritters.
5. Serve the fritters immediately with the lemon-dill sauce and extra lemon wedges.

**STORAGE:** Store the fritters in an airtight container in the fridge for up to 4 days. Reheat in a skillet or toaster oven at 350°F until crisp and warmed through. Avoid microwaving to keep the edges crispy.

**PER SERVING**
Protein: 14g
Carbohydrates: 10g
Fat: 27g

Gluten-Free
Grain-Free
**IF MODIFIED:**
Dairy-Free

# The Rachael Salad

SERVES 4 • PREP TIME: 25 MINUTES • TOTAL TIME: 25 MINUTES

Fun fact: Jennifer Aniston and I share a birthday—so naturally I figured we'd have some of the same great taste, including a love for this kind of salad. Inspired by the viral Jen Aniston Salad, I had to put my own spin on it, and trust me, this riff might just win a spot as your new go-to salad. What makes it shine is the combo of fresh herbs, crunchy nuts, savory feta, and the unexpected touch of sweetness from chopped dates.

FOR THE DRESSING

¼ cup extra-virgin olive oil
¼ cup lemon juice
1 tablespoon honey
1 garlic clove, grated
½ teaspoon sea salt
½ teaspoon freshly ground black pepper

FOR THE SALAD

3 cups shredded rotisserie chicken
1 (15-ounce) can chickpeas, drained and rinsed
1 cup crumbled feta (omit for dairy-free)
1 English cucumber, cut into ½-inch dice
½ cup ¼-inch-diced red onion
½ cup dates, chopped
⅓ cup packed fresh parsley leaves, chopped
⅓ cup packed fresh mint leaves, chopped
½ cup roasted pistachios
½ cup dry roasted almonds, chopped
¼ cup hemp seeds
½ teaspoon sea salt
½ teaspoon freshly ground black pepper

1. **Make the dressing:** In a jar or small bowl, combine the oil, lemon juice, honey, garlic, salt, and pepper and shake or whisk until well combined.
2. **Assemble the salad:** In a large bowl, combine the chicken, chickpeas, feta, cucumber, onion, dates, parsley, mint, pistachios, almonds, and hemp seeds. Sprinkle with the salt and pepper. Pour the dressing over the salad a little bit at a time, then toss until well combined. Serve immediately.

**STORAGE:** Store the dressing and salad components separately in airtight containers in the fridge for up to 4 days. Toss everything together just before serving to keep the salad fresh and crisp.

**PER SERVING**
Protein: 34g
Carbohydrates: 28g
Fat: 38g

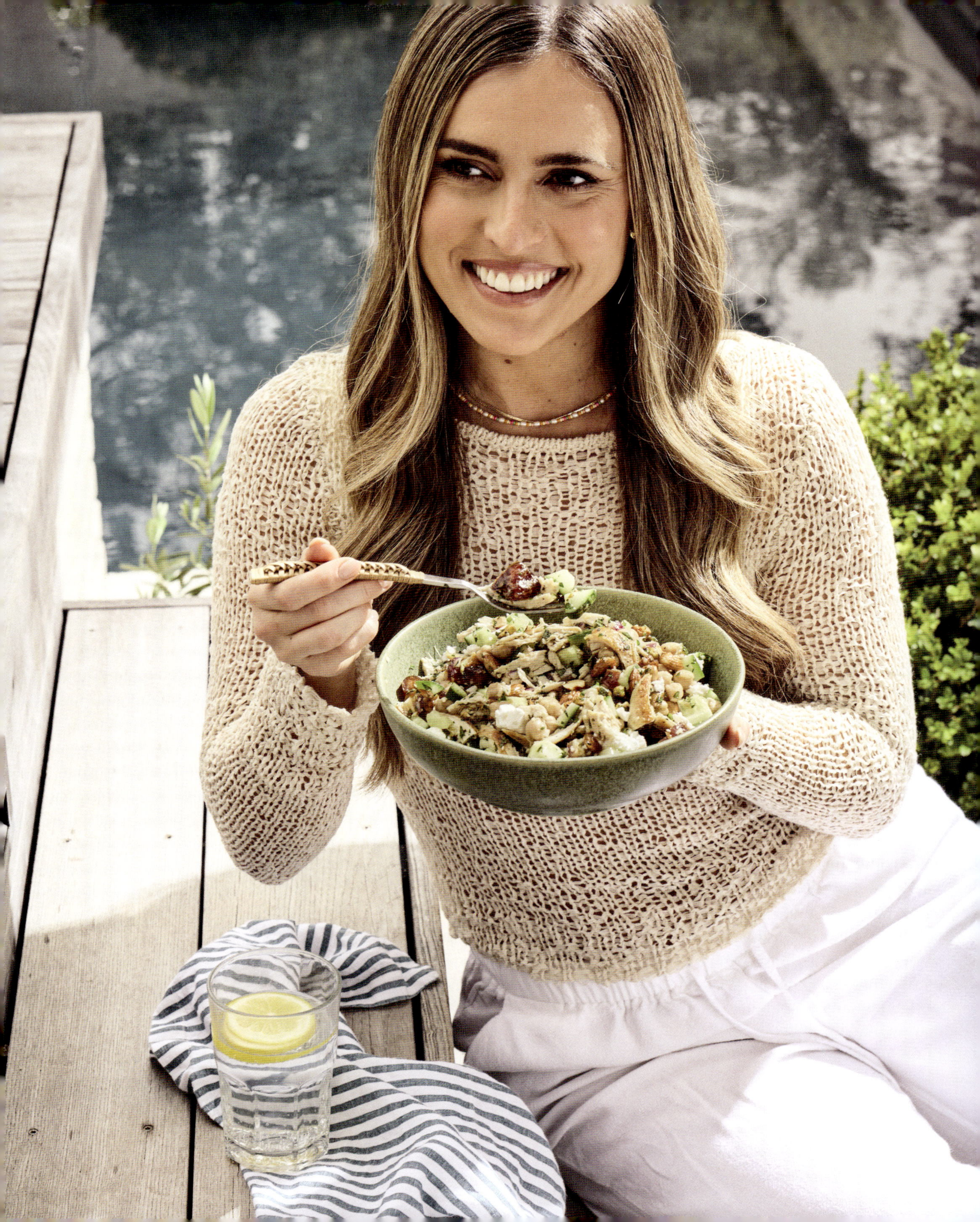

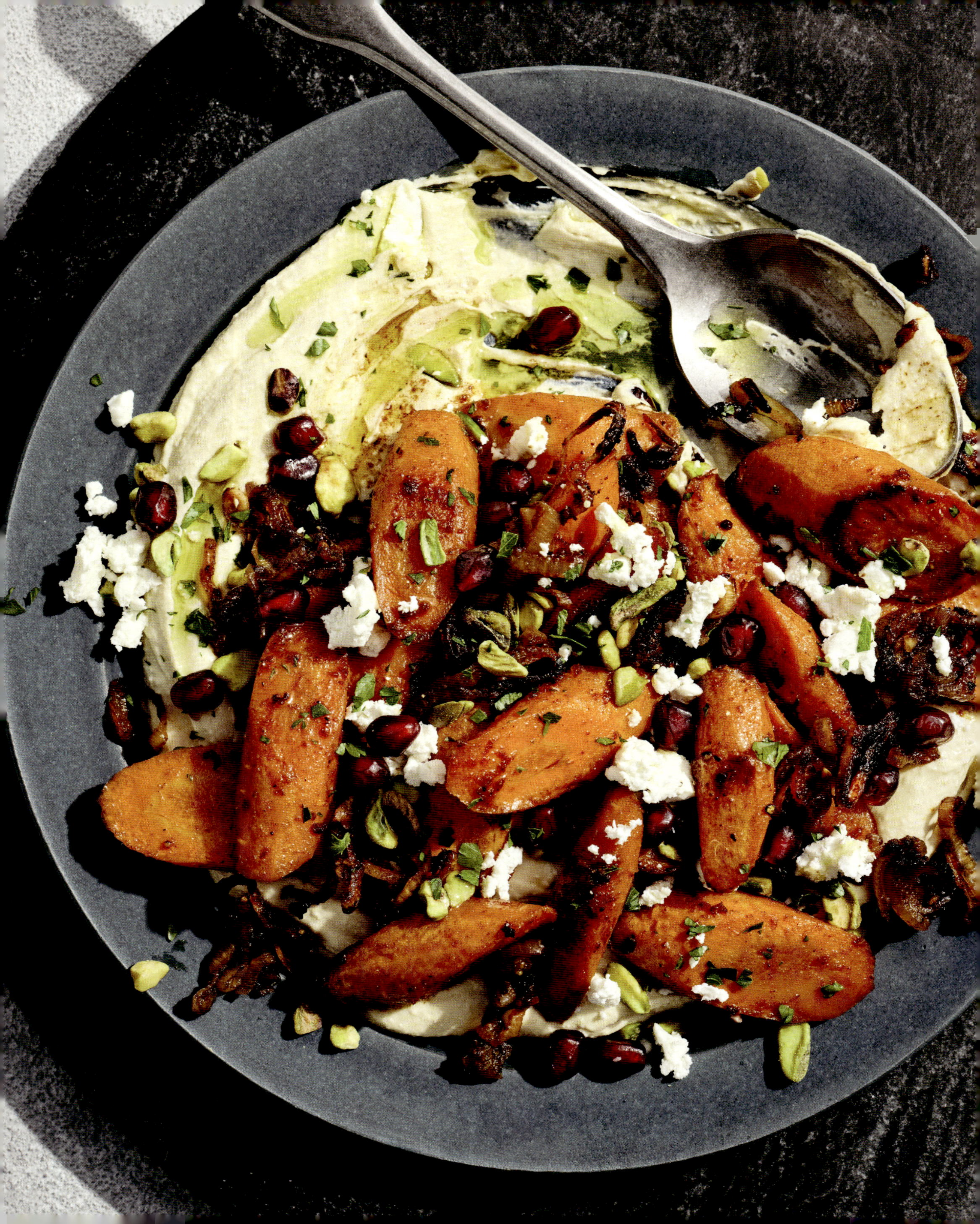

Gluten-Free
Grain-Free
No Added Sugar

# Moroccan-Spiced Carrots with Hummus

**SERVES 4 • PREP TIME: 10 MINUTES • COOK TIME: 30 MINUTES • TOTAL TIME: 40 MINUTES**

- 4 large carrots, sliced diagonally into 1-inch pieces
- 1 large shallot, thinly sliced
- 2 tablespoons extra-virgin olive oil, plus more for drizzling
- 1 tablespoon honey
- 1 teaspoon smoked paprika
- 1 teaspoon ground cumin
- ½ teaspoon ground cinnamon
- 1 teaspoon sea salt
- ½ teaspoon freshly ground black pepper
- 1 cup store-bought hummus
- ½ cup cottage cheese

**TOPPINGS**

- ½ cup crumbled feta
- ½ cup pistachios
- ¼ cup pomegranate seeds
- ¼ cup chopped fresh parsley

I love a dish that brings together big flavor and stunning presentation without much effort. These roasted spiced carrots do just that. They are sweet, smoky, and perfectly caramelized. The creamy hummus–cottage cheese base balances the warmth of the spices, while feta, pistachios, and pomegranate add the perfect mix of crunch, salt, and freshness. Serve as a side, or roast some chicken alongside the carrots for a well-rounded, protein-forward meal.

1. Preheat the oven to 400°F. Line a baking sheet with parchment paper.
2. In a large bowl, combine the carrots, shallot, oil, honey, paprika, cumin, cinnamon, salt, and pepper and toss until evenly coated. Spread on the baking sheet in a single layer, leaving as much room between the carrots as possible. Roast for 30 to 35 minutes, until the carrots are caramelized.
3. Meanwhile, in a food processor, blend the hummus and cottage cheese on high for 30 seconds, or until smooth.
4. On a large serving platter or plate, spread the hummus mixture. Top with the carrots, then sprinkle with the feta, pistachios, pomegranate seeds, and parsley. Drizzle more oil over the top. Serve warm or at room temperature.

**STORAGE:** Store in an airtight container in the fridge for up to 4 days. Reheat the carrots in a skillet or oven until warmed through, or enjoy them cold. Store hummus separately and add just before serving.

---

**PER SERVING**
Protein: 14g
Carbohydrates: 30g
Fat: 24g

Gluten-Free
Grain-Free
No Added Sugar

# Cheesy Bone Broth Mashed Potatoes

**SERVES 5 TO 6 • PREP TIME: 10 MINUTES • COOK TIME: 25 MINUTES • TOTAL TIME: 35 MINUTES**

If you're already a mashed potato fan, try this version: classic mashed potatoes, but with a hefty dose of protein. Bone broth adds deep, savory flavor, while whipped cottage cheese makes them impossibly creamy and cheesy. The result is a rich, velvety side that's just as nourishing as it is comforting. Perfect for pairing with any meal—or honestly, eating straight from the pan over the stove.

- 3 pounds Yukon Gold potatoes, peeled and cut into 1-inch pieces
- 2 cups chicken bone broth
- 1 cup full-fat cottage cheese
- 2 tablespoons ghee, plus more for serving
- 1 teaspoon sea salt
- ½ teaspoon freshly ground black pepper, plus more for garnish
- 2 tablespoons chopped fresh chives, for garnish

1. In a large saucepan, bring the potatoes and broth to a boil over medium-high heat. Cover, reduce the heat to medium, and simmer for 20 to 25 minutes, until the potatoes are fork-tender. Remove from the heat and mash the potatoes with a potato masher or fork.
2. Meanwhile, blend the cottage cheese in a food processor or blender for about 30 seconds, until smooth.
3. Stir the blended cottage cheese, ghee, salt, and pepper into the mashed potatoes, mixing until just combined. Be careful not to overmix, as this can make the potatoes gummy.
4. Garnish with chives, pepper, and a drizzle of melted ghee, if desired.

**STORAGE:** Store in an airtight container in the fridge for up to 4 days. Reheat gently on the stovetop or in the microwave, adding a splash of broth or milk to bring back the creamy texture.

**PER SERVING (FOR 6 SERVINGS)**
Protein: 10g
Carbohydrates: 40g
Fat: 7g

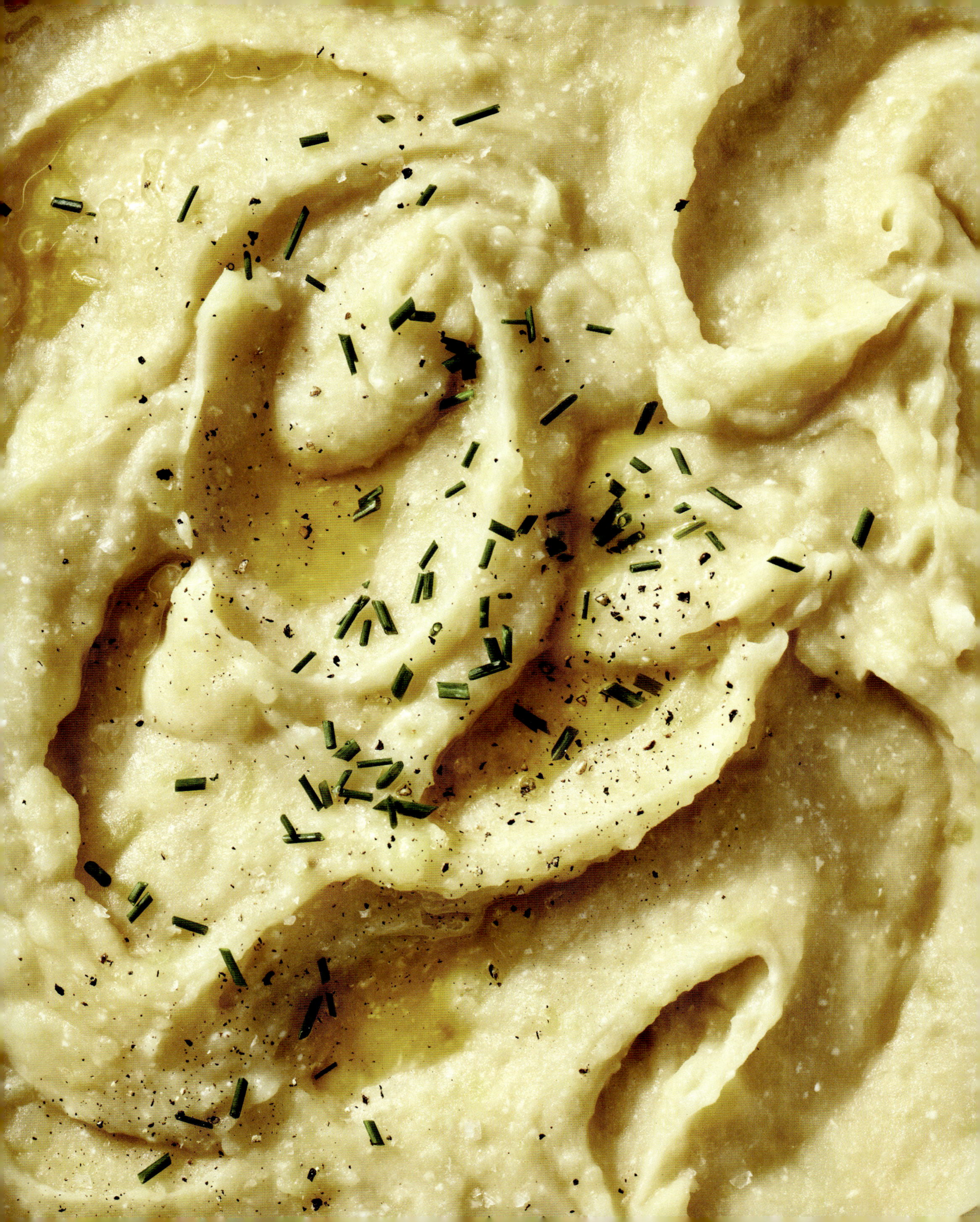

Dairy-Free
Gluten-Free
Grain-Free
No Added Sugar

# Sheet-Pan Greek Chicken and Chickpea Salad

**SERVES 4 TO 6 • PREP TIME: 15 MINUTES • COOK TIME: 20 MINUTES • TOTAL TIME: 35 MINUTES**

Mediterranean food is easily my favorite cuisine. It's fresh and light, with an emphasis on lean proteins and tons of veggies. It just leaves me feeling really good after a meal, no matter what it is. We also all love a sheet-pan meal, because it makes prep super easy—and it's a smart way to stretch meal prep across a couple of days. Just store everything in separate containers in the fridge, then toss it together when you're ready to eat.

**FOR THE CHICKEN AND CHICKPEAS**

- 2 teaspoons smoked paprika
- 2 teaspoons garlic powder
- ½ teaspoon ground cumin
- 2 teaspoons dried oregano
- 1½ teaspoons kosher salt
- 1 (15-ounce) can chickpeas, drained, rinsed, and patted dry
- 2 tablespoons extra-virgin olive oil
- 1½ pounds chicken breasts, cut into 1-inch cubes

**FOR THE SALAD**

- ¼ cup extra-virgin olive oil
- 2 tablespoons red wine vinegar
- 2 tablespoons lemon juice
- 1 teaspoon Dijon mustard
- 1 teaspoon dried oregano
- ½ teaspoon kosher salt
- ¼ cup minced red onion
- 1 English cucumber, diced
- 1 large red bell pepper, seeded and diced (or sub sliced cucumber for a similar fresh crunch)
- 1 cup cherry tomatoes, halved
- 4 cups baby arugula
- 4 cups chopped romaine lettuce
- ½ cup chopped fresh dill
- ½ cup chopped fresh cilantro
- Pepperoncini, drained and sliced, for garnish
- Crumbled feta, for garnish (optional)

---

**PER SERVING (FOR 4 SERVINGS)**
Protein: 42g
Carbohydrates: 21g
Fat: 17g

1. **Roast the chicken and chickpeas:** Preheat the oven to 425°F. Line a baking sheet with parchment paper for easy cleanup.
2. In a small bowl, mix the paprika, garlic powder, cumin, oregano, and salt. Place the chickpeas on one side of the baking sheet. Drizzle with 1 tablespoon of the oil and sprinkle with about one-third of the spice blend, tossing to coat. On the other side, add the chicken. Drizzle with the remaining 1 tablespoon oil, sprinkle with the remaining spice blend, and toss until evenly coated. Spread both the chickpeas and the chicken into even layers.
3. Roast for 10 minutes. Toss the chickpeas, and roast for another 10 to 15 minutes, until the chicken reaches an internal temperature of 165°F and the chickpeas are crispy.
4. **Make the salad:** Meanwhile, in a large mixing bowl, whisk together the oil, vinegar, lemon juice, mustard, oregano, and salt until emulsified. Add the onion, cucumber, bell pepper, and cherry tomatoes and toss to combine.
5. Just before serving, add the arugula, romaine, dill, and cilantro to the salad. Toss to combine. Divide the salad among bowls and top with the chicken and chickpeas. Garnish with pepperoncini and feta, if using.

**STORAGE:** To avoid a soggy salad, store the components separately in airtight containers in the fridge for up to 3 days. Keep the chicken and chickpeas together, the salad greens and veggies in a separate container, and the dressing in a small jar. Shake the dressing before using and toss everything together just before serving for a fresh, just-made taste.

**MAKE-AHEAD TIP:** *You can make the vinaigrette up to 5 days in advance. The chicken and chickpeas can also be prepped ahead and stored together for easy grab-and-go lunches or quick dinners.*

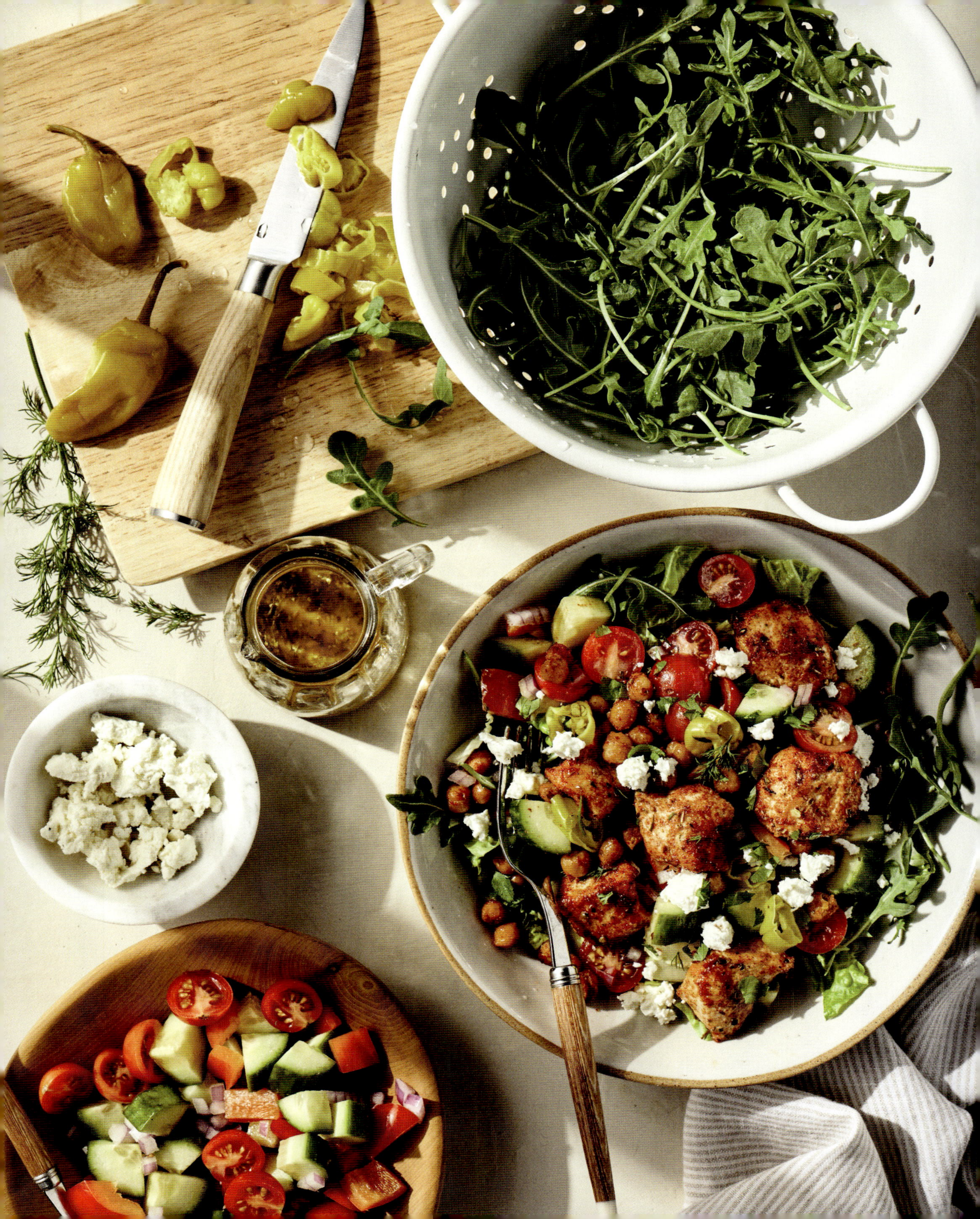

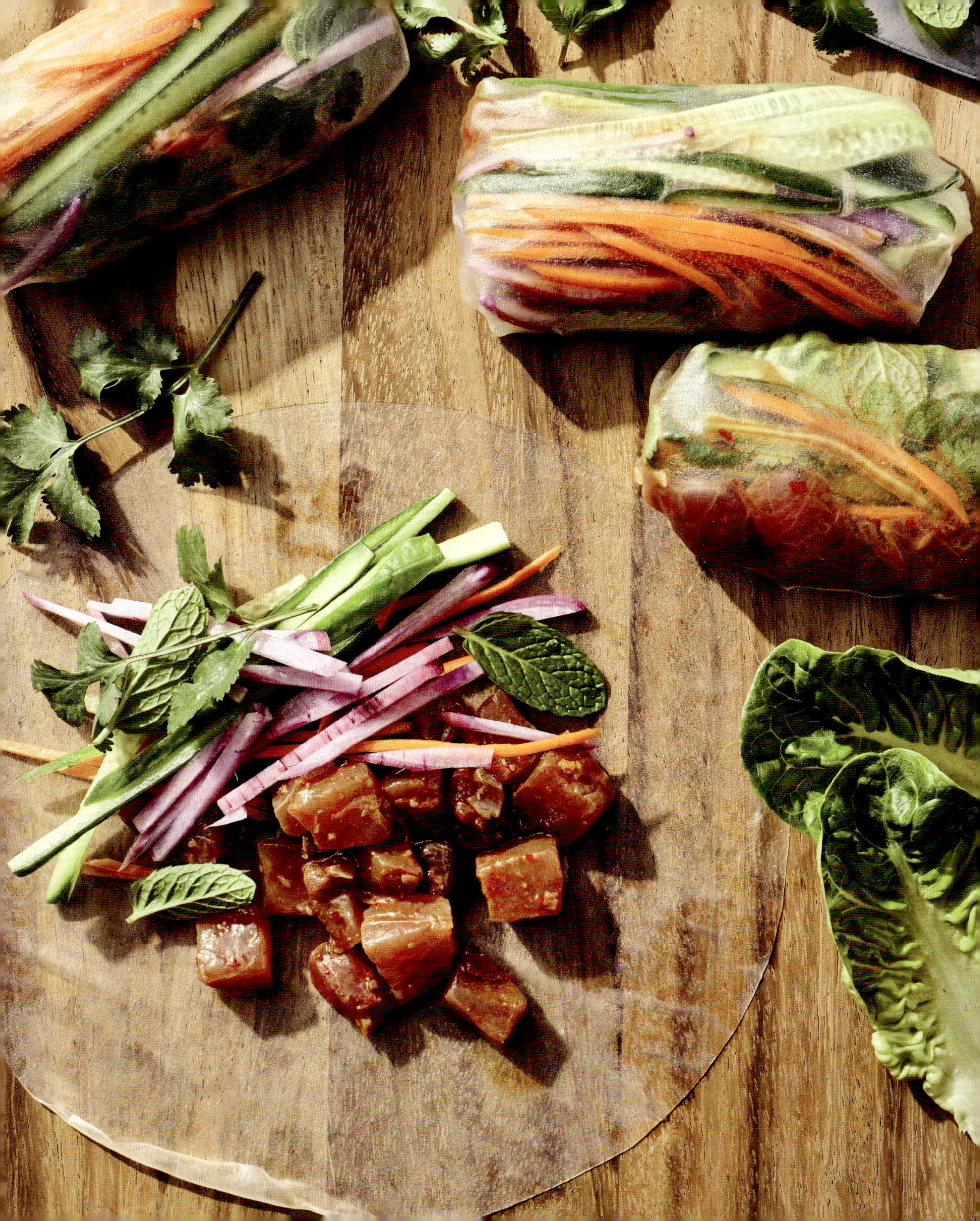

Dairy-Free
Gluten-Free
No Added Sugar

# Spicy Tuna Spring Rolls

SERVES 4 • PREP TIME: 20 MINUTES, PLUS 15 MINUTES MARINATING • TOTAL TIME: 35 MINUTES

Here, I've taken all my favorite things about a spicy tuna roll—protein-rich ahi tuna, crisp veggies, and that spicy garlic chili kick—and wrapped them up into a fresh spring roll. It's everything I love about sushi, just way easier (no rolling mats or sticky rice required). Perfect as a fresh appetizer or paired with a side for a light, satisfying meal.

FOR THE TUNA FILLING

1 pound sushi-grade wild ahi tuna

2 tablespoons garlic chili sauce, plus more for serving

2 tablespoons coconut aminos, plus more for serving

1 tablespoon toasted sesame oil

2 tablespoons lime juice

FOR THE SPRING ROLLS

4 spring roll wrappers

2 Persian cucumbers, julienned

1 large carrot, julienned

1 daikon radish (purple if you can find it), julienned

½ cup fresh mint leaves

½ cup fresh cilantro leaves

1 head Little Gem or romaine lettuce

1. **Make the tuna filling:** Dice the tuna into ½-inch pieces. In a medium bowl, whisk together the garlic chili sauce, coconut aminos, oil, and lime juice. Add the tuna and mix to coat. Cover and refrigerate for 15 to 20 minutes.
2. **Make the spring rolls:** Pour warm water into a pie plate or shallow baking dish. Working with one wrapper at a time, dip it into the water for 15 to 20 seconds, until softened. Gently shake off excess water and transfer to a clean cutting board. Fill with about ½ cup of the marinated tuna, 1 to 2 tablespoons each of cucumber, carrot, and radish, a few mint and cilantro leaves, and a small lettuce leaf. (Avoid overfilling so the roll seals properly.) Fold the bottom of the wrapper over the filling, then fold in the sides and roll tightly to seal.
3. Repeat with the remaining ingredients to make four spring rolls. Cut each roll in half and serve with additional garlic chili sauce and coconut aminos for dipping.

**STORAGE:** These are best enjoyed fresh, but leftovers can be stored in an airtight container in the fridge for up to 1 day. To keep the wrappers from drying out, place a damp paper towel over the rolls before sealing the container.

**PER SERVING**
Protein: 25g
Carbohydrates: 14g
Fat: 4g

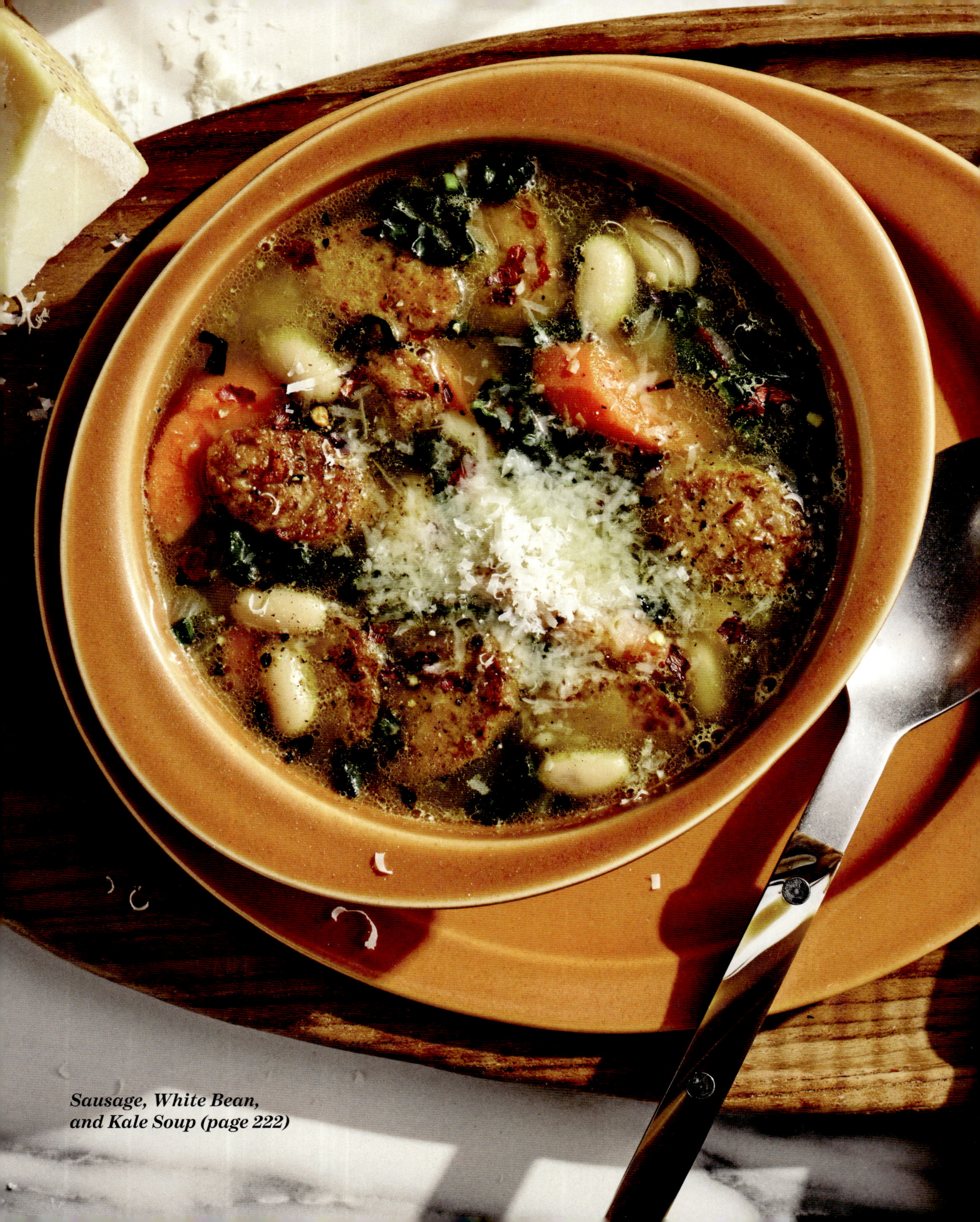

*Sausage, White Bean, and Kale Soup (page 222)*

218 **Slow Cooker Beef Stew**

221 **Creamy Tuscan Chicken Soup**

222 **Sausage, White Bean, and Kale Soup**

225 **Hearty Protein-Packed Chili**

226 **Golden Chicken Bone Broth**

228 **Roasted Butternut Squash Soup with Coconut-Lime Crema**

# Soups

Dairy-Free
Gluten-Free
Grain-Free
No Added Sugar

# Slow Cooker Beef Stew

SERVES 4 TO 6 • PREP TIME: 20 MINUTES • COOK TIME: 2½ TO 3 HOURS (DUTCH OVEN) OR 7 TO 8 HOURS (SLOW COOKER) • TOTAL TIME: 2 HOURS 50 MINUTES TO 3 HOURS 20 MINUTES (DUTCH OVEN) OR 7 HOURS 20 MINUTES TO 8 HOURS 20 MINUTES (SLOW COOKER)

I can't tell you how much I crave this stew the second the weather shifts. It's on my list of repeats for meal prep because it gets richer and more flavorful with time. Plus, the slow cooker does all the heavy lifting, leaving you with tender beef, rich broth, and warming veggies—aka everything you want in a stew.

2 pounds boneless beef chuck, cut into 1-inch cubes
1½ teaspoons sea salt
1 teaspoon freshly ground black pepper
2 tablespoons avocado oil
1 medium onion, sliced
1 celery stalk, thinly sliced crosswise
4 cloves garlic, minced
6 ounces cremini mushrooms, trimmed and thinly sliced
4 large carrots, sliced into ½-inch-thick rounds
3 medium Yukon Gold potatoes, cut into 1-inch cubes
2 cups beef bone broth
1 tablespoon Dijon mustard
1½ tablespoons tomato paste
2 tablespoons coconut aminos
2 tablespoons balsamic vinegar
1½ teaspoons fresh rosemary, finely chopped
1 bay leaf

1. Generously season the beef with salt and pepper. In a large sauté pan, heat the oil over medium heat. Add the beef and brown on all sides, 1 to 2 minutes per side. Transfer to a plate and let rest for 5 minutes.
2. In the same pan, add the onion, celery, garlic, and mushrooms. Sauté for 5 minutes, until softened. Remove from the heat and set aside.
3. In the slow cooker, combine the carrots, potatoes, broth, mustard, tomato paste, coconut aminos, vinegar, rosemary, and bay leaf. Stir to combine. Add the beef and vegetables, stir again, and cover. Cook on low for 7 to 8 hours or on high for 3 to 4 hours, until the beef is fork-tender.
4. **If using a Dutch oven instead of a slow cooker:** After browning the beef and sautéing the vegetables, add everything to a large Dutch oven. Bring the mixture to a gentle simmer over medium heat. Reduce the heat to low, cover, and cook for 2½ to 3 hours, until the beef is fork-tender. Stir occasionally and add a splash more broth if the stew gets too thick.
5. Remove the bay leaf from the stew and serve warm.

**STORAGE:** The stew will keep in an airtight container in the fridge for up to 4 days. Reheat gently on the stovetop or in the microwave.

---

**PER SERVING (FOR 4 SERVINGS)**
Protein: 34g
Carbohydrates: 40g
Fat: 18g

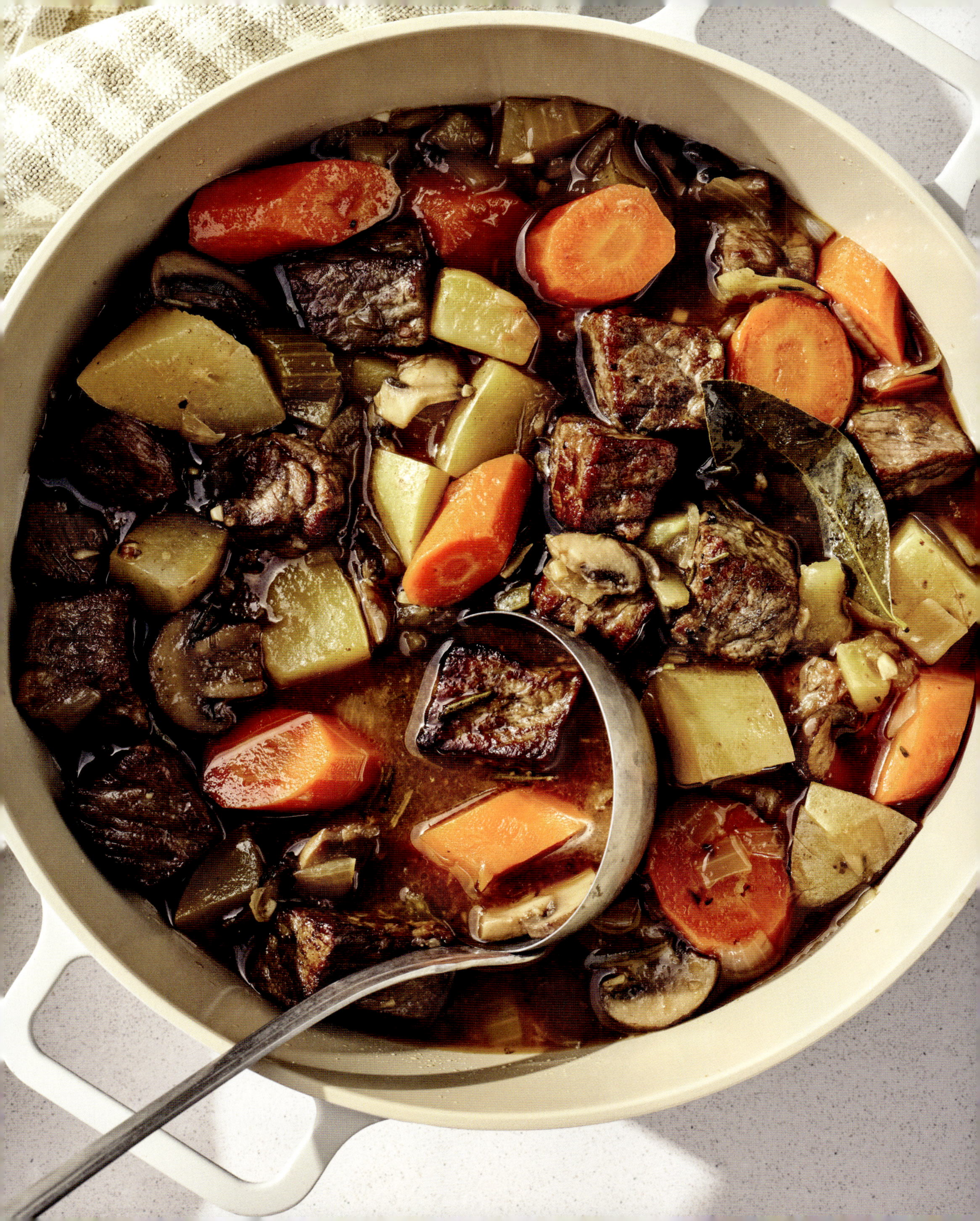

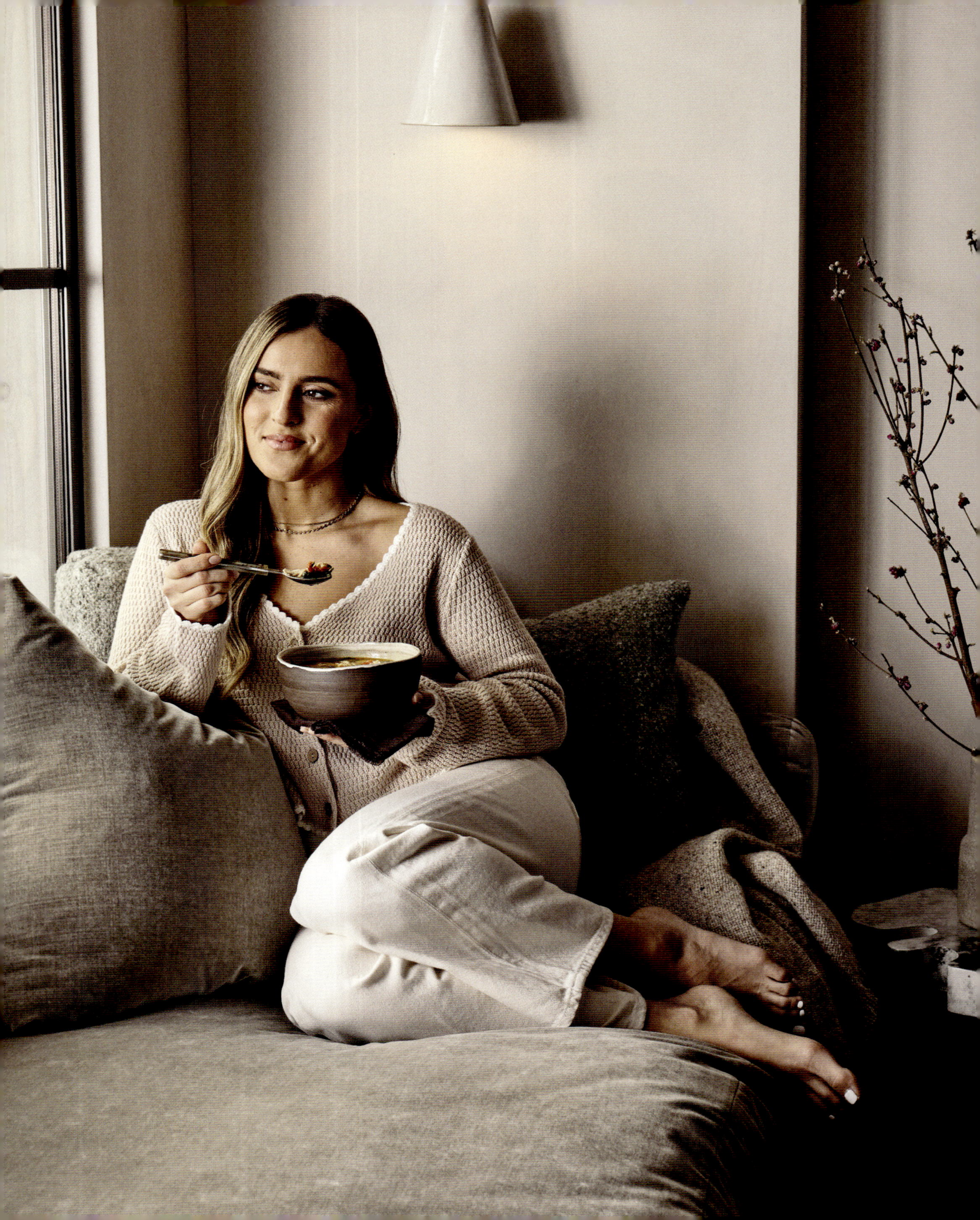

Dairy-Free
Gluten-Free
Grain-Free
No Added Sugar

# Creamy Tuscan Chicken Soup

**SERVES 5 • PREP TIME: 10 MINUTES • COOK TIME: 30 MINUTES • TOTAL TIME: 40 MINUTES**

With 50 grams of protein per serving, this soup brings major staying power. It's inspired by the same flavor profile as my Marry Me Chicken (page 160)—which you all already love. Rich, creamy, and loaded with sun-dried tomatoes, spinach, and tender chicken, it's comforting in all the right ways. This one's worth bookmarking for weeknights, meal prep, or when you're craving something satisfying *and* protein-forward.

**FOR THE CHICKEN**

2 pounds boneless chicken breasts
½ teaspoon sea salt
½ teaspoon freshly ground black pepper
½ teaspoon paprika
½ teaspoon garlic powder
1 tablespoon avocado oil
½ cup chicken bone broth

**FOR THE SOUP BASE**

1 tablespoon avocado oil
½ cup diced onion
3 cloves garlic, minced
4½ cups chicken bone broth
½ cup chopped sun-dried tomatoes
1 teaspoon Italian seasoning
½ teaspoon paprika
½ teaspoon crushed red pepper flakes
1 tablespoon arrowroot powder

**FINAL ADDITIONS**

1 (14-ounce) can full-fat coconut milk
3 cups baby spinach
½ cup jarred roasted red bell peppers, chopped
1 tablespoon nutritional yeast
Juice of ½ lemon
1 tablespoon chopped fresh basil or parsley, for garnish

1. **Cook the chicken:** Pat the chicken dry and season with the salt, black pepper, paprika, and garlic powder. In a large Dutch oven or heavy-bottomed pot, heat the oil over medium-high heat. Add the chicken and sear for 4 to 5 minutes per side, until golden brown. Pour in the broth, cover, and reduce the heat to medium-low. Let simmer for 8 to 10 minutes, until the chicken is cooked through. Remove the chicken and let rest for 5 minutes before shredding with two forks. Set aside. Pour the cooking liquid into a small bowl and reserve.
2. **Build the soup base:** In the same pot, heat the oil over medium heat. Add the onion and sauté for 4 to 5 minutes, until softened. Stir in the garlic and cook for another 30 seconds, until fragrant. Pour in the reserved cooking liquid and the remaining 4½ cups broth. Stir in the sun-dried tomatoes, Italian seasoning, paprika, red pepper flakes, and a pinch of salt and black pepper. Bring to a gentle simmer.
3. In a small bowl, whisk the arrowroot powder with 2 to 3 tablespoons warm broth until dissolved. Stir the slurry into the soup. Cover and simmer over medium-low heat for 5 to 10 minutes to thicken slightly.
4. **Add the final ingredients:** Return the chicken to the pot and stir in the coconut milk. Simmer for 2 to 3 minutes. Add the spinach, roasted red peppers, and nutritional yeast, stirring until the spinach wilts, 2 to 3 minutes. Squeeze in the lemon juice and stir to combine. Ladle into bowls and garnish with basil.

**STORAGE:** Store in an airtight container in the fridge for up to 4 days, or freeze for up to 2 months. Reheat gently on the stovetop or in the microwave, stirring occasionally. If the soup thickens, add a splash of broth or water to loosen.

**PER SERVING**
Protein: 50g
Carbohydrates: 8g
Fat: 17g

Gluten-Free
Grain-Free
No Added Sugar
**IF MODIFIED:**
Dairy-Free

# Sausage, White Bean, and Kale Soup

**SERVES 4 • PREP TIME: 10 MINUTES • COOK TIME: 45 MINUTES • TOTAL TIME: 55 MINUTES**

This hearty soup is on constant rotation in my house during soup season. But honestly, the broth is light enough to make it year-round. Blended white beans create a creamy (yet totally dairy-free) base, while Italian chicken sausage and kale bring the perfect balance of protein and greens. Whether you're making it ahead for the week or serving it fresh for a cozy dinner, this one never disappoints.

- 3 tablespoons extra-virgin olive oil
- 1 (4-pack, about 12 ounces) precooked Italian chicken sausage, sliced diagonally
- 1 medium yellow onion, diced
- 2 carrots, cut into ½-inch-thick rounds
- 1 tablespoon minced garlic
- 2 (15-ounce) cans white beans, drained and rinsed
- 4 cups chicken bone broth
- 1 bunch lacinato or curly kale, finely chopped
- 1 teaspoon sea salt
- ½ to 1 teaspoon red chili flakes, plus more for garnish
- Freshly ground black pepper
- Freshly grated Parmesan, for garnish (optional)

1. Heat 2 tablespoons of the oil in a large pot over medium heat. Add the chicken sausage and cook for 4 to 6 minutes per side, until seared and lightly browned. Transfer to a plate and set aside.
2. In the same pot, heat the remaining 1 tablespoon oil and add the onion, carrots, and garlic. Cover and sauté for 4 to 5 minutes, until softened.
3. Meanwhile, in a blender, combine one can of the beans with 2 cups of the broth. Blend for 30 seconds, or until smooth.
4. Pour the blended mixture into the pot and add the sausage, the remaining beans, remaining broth, kale, salt, chili flakes, and black pepper. Reduce the heat to medium-low, cover, and let simmer for 25 minutes. Serve immediately, garnished with Parmesan (if using), chili flakes, and additional black pepper.

**STORAGE:** Store in an airtight container in the fridge for up to 4 days, or freeze for up to 2 months. Reheat on the stovetop or in the microwave until hot, adding a splash of broth if needed.

---

**PER SERVING**
Protein: 33g
Carbohydrates: 33g
Fat: 20g

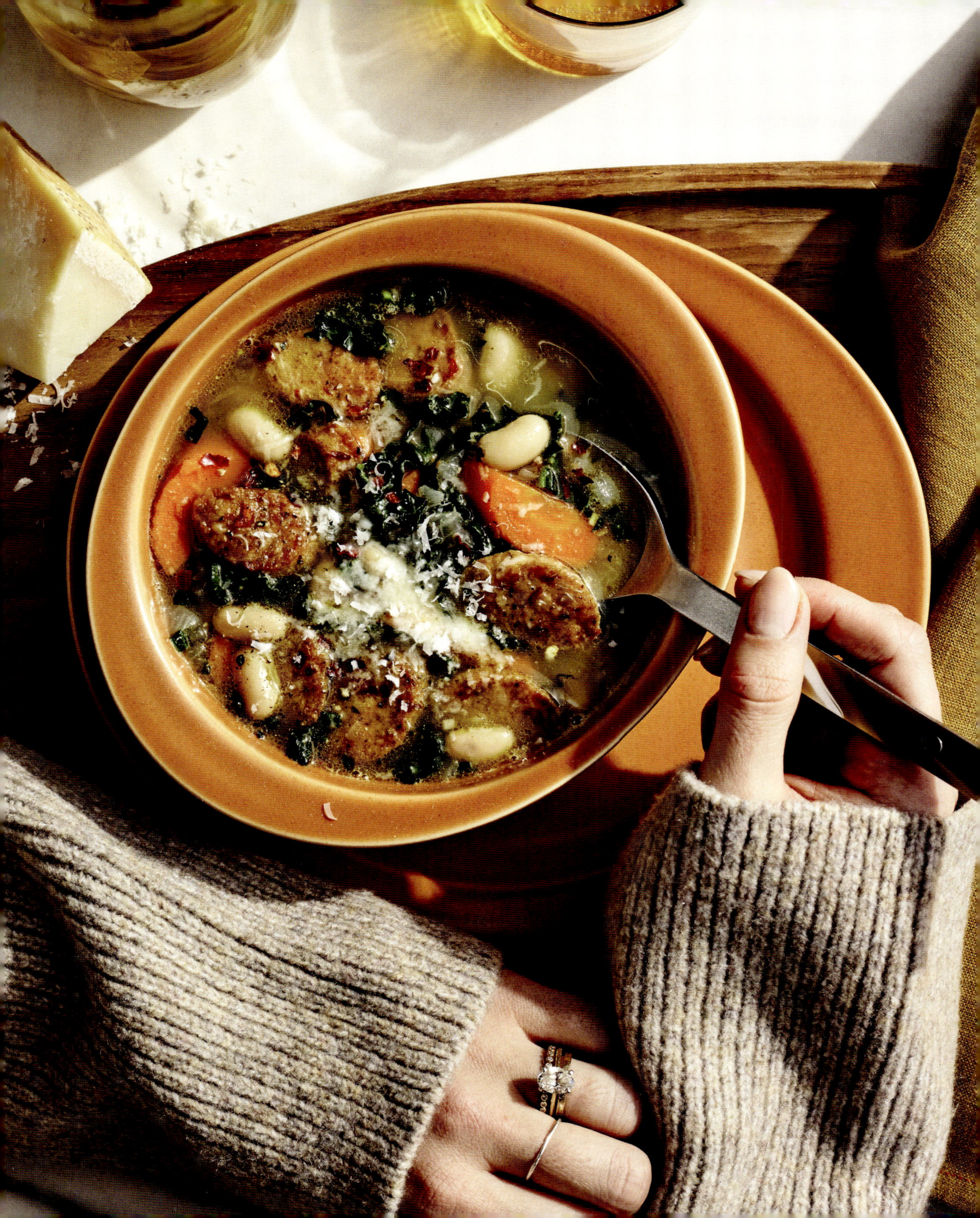

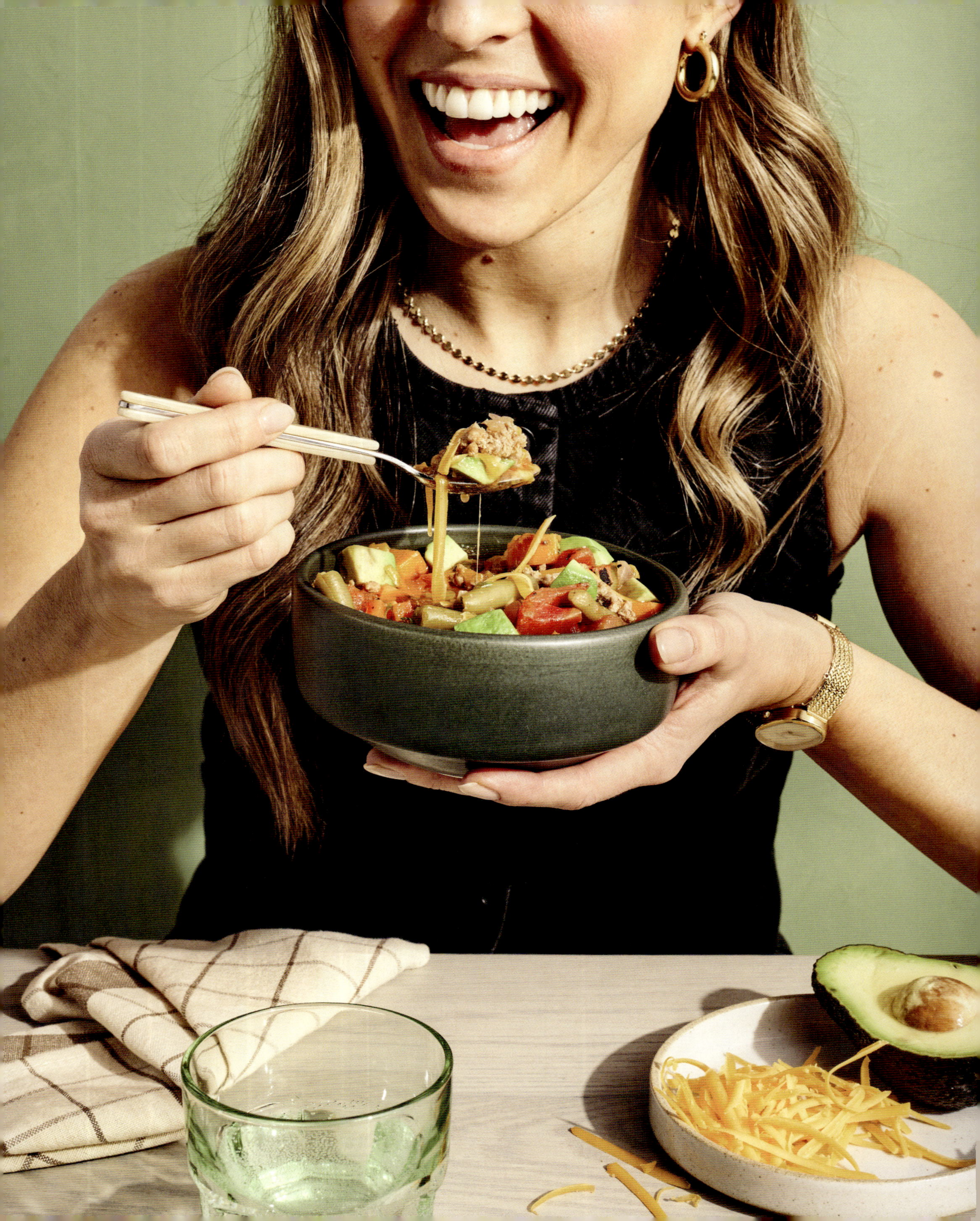

Dairy-Free
Gluten-Free
Grain-Free
No Added Sugar

# Hearty Protein-Packed Chili

**SERVES 4 • PREP TIME: 15 MINUTES • COOK TIME: 30 MINUTES • TOTAL TIME: 45 MINUTES**

- 2 tablespoons avocado oil
- ½ red onion, diced
- 1 pound ground turkey (or preferred ground protein)
- ½ teaspoon chili powder
- ½ teaspoon ground cumin
- ½ teaspoon ground oregano
- ½ teaspoon sea salt
- ¼ teaspoon garlic powder
- ¼ teaspoon red chili flakes
- ⅛ teaspoon paprika
- 1 (15-ounce) can fire-roasted tomatoes
- 3 tablespoons tomato paste
- 2½ cups chicken or beef bone broth
- 1 medium sweet potato, peeled and cut into ½-inch dice
- 1 red bell pepper, seeded and diced (1 cup diced poblano, zucchini, or corn work too)
- 1 (14.5-ounce) can chopped green beans
- 1 cup spinach, chopped (optional)
- Optional toppings: sliced avocado, sour cream, shredded cheese of choice or nutritional yeast, sliced jalapeño, chopped fresh chives, tortilla chips

**PER SERVING**
Protein: 30g
Carbohydrates: 15g
Fat: 10g

This is the chili I've been making the longest—since college, actually—and it's one I come back to again and again. Everything simmers together in one pot, making it a super easy option for busy weeks. It also reheats like a dream, which is why I keep it in heavy rotation when I'm prepping meals ahead.

1. Heat the oil in a medium pot over medium heat. Add the onion and sauté for 2 to 3 minutes, until softened. Add the ground turkey and cook for 2 to 3 minutes, breaking it apart with a wooden spoon as it browns. Stir in the chili powder, cumin, oregano, salt, garlic powder, chili flakes, and paprika, mixing until well combined.
2. Pour in the tomatoes, tomato paste, and broth, stirring to combine. Reduce the heat to medium-low and simmer for 15 minutes.
3. Add the sweet potato, bell pepper, and green beans, cover, and cook for 10 to 15 minutes longer, until the potatoes are tender. Stir in the spinach, if using, letting it wilt into the chili. Serve immediately, topped with avocado, sour cream, cheese, jalapeño, chives, and tortilla chips, if desired.

**STORAGE:** Store in an airtight container in the fridge for up to 5 days or freeze for up to 3 months. Reheat on the stovetop or in the microwave, stirring occasionally, until warmed through.

Dairy-Free
Gluten-Free
Grain-Free
No Added Sugar

# Golden Chicken Bone Broth

MAKES 10 CUPS (10 SERVINGS) • PREP TIME: 5 MINUTES • COOK TIME: 6 TO 8 HOURS IN DUTCH OVEN OR 14 TO 16 HOURS IN SLOW COOKER • TOTAL TIME: 6 TO 16 HOURS

- 2 pounds chicken bones (see Note)
- 1 pound chicken feet (see Note, optional)
- 1 onion, quartered
- 1 large carrot, cut into 2-inch chunks
- 1 celery stalk, halved
- 1 (2- to 3-inch) piece fresh ginger, peeled and halved
- 1 (2- to 3-inch) piece turmeric, halved
- 1 tablespoon whole black peppercorns
- 2 sprigs fresh rosemary or thyme
- 12 cups water
- 1 tablespoon apple cider vinegar
- 1 teaspoon sea salt, plus more to taste

I'm a big fan of making homemade bone broth—it's easier than you think and so worth it. It's rich, golden, and full of flavor, with about 12 grams of protein per cup. I love sipping it between meals or pairing it with lunch or dinner to help stay full and nourished. Thanks to the collagen and minerals from the slow-simmered bones, it's a great support for gut health, immunity, skin, and joints. And hey, if chicken feet aren't your thing, they're totally optional.

1. In a slow cooker, combine the chicken bones, chicken feet (if using), onion, carrot, celery, ginger, turmeric, peppercorns, rosemary, and water. Cover and cook on low for 14 to 16 hours.
2. **If using a Dutch oven instead of a slow cooker:** Combine the chicken bones, chicken feet (if using), onion, carrot, celery, ginger, turmeric, peppercorns, rosemary, and water in a large Dutch oven. Bring to a simmer over medium heat, then reduce to low. Cover with the lid slightly ajar and simmer gently for 6 to 8 hours, checking occasionally and skimming any foam or impurities from the surface.
3. Using a fine-mesh sieve over a large bowl, strain out all the solids, leaving only the liquid in the bowl. Season the broth with the vinegar and salt, adding more as needed to taste. Serve immediately.

**STORAGE:** Store in airtight jars or containers in the fridge for up to 5 days, or freeze for up to 3 months. Reheat on the stovetop until hot. Shake or stir before serving, as natural separation may occur.

**PER SERVING (1 CUP)**
Protein: 12g
Carbohydrates: 1g
Fat: 3g

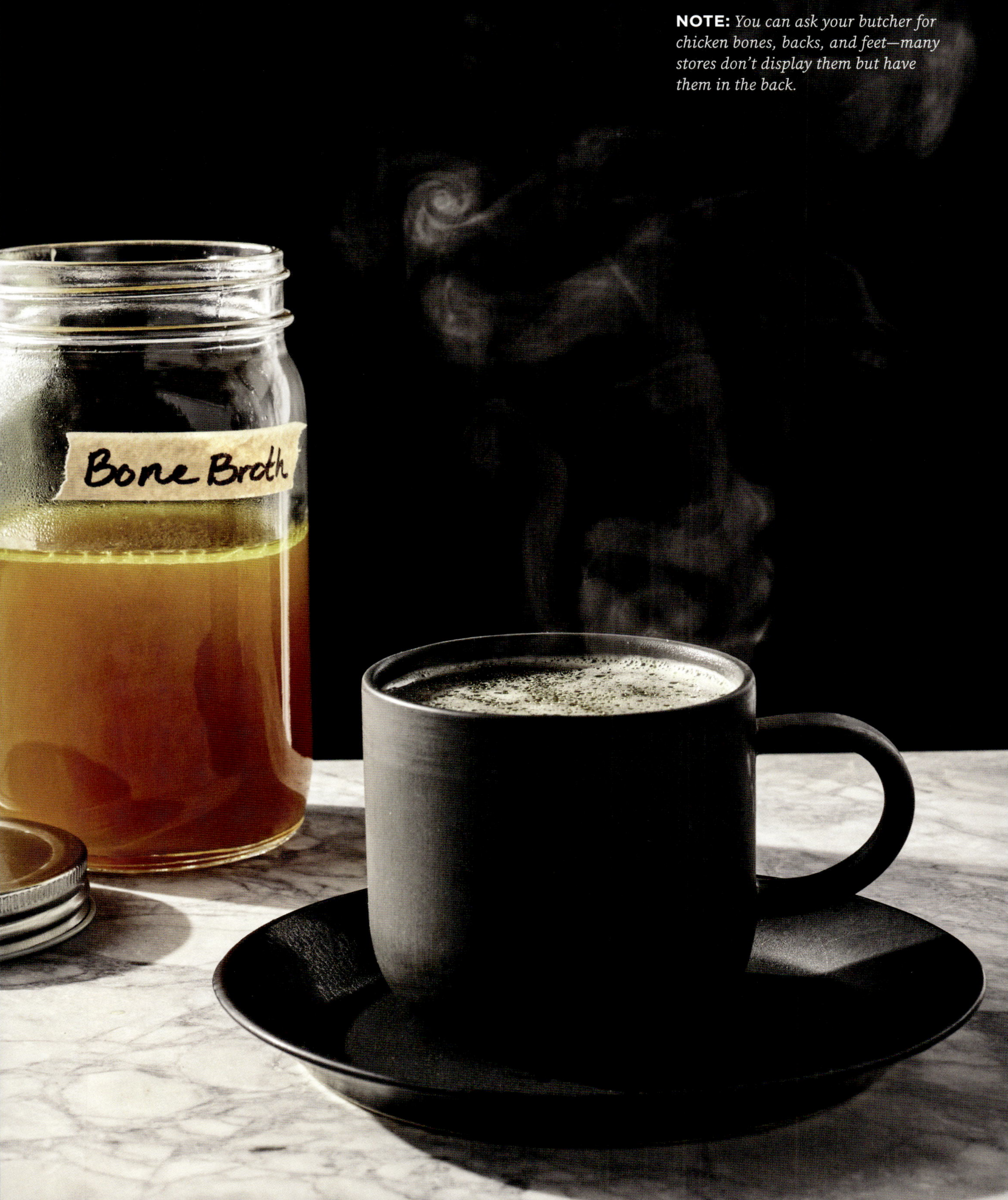


**NOTE:** *You can ask your butcher for chicken bones, backs, and feet—many stores don't display them but have them in the back.*

Gluten-Free
Grain-Free
No Added Sugar
**IF MODIFIED:**
Dairy-Free

# Roasted Butternut Squash Soup with Coconut-Lime Crema

SERVES 4 • PREP TIME: 15 MINUTES • COOK TIME: 45 MINUTES • TOTAL TIME: 1 HOUR

This recipe is sure to impress—and not just on flavor. It's surprisingly high in protein, super filling, and hits all the right notes with warm roasted veggies and cozy spices. The citrusy kick from the coconut-lime crema is the cherry on top. This is my subtle urge for you to try this one!

FOR THE SOUP

- 1 medium butternut squash, peeled and seeded
- 1 red bell pepper, seeded and diced (or 1 cup diced carrots, fennel, or sweet potato)
- 1 small white onion, diced
- 3 to 4 garlic cloves, unpeeled
- 2 tablespoons extra-virgin olive oil
- Sea salt and freshly ground black pepper
- Leaves from 4 sprigs fresh thyme
- ¼ cup pumpkin seeds, for garnish
- 4 cups bone broth, plus more if needed
- 1 (15-ounce) can white beans, drained and rinsed
- ½ cup cottage cheese (optional)
- ½ cup collagen peptides
- 1 tablespoon chopped fresh sage
- ½ teaspoon ground turmeric

FOR THE COCONUT-LIME CREMA

- ½ cup (5.4-ounce can) full-fat coconut cream
- 1 tablespoon grated lime zest
- 1 tablespoon lime juice
- ¼ teaspoon sea salt
- ¼ cup toasted pumpkin seeds, for garnish
- ½ cup crumbled feta, for serving (optional)

---

**PER SERVING**
Protein: 30g
Carbohydrates: 34g
Fat: 16g

1. **Make the soup:** Preheat the oven to 425°F. Line a baking sheet with parchment paper.
2. Combine the butternut squash, bell pepper, onion, garlic, oil, 1 teaspoon salt, and ¼ teaspoon black pepper on the baking sheet and toss to coat evenly. Sprinkle the thyme leaves over the vegetables. Roast for 35 to 40 minutes, until the squash is very tender. Let cool for 5 minutes. Squeeze the roasted garlic cloves out of their skins (discard the skins) and add the garlic flesh to the vegetables.
3. In a dry skillet over medium heat, toast the pumpkin seeds for 2 to 3 minutes, stirring frequently, until golden and fragrant. Set aside.
4. **For an immersion blender:** In a large pot or Dutch oven, combine the roasted vegetables, broth, beans, cottage cheese (if using), collagen peptides, sage, turmeric, 1 teaspoon salt, and ¼ teaspoon pepper. Blend with an immersion blender until smooth. (Or combine the ingredients in a stand blender, working in batches if needed, and blend until smooth.) Adjust with additional broth, if desired. Bring the soup to a simmer over medium heat for 5 to 10 minutes, stirring occasionally, until fully heated through.
5. **Make the coconut-lime crema:** In a medium bowl, whisk together the coconut cream, lime zest, lime juice, and salt until well combined.
6. To serve, ladle the soup into bowls and top with a drizzle of coconut-lime crema, pumpkin seeds, and feta, if using.

**STORAGE:** Store in an airtight container in the fridge for up to 5 days, or freeze for up to 2 months. Reheat on the stovetop over low heat or in the microwave until warmed through. Store crema separately and add just before serving.

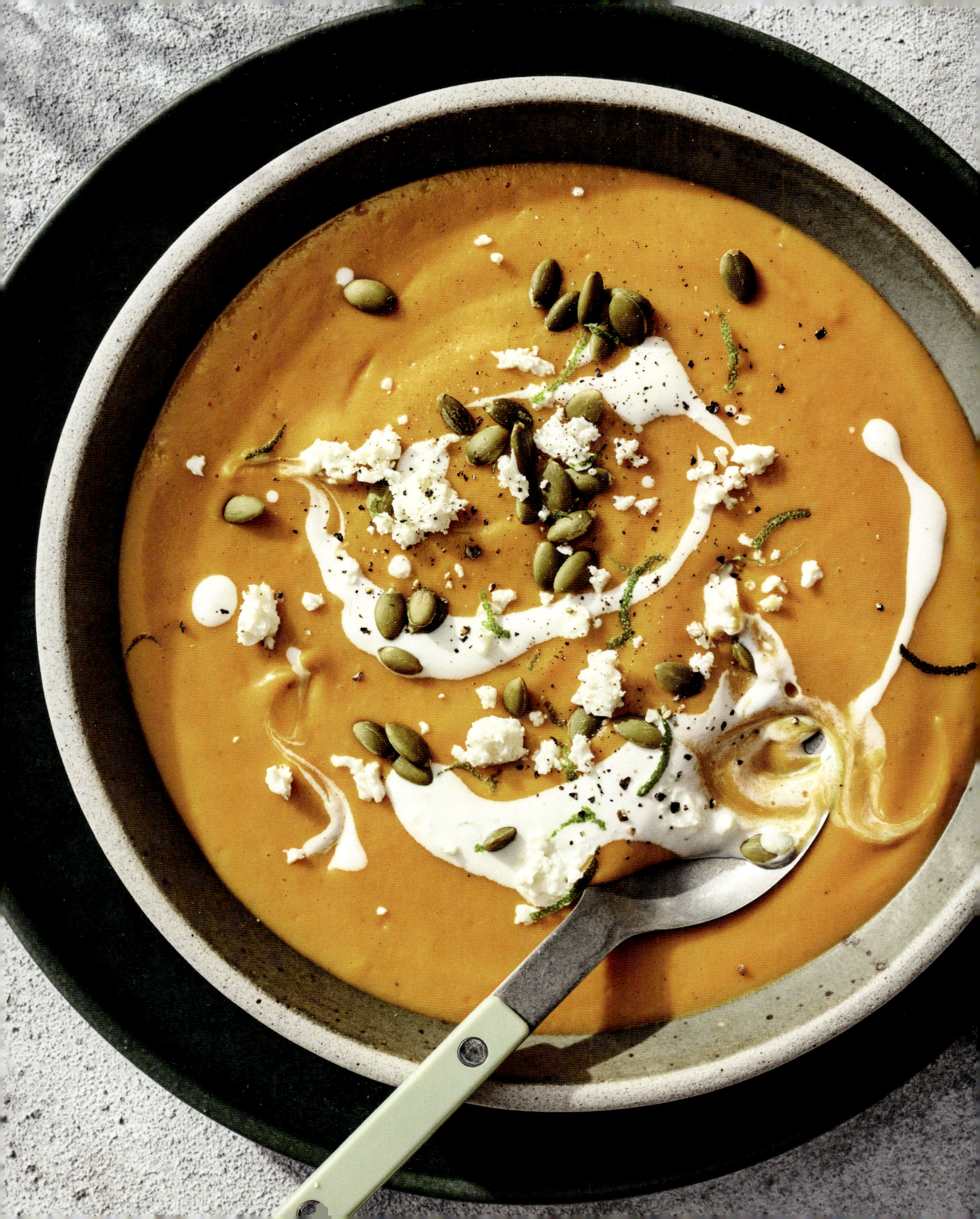

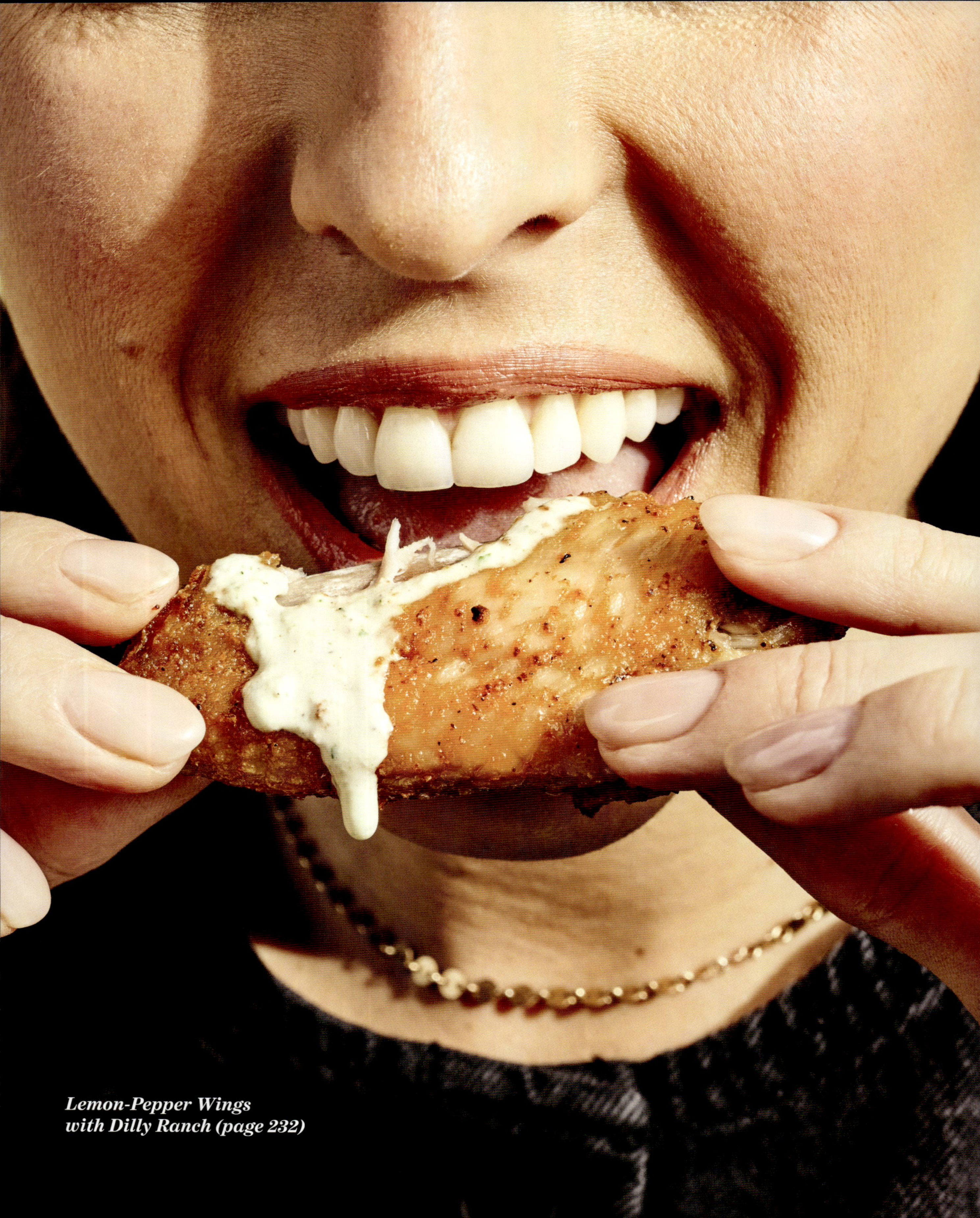

*Lemon-Pepper Wings*
*with Dilly Ranch* *(page 232)*

232 **Lemon-Pepper Wings with Dilly Ranch**

234 **Birthday Cake Bliss Balls**

237 **Game-Day Buffalo Chicken Dip**

238 **Savory Beefy Queso Dip**

241 **Crispy Ranch Air-Fryer Chickpeas**

242 **Savory Cottage Cheese Bowls**

245 **Avocado Whipped Feta**

246 **Banana Bread Protein Muffins**

248 **Magic Shell Yogurt Bowl**

# Satisfying Snacks

Gluten-Free
Grain-Free
**IF MODIFIED:**
Dairy-Free

# Lemon-Pepper Wings with Dilly Ranch

**SERVES 4 • PREP TIME: 20 MINUTES • COOK TIME: 20 MINUTES • TOTAL TIME: 40 MINUTES**

**FOR THE WINGS**

- 2 pounds chicken wings
- 1 tablespoon baking powder
- 1 teaspoon garlic powder
- 1 teaspoon onion powder
- 1 teaspoon smoked paprika
- 1 teaspoon sea salt
- ½ teaspoon freshly ground black pepper
- Avocado oil spray

These wings are going head-to-head with my Honey Glazed Garlic Chicken Wings from my first cookbook—and honestly, I can't pick a winner. You'll just have to make both and decide for yourself. Baked or air-fried until golden and crispy, they get tossed in a buttery lemon-pepper sauce that gives them an incredibly mouthwatering, citrusy finish. And because wings deserve a proper dip, the dairy-free dilly ranch ties it all together. **Pro tip:** Double the ranch and use it throughout the week with sliced veggies or alongside anything spicy. Because everything's better with a little ranch, right?

1. **Prep the wings:** Pat the chicken wings dry with paper towels. In a large bowl, toss them with the baking powder, garlic powder, onion powder, paprika, salt, and pepper until well coated.

COOK THE WINGS

2. **Oven method:** Preheat the oven to 400°F. Line a baking sheet with a wire rack and lightly spray with avocado oil. Arrange the wings in a single layer on the rack and spray with more avocado oil. Bake for 20 minutes. Flip the wings and bake for another 20 to 25 minutes, until crispy and the internal temperature reaches 165°F.
3. **Air-fryer method:** Preheat the air fryer to 375°F. Lightly spray the wings with avocado oil, then arrange the wings in a single layer in the basket. Cook for 10 minutes, shake the basket, and cook for another 10 minutes, until crispy and cooked through.

---

**PER SERVING**
Protein: 45g
Carbohydrates: 8g
Fat: 44g

FOR THE LEMON-PEPPER SAUCE

2 tablespoons ghee (or vegan butter for dairy-free), slightly melted

1 tablespoon extra-virgin olive oil

1 tablespoon grated lemon zest (2 lemons), plus more for garnish

2 tablespoons fresh lemon juice

1 small clove garlic, minced

1 teaspoon honey

½ teaspoon sea salt

1 teaspoon freshly ground black pepper

FOR THE DAIRY-FREE DILLY RANCH

½ cup raw cashews, soaked in boiling water for 10 minutes, then drained

1 tablespoon fresh lemon juice, plus more for serving

1 teaspoon apple cider vinegar

1 clove garlic, minced

¼ teaspoon onion powder

¼ teaspoon sea salt, plus more for garnish

¼ teaspoon freshly ground black pepper

3 tablespoons fresh herbs (dill, parsley, chives), finely chopped

MAKE THE SAUCE

4. **For the lemon-pepper sauce:** In a large bowl, whisk together the ghee, olive oil, lemon zest, lemon juice, garlic, honey, salt, and pepper.

   **For the ranch:** In a blender, combine the cashews, lemon juice, vinegar, garlic, onion powder, salt, and pepper. Blend on high for 30 seconds, until smooth. If needed, add water, 1 tablespoon at a time, to thin to your desired consistency. Transfer to a small bowl and stir in the herbs. Taste and adjust seasoning with more lemon juice, salt, or pepper as needed.

5. Once the wings are hot and crispy, transfer to the bowl with the lemon-pepper sauce and toss to coat. Garnish with extra lemon zest and pepper, if desired. Serve immediately with the ranch on the side.

**STORAGE:** Store wings in an airtight container in the fridge for up to 4 days. Reheat in the oven or air fryer at 375°F for 6 to 8 minutes, until crisp and warmed through. Store ranch separately and serve chilled.

Dairy-Free
Gluten-Free
Grain-Free

# Birthday Cake Bliss Balls

**MAKES 12 BALLS • PREP TIME: 15 MINUTES, PLUS 30 MINUTES CHILLING • TOTAL TIME: 45 MINUTES**

Some people go for cake pops—I'll happily take these birthday cake bliss balls instead. They're a little more dense, a lot more functional, and way easier to make. No baking required—just mix, roll, and stash in the fridge or freezer for a quick grab-and-go treat. And yes, rainbow sprinkles are non-negotiable!

**½ cup cashew butter (or almond butter)**
**½ cup vanilla protein powder**
**⅓ cup almond flour**
**3½ tablespoons maple syrup (or honey)**
**1 tablespoon coconut milk or almond milk**
**1 teaspoon vanilla extract**
**¼ teaspoon almond extract**
**Pinch of sea salt**
**2 tablespoons naturally colored rainbow sprinkles, plus more for rolling**
**Shredded desiccated coconut, for rolling, optional**

1. Line a plate or small baking sheet with parchment paper.
2. In a medium bowl, combine the cashew butter, protein powder, almond flour, maple syrup, coconut milk, vanilla, almond extract, and salt and mix into a dough consistency. Add the sprinkles and mix until incorporated.
3. Scoop heaping tablespoons of the dough and roll into balls; you should have 12 balls. Roll each ball in the additional sprinkles and coconut, if using.
4. Refrigerate for 30 minutes, until the dough is set. At this point, you can enjoy them right away or transfer to an airtight container. Store in the fridge for up to 1 week, or freeze for up to 3 months. They're just as good straight from the freezer!

---

**PER SERVING (1 BALL)**
Protein: 5g
Carbohydrates: 8g
Fat: 4g

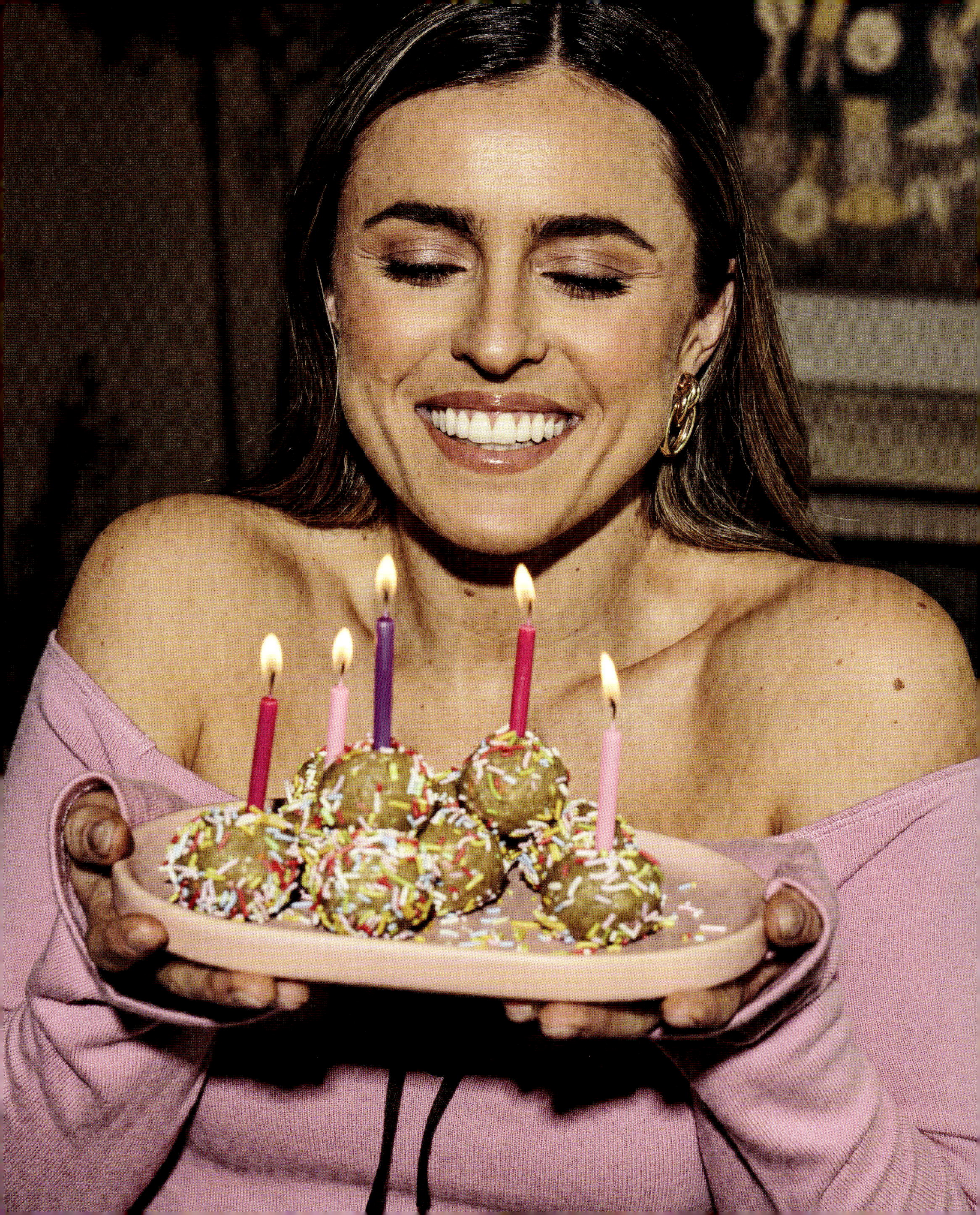

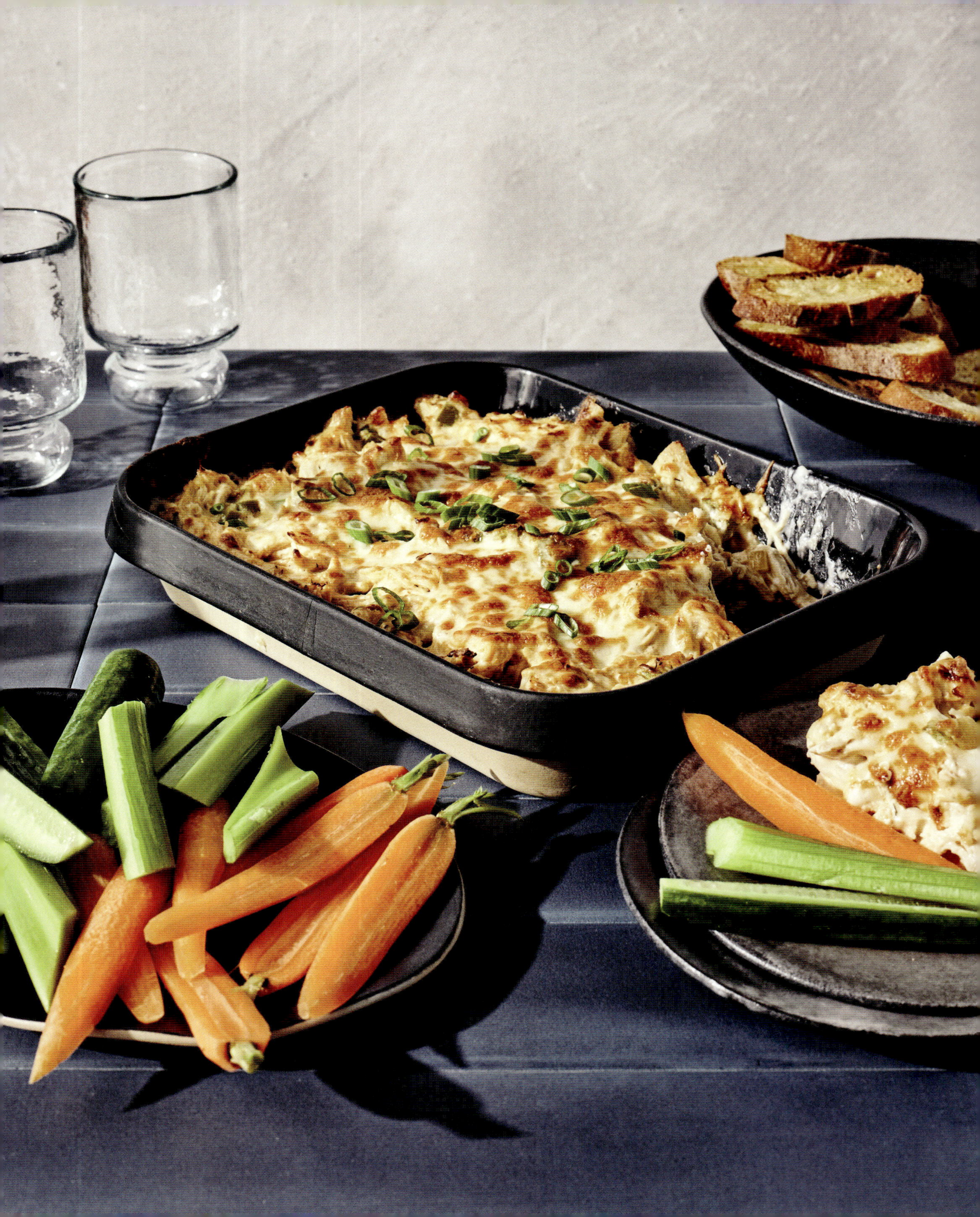

Gluten-Free
Grain-Free
No Added Sugar
**IF MODIFIED:**
Dairy-Free

# Game-Day Buffalo Chicken Dip

**SERVES 10 • PREP TIME: 15 MINUTES • COOK TIME: 30 MINUTES • TOTAL TIME: 45 MINUTES**

- **1 tablespoon ghee or avocado oil**
- **½ cup diced yellow onion**
- **1 (4-ounce) can green chilies**
- **½ teaspoon garlic powder**
- **½ teaspoon onion powder**
- **¼ teaspoon dried dill**
- **1 cup (8 ounces) cream cheese (or dairy-free cream cheese)**
- **3 to 4 cups shredded Buffalo chicken (from Buffalo Chicken Baked Tacos, page 148)**
- **1¼ cups shredded cheese (or dairy-free shredded cheese)**
- **3 green onions, white and green parts, chopped, for garnish**
- **For serving (optional): tortilla chips, toasted baguette slices, raw carrots, bell peppers, cucumber, celery**

This is the ultimate game-day dip—hot, creamy, and memorable for its bold, spicy flavor. You can easily prep it with leftovers from my Buffalo Chicken Baked Tacos (page 148) so you get two epic meals in one, or make the Buffalo chicken fresh; it's that good. Baked until golden and bubbly, the dip pairs perfectly with crunchy veggies, tortilla chips, or toasted baguette slices. Just a heads-up: You'll be looking for excuses to make this one on repeat.

1. Preheat the oven to 400°F. Lightly grease an 10 x 8-inch baking dish.
2. In a medium skillet, heat the ghee over medium heat. Add the onion and sauté for 4 to 5 minutes, until softened. Reduce the heat to medium-low and stir in the green chilies, garlic powder, onion powder, and dried dill. Add the cream cheese and stir until fully melted and combined. Mix in the chicken and 1 cup of the cheese, stirring until everything is evenly incorporated.
3. Transfer the chicken mixture to the baking dish and spread evenly. Top with the remaining ¼ cup cheese. Bake for 25 minutes, until hot and bubbling around the edges, then broil for 2 to 3 minutes, until the top is golden and bubbly. Keep a close eye to prevent burning.
4. Garnish with green onions and serve immediately with chips, baguette slices, and/or raw veggies.

**STORAGE:** Store in an airtight container in the fridge for up to 4 days. Reheat in the microwave or in a 350°F oven until hot and bubbly. Stir before serving.

**PER SERVING (FOR 10 SERVINGS)**
Protein: 26g
Carbohydrates: 2g
Fat: 18g

**NOTE**: *Make 2 servings of the shredded Buffalo chicken from the Buffalo Chicken Baked Tacos (page 148), using one serving for the tacos and one serving for this dip.*

Dairy-Free
Gluten-Free
Grain-Free
No Added Sugar

# Savory Beefy Queso Dip

SERVES 4 TO 6 • PREP TIME: 30 MINUTES, INCLUDING SOAKING THE CASHEWS • COOK TIME: 10 MINUTES • TOTAL TIME: 40 MINUTES

FOR THE QUESO

**1½ cups raw cashews**

**2 cups boiling water, for soaking**

**1 cup unsweetened almond milk**

**¼ cup nutritional yeast**

**1 clove garlic, smashed**

**1 jalapeño, seeded and diced**

**½ teaspoon apple cider vinegar**

**½ teaspoon ground turmeric**

**½ teaspoon paprika**

**½ teaspoon onion powder**

**1 teaspoon sea salt**

FOR THE BEEF

**1 tablespoon extra-virgin olive oil**

**1 pound ground beef**

**2 tablespoons taco seasoning (I like Siete)**

**1 (10-ounce) can diced tomatoes with green chilies**

**For serving: ¼ cup chopped cilantro, sliced fresh or pickled jalapeños (optional), grain-free tortilla chips**

This creamy, rich queso dip delivers everything you love about a classic queso—just without the dairy. Made with cashews, nutritional yeast, and warm spices, it's rich, savory, and sneakily high in protein thanks to grass-fed beef. And if you're wondering whether a dairy-free queso can actually hold up—Bridger has signed off on it and given it his approval, which is a big deal: You know it's legit. Serve it warm with tortilla chips or fresh veggies, or scoop it over any Tex-Mex dish.

1. **Make the queso:** In a heatproof bowl or large glass, cover the cashews with the boiling water and soak for 30 minutes. Drain. In a blender, combine the cashews, almond milk, nutritional yeast, garlic, jalapeño, vinegar, turmeric, paprika, onion powder, and salt. Blend on high for 30 seconds, or until smooth and creamy. Set aside.
2. **Cook the beef:** In a large skillet, heat the oil over medium heat. Add the ground beef and taco seasoning and cook for 7 to 8 minutes, until browned and cooked through. Stir in the tomatoes and green chilies and cook for another 2 to 3 minutes, until some of the liquid has evaporated.
3. Reduce the heat to low and stir in the cashew queso. Cook for 1 to 2 minutes, just until warmed through.
4. Transfer the beef mixture to a serving bowl and top with the cilantro and jalapeños, if using. Serve warm with tortilla chips.

**STORAGE:** Store in an airtight container in the fridge for up to 4 days. Reheat gently on the stovetop or in the microwave, stirring occasionally, adding a splash of almond milk or broth if the dip is thick.

---

**PER SERVING (FOR 6 SERVINGS)**
Protein: 24g
Carbohydrates: 16g
Fat: 25g

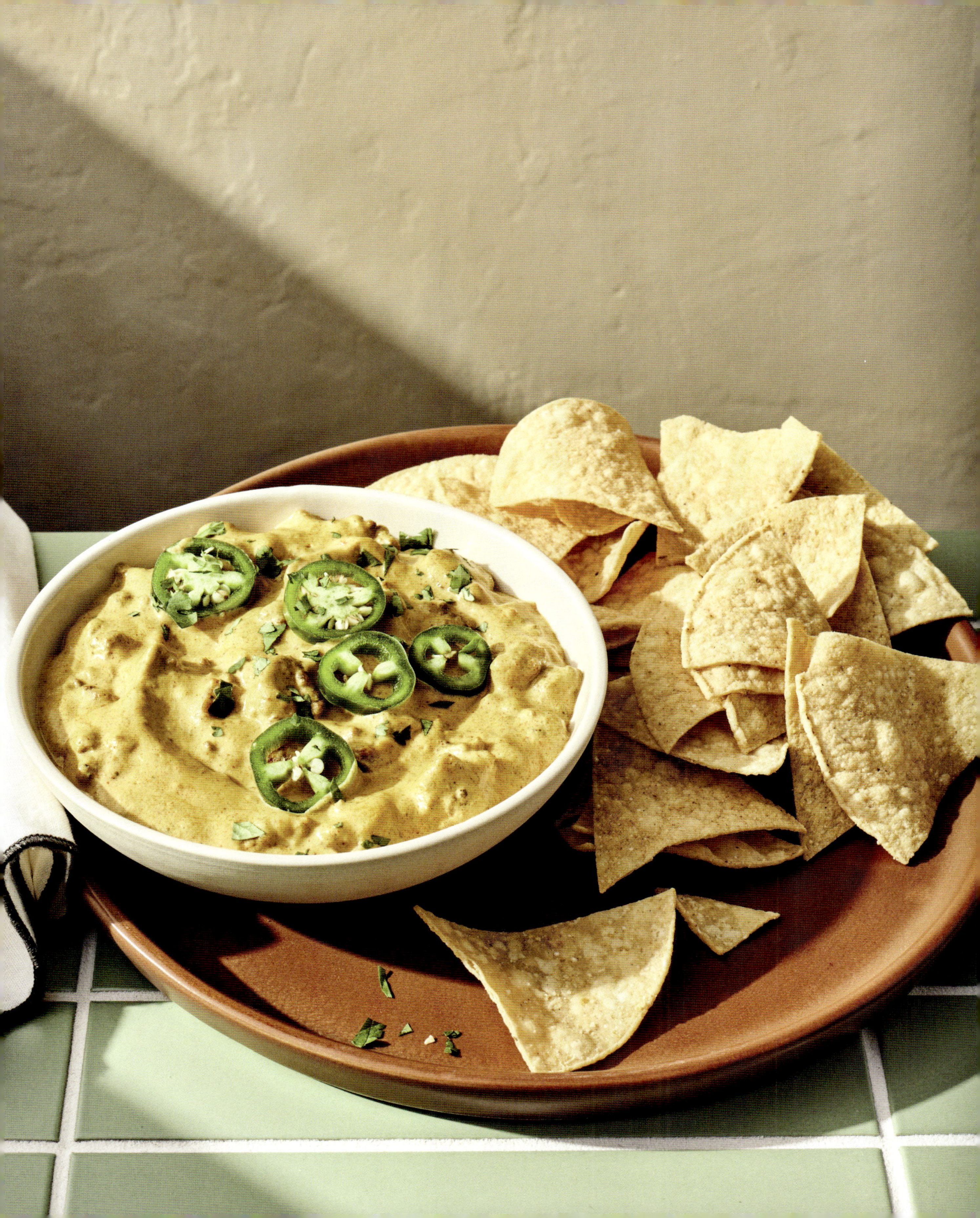

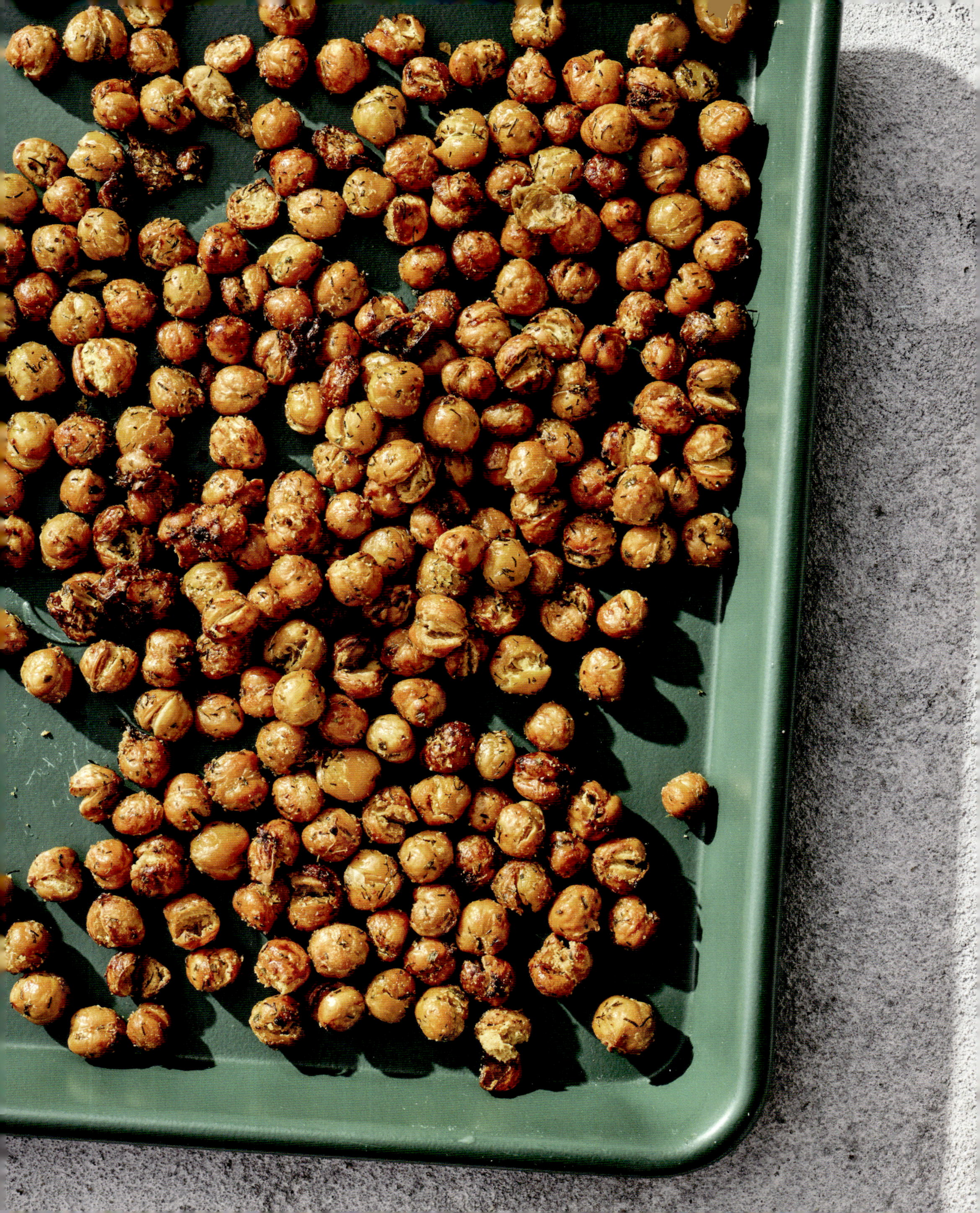

Dairy-Free
Gluten-Free
Grain-Free
No Added Sugar

# Crispy Ranch Air-Fryer Chickpeas

**SERVES 2 • PREP TIME: 5 MINUTES • COOK TIME: 15 MINUTES • TOTAL TIME: 20 MINUTES**

- 1 (15-ounce) can chickpeas, drained and rinsed
- 1 tablespoon extra-virgin olive oil
- ½ teaspoon dried dill
- ½ teaspoon dried parsley
- ¼ teaspoon garlic powder
- ¼ teaspoon onion powder
- ¼ teaspoon sea salt

These light and crunchy chickpeas are the perfect high-protein snack. Seasoned with savory ranch-inspired herbs, they turn irresistibly crispy in the air fryer in just minutes. Sprinkle over salads, grain bowls, or soups—or enjoy them straight from the bowl. Store in an airtight container to keep crisp for days—they're meal-prep friendly and a solid pick for anytime snacking.

1. Preheat the air fryer to 400°F. In a medium bowl, combine the chickpeas, oil, dill, parsley, garlic powder, onion powder, and salt. Toss until the chickpeas are evenly coated.
2. Transfer the chickpeas to the air fryer basket in a single layer. Air-fry for 6 minutes, shake the basket, then continue cooking for 6 to 8 minutes more, until crispy and golden brown. Let cool for 5 minutes before serving.

**STORAGE:** Store in an airtight container at room temperature for up to 3 days. For maximum crunch, let them cool completely before sealing. If they lose crispiness, pop them back in the air fryer for 2 to 3 minutes.

**PER SERVING**
Protein: 11g
Carbohydrates: 25g
Fat: 10g

Gluten-Free
Grain-Free
No Added Sugar

# Savory Cottage Cheese Bowls

**SERVES 2 • PREP TIME: 20 MINUTES, INCLUDING 10 MINUTES CHILLING • COOK TIME: 6 MINUTES • TOTAL TIME: 25 MINUTES**

- 2 large eggs
- 1 (16-ounce) container full-fat cottage cheese
- 1 ripe avocado, sliced
- 1 cup cherry tomatoes, halved
- 2 Persian cucumbers, sliced
- ¼ cup sunflower seeds
- 1 tablespoon hemp seeds
- 1 tablespoon sesame seeds (I like using both black and white)
- Extra-virgin olive oil, for serving
- Flaky salt, for garnish

I love a snack that takes almost no effort but still hits every note—creamy, crunchy, savory, and seriously good. This bowl is not only a terrific high-protein snack, it's incredible for busy mornings or a quick lunch. I love how the creamy cottage cheese is balanced with crunchy seeds and perfectly jammy eggs. It's simple, full of protein, and exactly the kind of snack that holds you over to the next meal.

1. In a small saucepan, bring 2 to 3 inches of water (enough to cover the eggs) to a boil over high heat. Add the eggs and cook for 6 to 7 minutes, depending on how jammy you like them. Meanwhile, prepare an ice bath in a small bowl. Transfer the eggs to the ice bath and chill for 10 to 15 minutes. Peel the eggs and slice in half.
2. Divide the cottage cheese between two bowls. Top each with egg halves, avocado, tomatoes, cucumbers, sunflower seeds, hemp seeds, and sesame seeds. Garnish with a drizzle of oil and flaky salt. Serve immediately.

**PER SERVING**
Protein: 41g
Carbohydrates: 22g
Fat: 36g

**TIP**: *To peel a hard-boiled egg, crack it on a hard surface and roll it on the surface with your entire palm. Cup the egg with a spoon and find an opening within the shell. Twist the spoon inside to remove the shell entirely.*

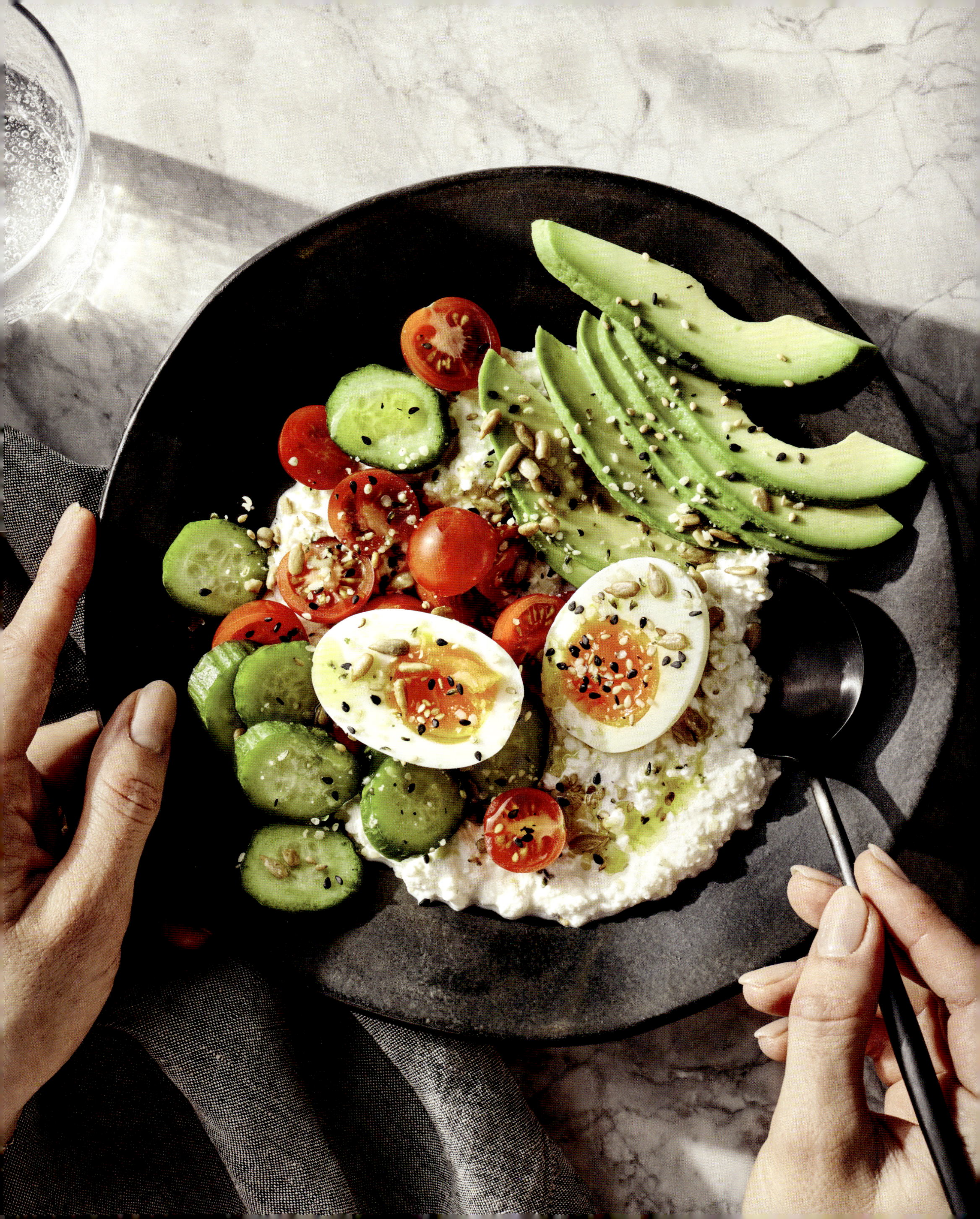

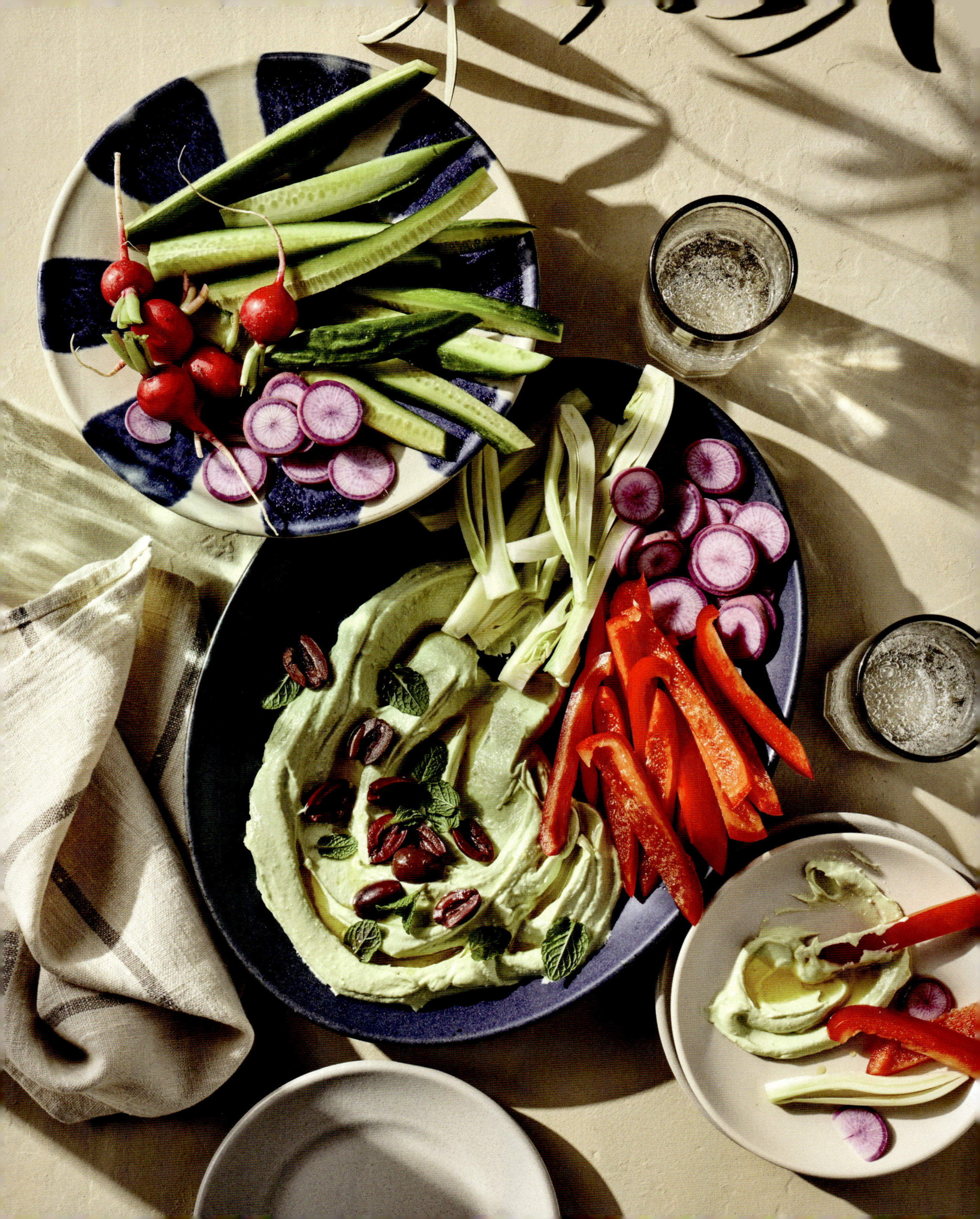

Gluten-Free
Grain-Free

# Avocado Whipped Feta

**SERVES 4 • PREP TIME: 15 MINUTES • TOTAL TIME: 15 MINUTES**

**8 ounces feta**

**⅓ cup full-fat plain Greek yogurt**

**3 tablespoons extra-virgin olive oil**

**1 ripe avocado**

**1 clove garlic, smashed**

**Savory toppings: kalamata olives, extra-virgin olive oil, finely chopped fresh mint**

**Sweet toppings: raw honey, crushed pistachios**

**For serving: fresh veggies, pita bread, crackers, toasted sourdough baguette**

If you've had whipped feta before, you know it's next-level creamy and instantly makes anything you dip into it better. I add full-fat Greek yogurt to bump up the protein and avocado for even more richness. It's ultra-smooth, super versatile, and easy to customize—go sweet with honey and pistachios or savory with olives and mint. Either way, it's a guaranteed crowd-pleaser.

1. In the bowl of a food processor, combine the feta, yogurt, oil, avocado, and garlic and process for 30 seconds, or until smooth and creamy.
2. Transfer to a serving platter or bowl, top with desired toppings, and serve immediately with dippers of choice.

---

**PER SERVING**
Protein: 7g
Carbohydrates: 5g
Fat: 19g

**NOTE:** *This dip is best served fresh, as avocado can discolor slightly over time. If you're prepping ahead, add a teaspoon of lemon juice to help maintain its vibrant color.*

Dairy-Free
Gluten-Free
Grain-Free

# Banana Bread Protein Muffins

**SERVES 12 • PREP TIME: 15 MINUTES • COOK TIME: 15 MINUTES, PLUS 15 MINUTES COOLING • TOTAL TIME: 45 MINUTES**

- Avocado oil spray
- 3 very ripe bananas (about 1 cup mashed)
- 3 large eggs
- ¼ cup almond milk
- ¼ cup coconut oil, melted and cooled to room temperature
- 2 tablespoons maple syrup
- 2 tablespoons coconut sugar
- 1 teaspoon vanilla extract
- 1¾ cups almond flour, sifted
- ½ cup vanilla protein powder
- 1 teaspoon baking powder
- ½ teaspoon baking soda
- ½ teaspoon ground cinnamon
- ¼ teaspoon sea salt
- ½ cup walnuts, toasted and chopped
- ½ cup dairy-free dark chocolate chips, plus more for topping if you like
- 5 tablespoons hemp seeds

You know when you're running out the door and wish you had something quick and comforting to bite into? These are made for that moment—especially if you've got littles—because everyone can enjoy them on the go. Hayes is obsessed with them, which makes my mornings ten times easier. But if you're not in a rush, they're just as good warm with a swipe of ghee or nut butter and a cup of tea. Basically, they fit whatever kind of morning you're having.

1. Preheat the oven to 350°F. Grease a 12-cup muffin tin with avocado oil spray.
2. In a large bowl, combine the bananas, eggs, almond milk, coconut oil, maple syrup, coconut sugar, and vanilla. Mix until smooth. Add the almond flour, protein powder, baking powder, baking soda, cinnamon, and salt. Stir until just combined. Fold in the walnuts, chocolate chips, and 3 tablespoons of the hemp seeds.
3. Divide the batter evenly among the muffin cups, filling each about three-fourths full. Sprinkle the remaining 2 tablespoons hemp seeds over the tops, along with extra chocolate chips, if desired. Bake for 15 to 20 minutes, until golden brown and a toothpick inserted in the middle comes out clean. Let the muffins cool for 15 minutes before serving.

**STORAGE:** Store in an airtight container at room temperature for up to 3 days, or in the fridge for up to 5 days. Freeze for up to 2 months. Reheat in the microwave or toaster oven, if desired.

**PER SERVING**
Protein: 10g
Carbohydrates: 15g
Fat: 21g

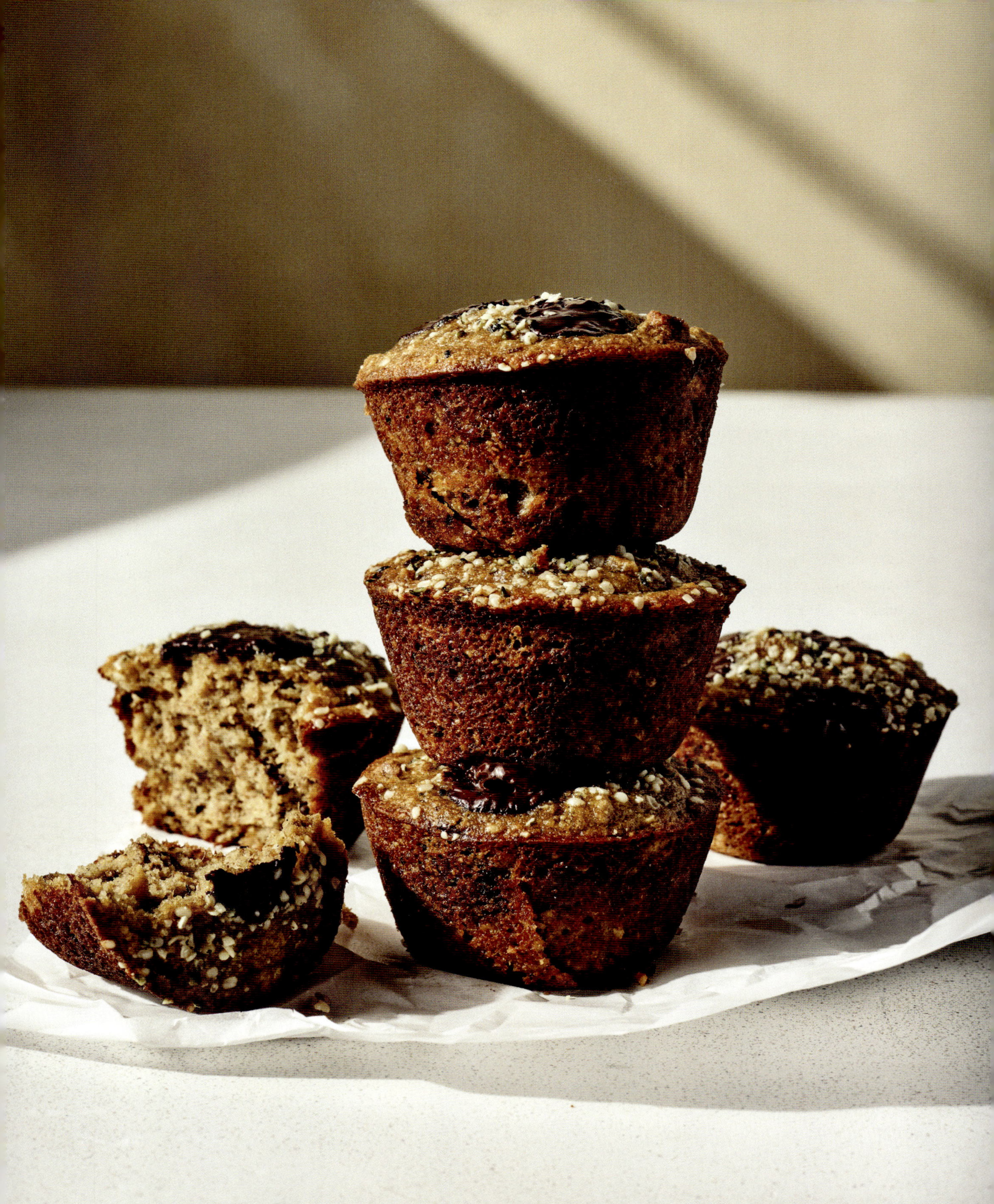

Gluten-Free
Grain-Free
**IF MODIFIED:**
Dairy-Free

# Magic Shell Yogurt Bowl

**SERVES 1 • PREP TIME: 10 MINUTES, PLUS 15 MINUTES CHILLING • TOTAL TIME: 25 MINUTES**

Thick, creamy yogurt mixed with vanilla protein powder gets topped with a drizzle of melted chocolate that hardens into a crackly shell, the kind we all loved as kids. It's sweet, salty, creamy, crunchy—basically, dessert disguised as a snack that will keep you on track. One bite and you'll be hooked.

**½ cup unsweetened full-fat plain Greek yogurt (or coconut yogurt for dairy-free)**
**3 tablespoons vanilla protein powder**
**¼ teaspoon ground cinnamon**
**1 tablespoon unsweetened peanut butter (or preferred nut butter)**
**2 tablespoons dairy-free dark chocolate chips**
**Flaky salt**

1. In a small bowl, mix the yogurt, protein powder, and cinnamon until fully combined. Smooth the top of the yogurt with the back of a spoon. Spread the peanut butter into a thin layer over the yogurt. To melt the chocolate, microwave in a small bowl in 20-second intervals, stirring between each, until smooth. Or melt in a double boiler over low heat, stirring frequently, until fully melted. Pour the melted chocolate evenly over the top, spreading it into a thin layer to cover the surface completely.
2. Chill in the fridge for 15 minutes to 1 hour, until the chocolate is hardened. Sprinkle with flaky salt and serve immediately.

**PER SERVING**
Protein: 35g
Carbohydrates: 20g
Fat: 23g

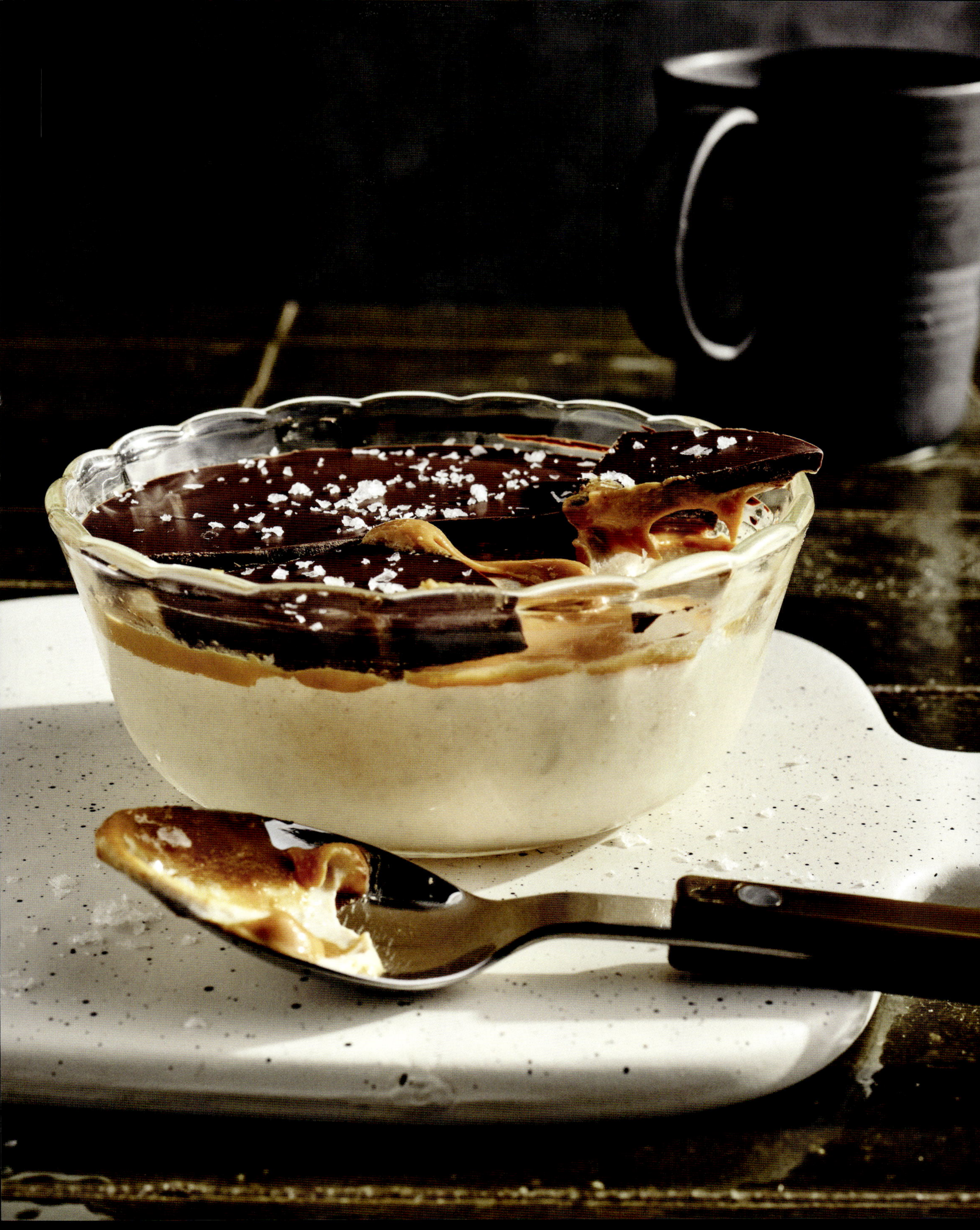

# Yes, There's Protein in Dessert

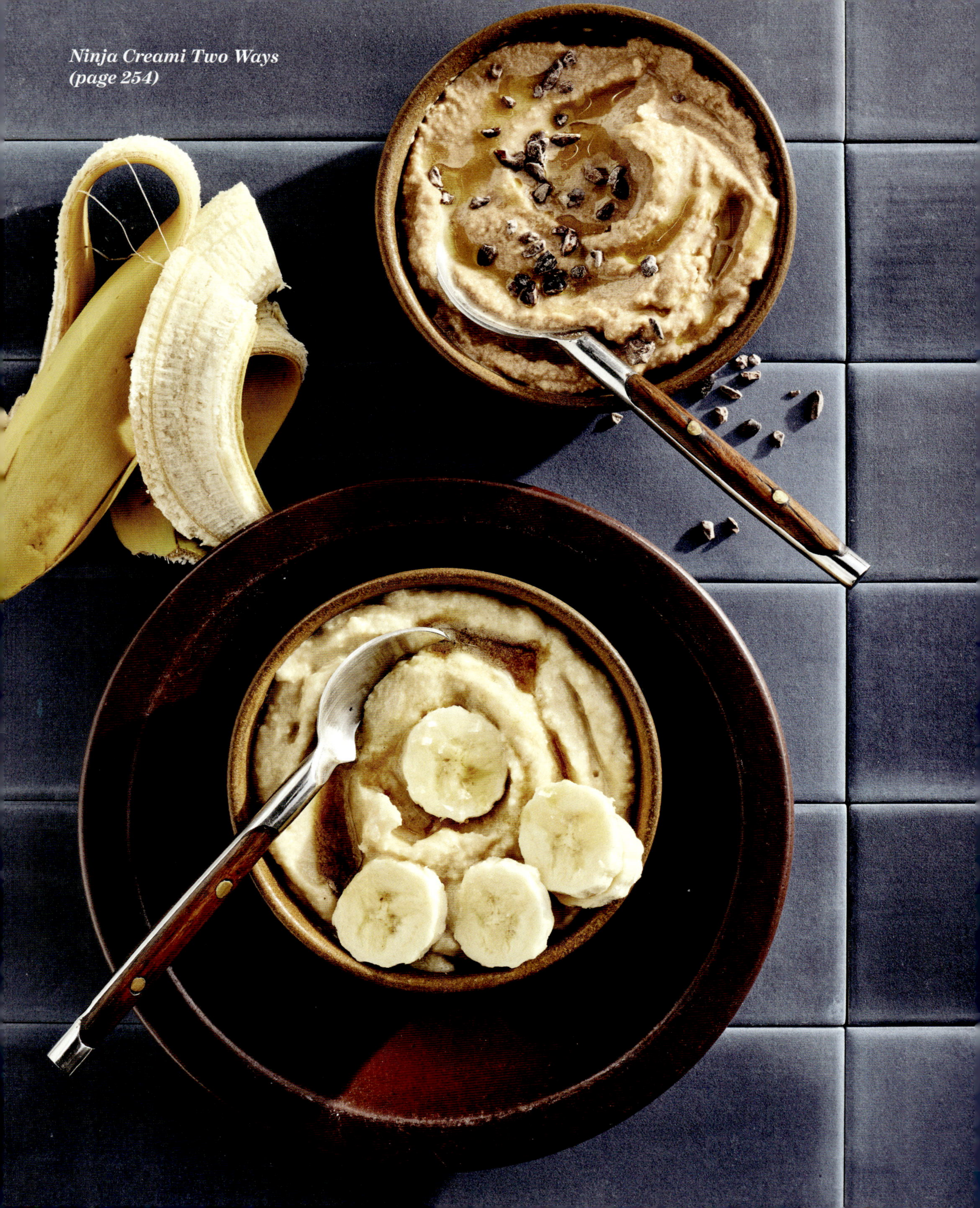

*Ninja Creami Two Ways*
*(page 254)*

254 **Ninja Creami Ice Cream Two Ways**

257 **Chocolate-Coconut Caramel Tart**

258 **Fudge Brownies**

261 **Raspberry-Vanilla Protein Mug Cake**

262 **Sweet and Salty Candy Bark**

265 **Mini Apple Tarts**

266 **Peppermint Patties**

269 **Protein Muddy Buddies**

270 **Brown Butter–Chocolate Chip Cookies**

273 **Strawberry Cheesecake Pudding**

# Desserts

Dairy-Free
Gluten-Free
Grain-Free

# Ninja Creami Two Ways

## *Double Chocolate Ice Cream*

**SERVES 1 • PREP TIME: 15 MINUTES, PLUS 12 HOURS FREEZING • TOTAL TIME: 12 HOURS 15 MINUTES**

- 1 cup almond or cashew milk (plus an additional 2 to 3 tablespoons if using a traditional blender)
- ¼ cup chocolate protein powder (dairy-free if preferred)
- 2 tablespoons unflavored collagen peptides
- 2 tablespoons maple syrup
- 2 tablespoons cacao nibs, plus more for garnish
- Optional toppings: extra-virgin olive oil, flaky salt

Okay here's the thing—people love ice cream. So I created two flavor combos that taste just as indulgent as the real thing, but with better (and fewer) ingredients and a solid dose of protein. Whether you're into deep chocolatey richness or craving that salty-sweet caramel fix, these frozen treats deliver. No Ninja Creami? No problem—a high-speed blender works just as well.

1. **To make in a Ninja Creami:** Warm the Ninja Creami container by briefly rinsing it with hot water. In the container, whisk together the almond milk, protein powder, collagen peptides, and maple syrup until smooth. You can also use an electric hand frother to do this. Place the container in the freezer and freeze for at least 12 hours.
2. Let sit at room temperature for 10 minutes. Place the container in the Ninja Creami and run on the full Light Ice Cream cycle. Scrape down the sides and add the cacao nibs, then place back in the machine and run on the Mix-In cycle.
3. Serve immediately, topped with extra cacao nibs, a drizzle of oil, and flaky salt.
4. **To make in a high-powered blender:** Whisk together the 1 cup almond milk, protein powder, collagen peptides, and maple syrup. Pour the mixture into a silicone ice cube tray and freeze for at least 12 hours.
5. Let the cubes sit at room temperature for 10 minutes. Fill a blender with warm water and let stand for 2 to 3 minutes, then discard the water. Add the frozen cubes and 1 tablespoon almond milk to the blender and blend on high for 1 minute, or until smooth and creamy. Add 1 to 2 tablespoons almond milk if needed to blend. Stir in the cacao nibs. Serve immediately, topped with additional cacao nibs, oil, and flaky salt.

**PER SERVING**
Protein: 34g
Carbohydrates: 37g
Fat: 11g

Dairy-Free
Gluten-Free
Grain-Free

# Ninja Creami Two Ways

## *Salted Caramel–Banana Ice Cream*

SERVES 1 • PREP TIME: 15 MINUTES, PLUS 12 HOURS FREEZING • TOTAL TIME: 12 HOURS 15 MINUTES

- 1 cup almond or cashew milk (plus an additional 2 to 3 tablespoons if using a traditional blender)
- ¼ cup vanilla protein powder (dairy-free if preferred)
- 2 tablespoons unflavored collagen peptides
- 3 tablespoons maple syrup
- ½ ripe banana
- ½ teaspoon sea salt
- Optional toppings: banana slices, maple syrup, flaky salt

Okay here's the thing—people love ice cream. So I created two flavor combos that taste just as indulgent as the real thing, but with better (and fewer) ingredients and a solid dose of protein. Whether you're into deep chocolatey richness or craving that salty-sweet caramel fix, these frozen treats deliver. No Ninja Creami? No problem—a high-speed blender works just as well.

1. **To make in a Ninja Creami:** Combine the almond milk, protein powder, collagen peptides, maple syrup, banana, and salt in a blender and blend until smooth. Pour into a Ninja Creami container and freeze for at least 12 hours.
2. Remove from the freezer and let sit at room temperature for 10 minutes. Place the container in the Ninja Creami and run on the full Light Ice Cream cycle.
3. Serve immediately, topped with sliced banana, a drizzle of maple syrup, and flaky salt.
4. **To make in a high-powered blender:** Blend together the 1 cup almond milk, the protein powder, collagen peptides, maple syrup, banana, and salt until smooth. Pour into a silicone ice cube tray and freeze for at least 12 hours. Remove from the freezer and let sit at room temperature for 10 minutes.
5. Fill a blender container with warm water and let stand for 2 to 3 minutes, then discard the water. Add the frozen cubes and 1 tablespoon almond milk to the blender and blend on high for 1 minute, or until smooth and creamy. Add 1 to 2 tablespoons almond milk if needed to blend. Serve immediately, topped with sliced banana, maple syrup, and flaky salt.

---

**PER SERVING**
Protein: 40g
Carbohydrates: 44g
Fat: 5g

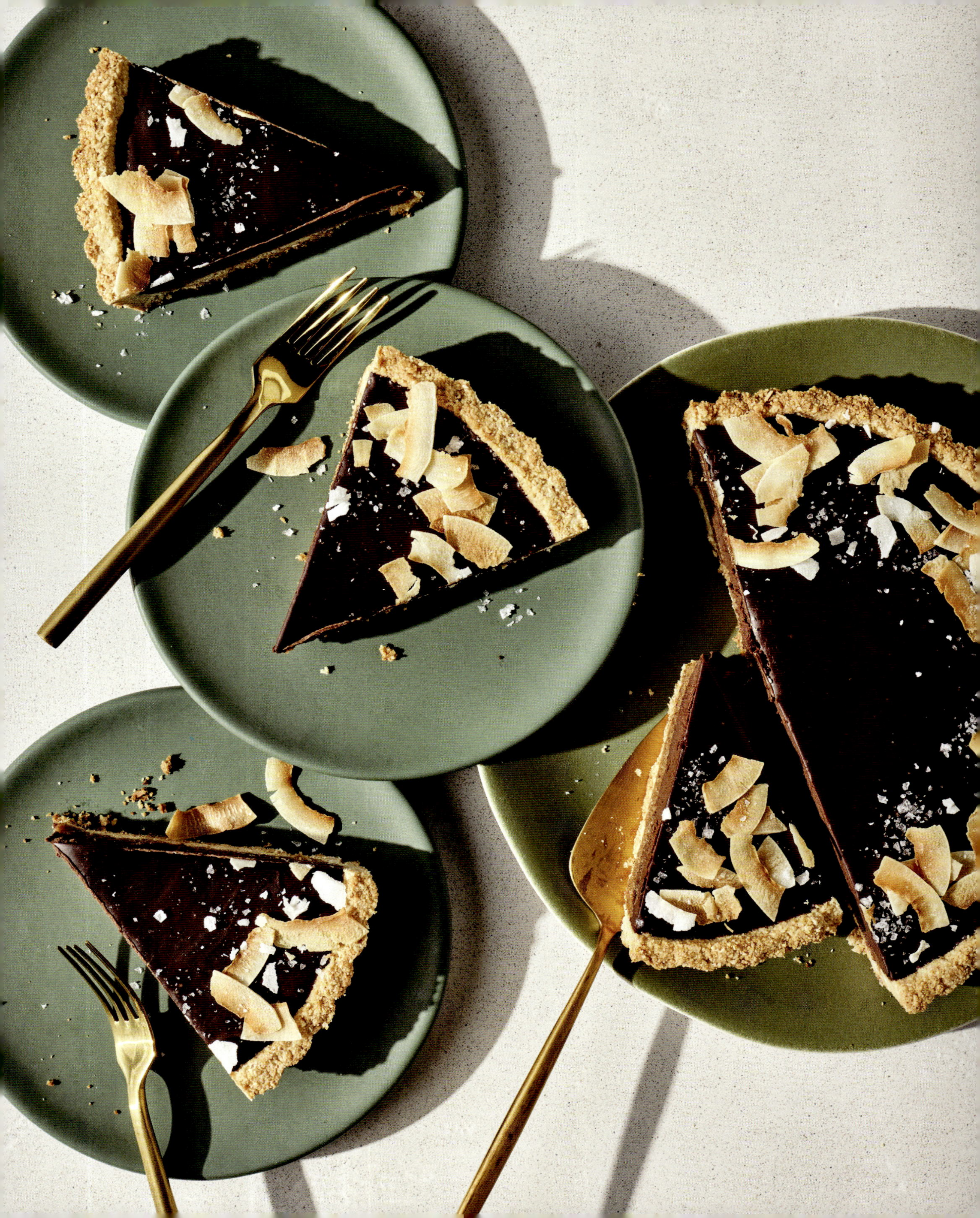

Dairy-Free
Gluten-Free
Grain-Free

# Chocolate-Coconut Caramel Tart

**SERVES 8 TO 12 • PREP TIME: 20 MINUTES, PLUS COOLING AND CHILLING • COOK TIME: 15 MINUTES • TOTAL TIME: 2 HOURS 30 MINUTES**

If you ever want to wow a group, this tart is your ticket. A crisp almond-coconut crust, gooey date caramel, and rich chocolate ganache come together in one show-stopping slice. It looks impressive but couldn't be easier to make—and tastes like something you'd buy at a bakery (but better). Just chill, slice, and top with coconut and flaky salt for the ultimate finish.

**FOR THE CRUST**

1 cup almond flour

½ cup dairy-free vanilla protein powder

¼ cup unsweetened desiccated coconut

1 tablespoon coconut flour

¼ cup coconut oil, melted

2 tablespoons almond butter

3 tablespoons maple syrup

½ teaspoon sea salt

**FOR THE CARAMEL LAYER**

10 pitted Medjool dates, soaked in hot water for 30 minutes and drained

¼ cup almond butter

¼ cup coconut oil, melted

1 teaspoon vanilla extract

½ teaspoon sea salt

**FOR THE CHOCOLATE TOPPING**

8 ounces dairy-free dark chocolate, finely chopped, or chocolate chips (about 1⅓ cups)

¾ cup canned coconut milk

¼ cup plus 2 tablespoons unflavored collagen powder

1 teaspoon vanilla extract

¼ teaspoon sea salt

Optional toppings: flaky salt, toasted coconut flakes

1. **Make the crust:** Preheat the oven to 350°F. In a medium bowl, combine the almond flour, protein powder, coconut, coconut flour, coconut oil, almond butter, maple syrup, and salt. Stir until the mixture resembles wet sand. Press the crust into a 9-inch tart pan, using your fingers to flatten the bottom and press up the sides. Bake for 15 to 18 minutes, until firm and golden brown around the edges. Set aside to cool completely, about 30 minutes (or place in the fridge to speed things up).
2. **Make the caramel layer:** Meanwhile, in a food processor, combine the dates, almond butter, coconut oil, vanilla, and salt. Process until smooth and creamy. Spread the caramel in the bottom of the cooled tart shell, using a spatula to create an even layer.
3. **Make the chocolate topping**: Place the chocolate in a medium heatproof bowl. In a small saucepan, heat the coconut milk over medium-low heat for 3 to 4 minutes, until just simmering. Remove from the heat and whisk in the collagen powder, vanilla, and salt until fully combined. Pour the coconut milk mixture over the chocolate and let sit for 1 minute. Stir until the chocolate is fully melted and smooth.
4. **Assemble the tart:** Pour the chocolate mixture over the caramel layer in the tart shell and smooth the top with a spatula. Refrigerate for at least 2 hours, until fully set.
5. Serve chilled, topped with flaky salt and coconut flakes.

**STORAGE:** Store in an airtight container in the fridge for up to 5 days. For the best texture, let it sit at room temperature for 10 to 15 minutes before serving.

**PER SERVING (FOR 8 SERVINGS)**
Protein: 16g
Carbohydrates: 26g
Fat: 35g

Dairy-Free
Gluten-Free
Grain-Free

# Fudge Brownies

**MAKES 9 BARS • PREP TIME: 15 MINUTES, PLUS 45 MINUTES COOLING • COOK TIME: 30 MINUTES • TOTAL TIME: 1 HOUR 30 MINUTES**

I'm a firm believer that everyone needs a ride-or-die brownie recipe, and *this* is mine. It's rich, it's fudgy, and it's got a hidden helping of collagen you'd never guess was there. Keep this one in your back pocket. Trust me!

**⅓ cup coconut oil, plus more for greasing the baking dish**
**1 cup dairy-free dark chocolate chips, plus more for topping**
**¾ cup collagen peptides**
**2 large eggs, at room temperature**
**¼ cup coconut sugar**
**¼ cup maple syrup**
**⅓ cup cacao powder**
**¼ cup almond flour**
**¼ teaspoon baking soda**
**Pinch of flaky salt**

1. Preheat the oven to 350°F. Line a 6 x 6-inch baking dish (see Tip) with parchment paper and lightly grease the parchment with coconut oil.
2. In a small saucepan, melt the ⅓ cup coconut oil and ⅔ cup of the chocolate chips over low heat, stirring occasionally, for 3 to 4 minutes, until the chocolate melts. Remove from the heat and whisk in the collagen peptides, ¼ cup at a time. Set aside to cool for 15 minutes.
3. Meanwhile, in a medium bowl, whisk the eggs and coconut sugar for 30 seconds, until well combined. Whisk in the maple syrup, then stir in the cooled chocolate mixture until just combined. Sift in the cacao powder, almond flour, and baking soda and mix until just combined. Be careful not to overmix or the brownies will be tough. Fold in the remaining ⅓ cup chocolate chips and gently mix.
4. Pour the batter into the baking dish and spread evenly. Top with additional chocolate chips and a pinch of flaky salt. Bake for 30 to 32 minutes, until the edges look set but the center is still slightly soft. Let cool for 30 minutes before slicing and serving.

**STORAGE:** Store in an airtight container at room temperature for up to 3 days, or in the fridge for up to 5 days. For a fudgier texture, enjoy chilled; for a softer bite, let them come to room temperature before serving.

---

**PER SERVING (1 BAR)**
Protein: 10g
Carbohydrates: 18g
Fat: 15g

**TIP:** *Since 6 x 6-inch pans aren't common, you can use an 8 x 8-inch pan for slightly thinner brownies. Adjust baking time to 25 to 28 minutes to prevent overbaking.*

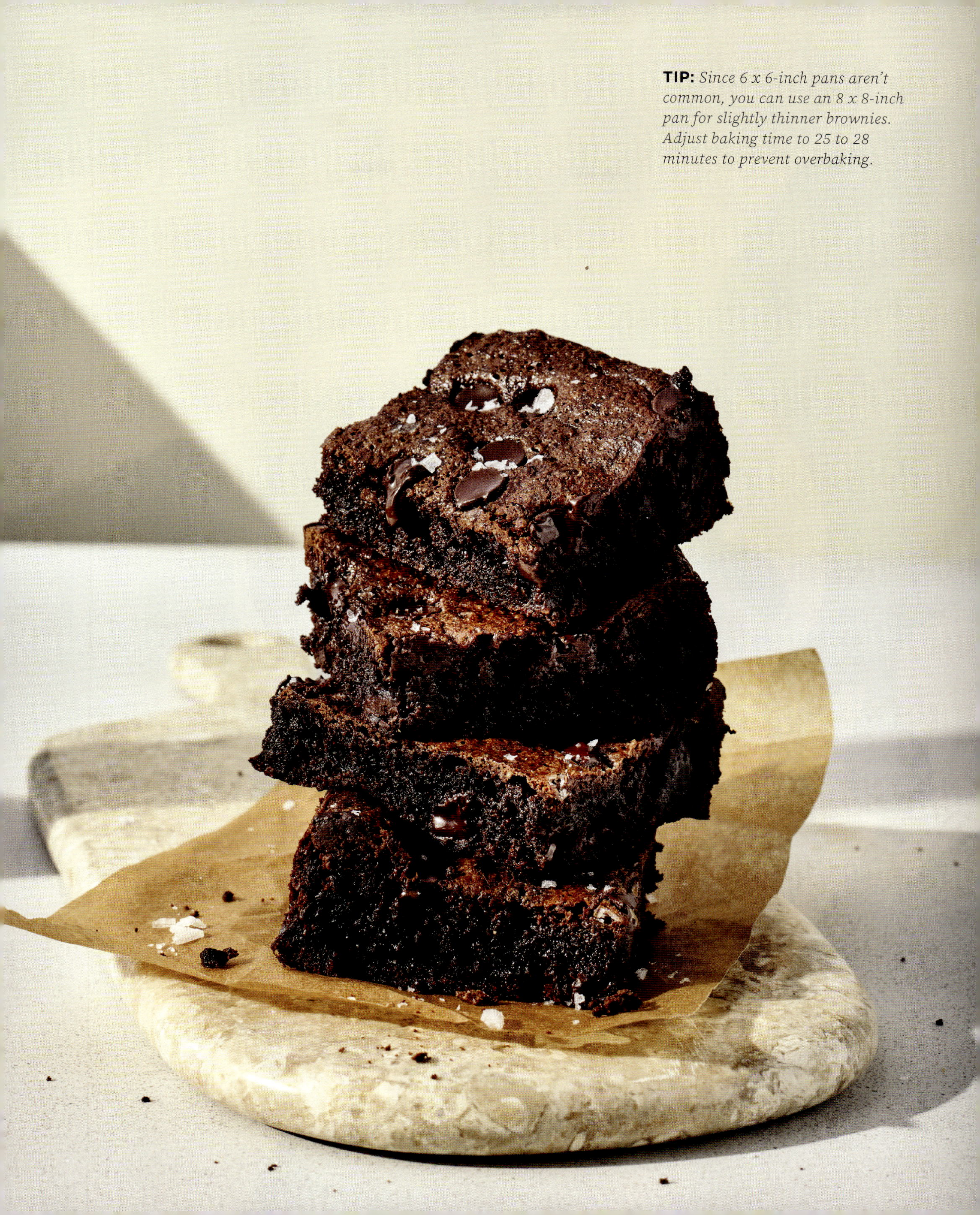

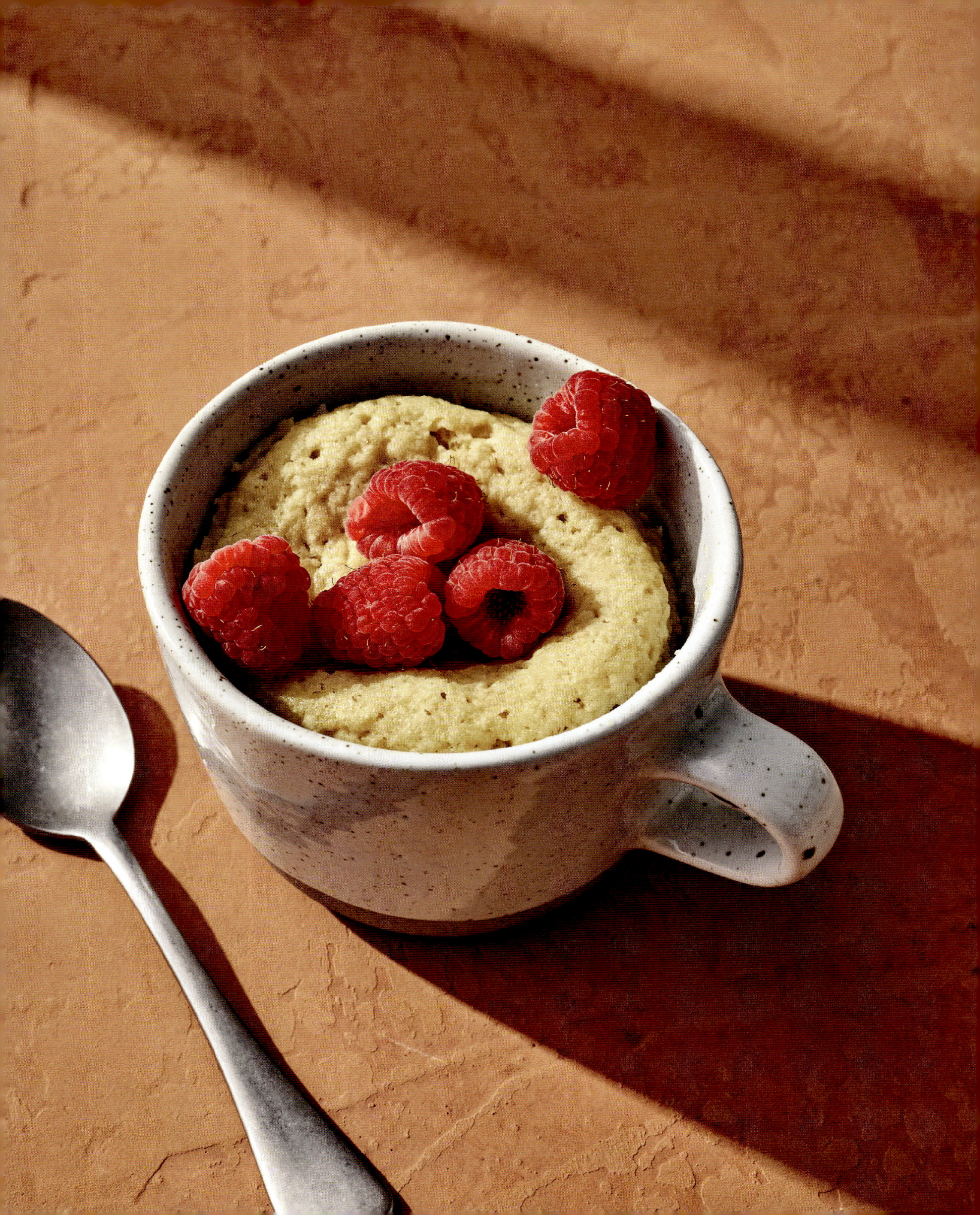

Dairy-Free
Gluten-Free
Grain-Free

# Raspberry-Vanilla Protein Mug Cake

**SERVES 1 • PREP TIME: 2 MINUTES • COOK TIME: 2 MINUTES • TOTAL TIME: 4 MINUTES**

Avocado oil spray
1½ tablespoons coconut flour
2 tablespoons vanilla protein powder
3 tablespoons unsweetened applesauce
1 large egg, beaten
1½ teaspoons maple syrup
1 teaspoon vanilla extract
½ teaspoon baking powder
¼ teaspoon sea salt
¼ cup fresh or frozen raspberries, plus more for garnish
For serving (optional): yogurt or coconut whipped cream

Mug cakes got me through college. With little time and barely any kitchen space, I became a pro at whipping up quick, single-serve treats in the microwave. I tested tons of different flavor combos, but this one always stood out—the sweet, jammy raspberries, warm vanilla tones, and soft, cake-like texture make it feel like a real dessert (minus the effort). Just a few high-quality ingredients and 4 minutes later, you've got a sweet treat that tastes like it took way longer. Top it with yogurt or coconut whip, and you're golden!

1. Spray a 16-ounce mug with avocado oil. In a medium bowl, combine the coconut flour, protein powder, applesauce, egg, maple syrup, vanilla, baking powder, and salt. Gently fold in the raspberries. Pour the batter into the mug and top with additional raspberries.
2. Microwave until the cake is set, 1½ to 2 minutes, depending on the strength of your microwave. Serve immediately, with a drizzle of yogurt or coconut whipped cream.

**PER SERVING**
Protein: 20g
Carbohydrates: 23g
Fat: 7g

Dairy-Free
Gluten-Free
Grain-Free

# Sweet and Salty Candy Bark

**MAKES 8 TO 12 PIECES • PREP TIME: 15 MINUTES, PLUS 1 HOUR FREEZING • TOTAL TIME: 1 HOUR 15 MINUTES**

I have a thing for re-creating iconic candy bar flavors, but with better-for-you desserts—and this chocolate bark just might be my best yet. The chewy, caramel-like dates, creamy peanut butter, crunchy roasted peanuts, and rich dark chocolate hit *every* sweet-and-salty craving. A sprinkle of flaky salt on top brings it all together. Best part? No baking required. Just layer, freeze, and break into pieces. Keep a stash in the freezer and thank me later.

**FOR THE CARAMEL LAYER**

16 large pitted Medjool dates

½ cup unsweetened creamy peanut butter

½ cup vanilla protein powder

2 tablespoons coconut oil, melted

**FOR THE CHOCOLATE LAYER**

⅓ cup dairy-free dark chocolate chips

1 tablespoon coconut oil

**TOPPINGS**

¼ cup roasted peanuts, chopped

1 tablespoon flaky salt

1. **Make the caramel layer:** Line a baking sheet with parchment paper. Slice the dates in half lengthwise and arrange them, skin side down and side by side, on the parchment to form a rectangular base. Place another piece of parchment over the dates to prevent sticking. Use your hands, the bottom of a measuring cup, or a rolling pin to press the dates into a thin, even layer, about ¼ inch thick.
2. In a medium bowl, stir together the peanut butter, protein powder, and coconut oil until smooth. Spread the peanut butter mixture evenly over the dates, covering them completely.
3. **Make the chocolate layer:** Combine the chocolate chips and coconut oil in a small microwave-safe bowl. Microwave in 30-second increments, stirring in between, until the chocolate and oil are fully melted and smooth. If you prefer to do this on the stovetop, heat the chocolate chips and coconut oil in a small saucepan over low heat, stirring continuously for 2 to 3 minutes, until fully melted and smooth. Immediately remove from the heat to prevent burning.
4. **Assemble the bars**: Pour the chocolate over the peanut butter layer and use a spatula or butter knife to spread it evenly. Sprinkle the top with peanuts and flaky salt.
5. Transfer the baking sheet to the freezer and freeze for at least 1 hour, until firm.
6. Once set, transfer the bark to a cutting board and slice into 3 x 1-inch candy-bar-size pieces. Serve immediately

**TIP:** *For added crunch and flavor, mix in unsweetened coconut flakes, sunflower seeds, or extra roasted peanuts before adding the chocolate layer.*

**STORAGE:** Store in an airtight container in the freezer for up to 3 months.

**PER SERVING (FOR 10 SERVINGS)**
Protein: 7g
Carbohydrates: 15g
Fat: 11g

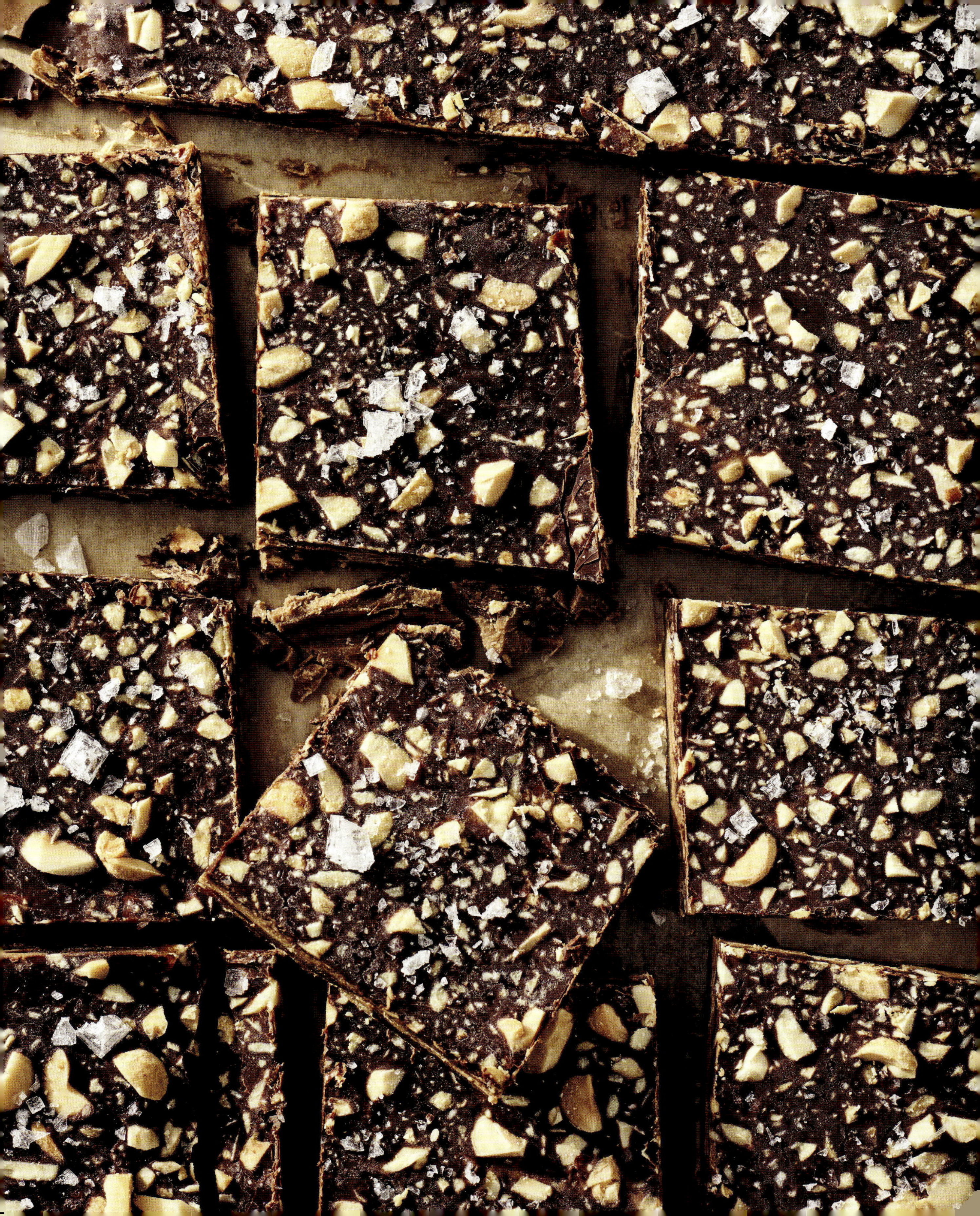

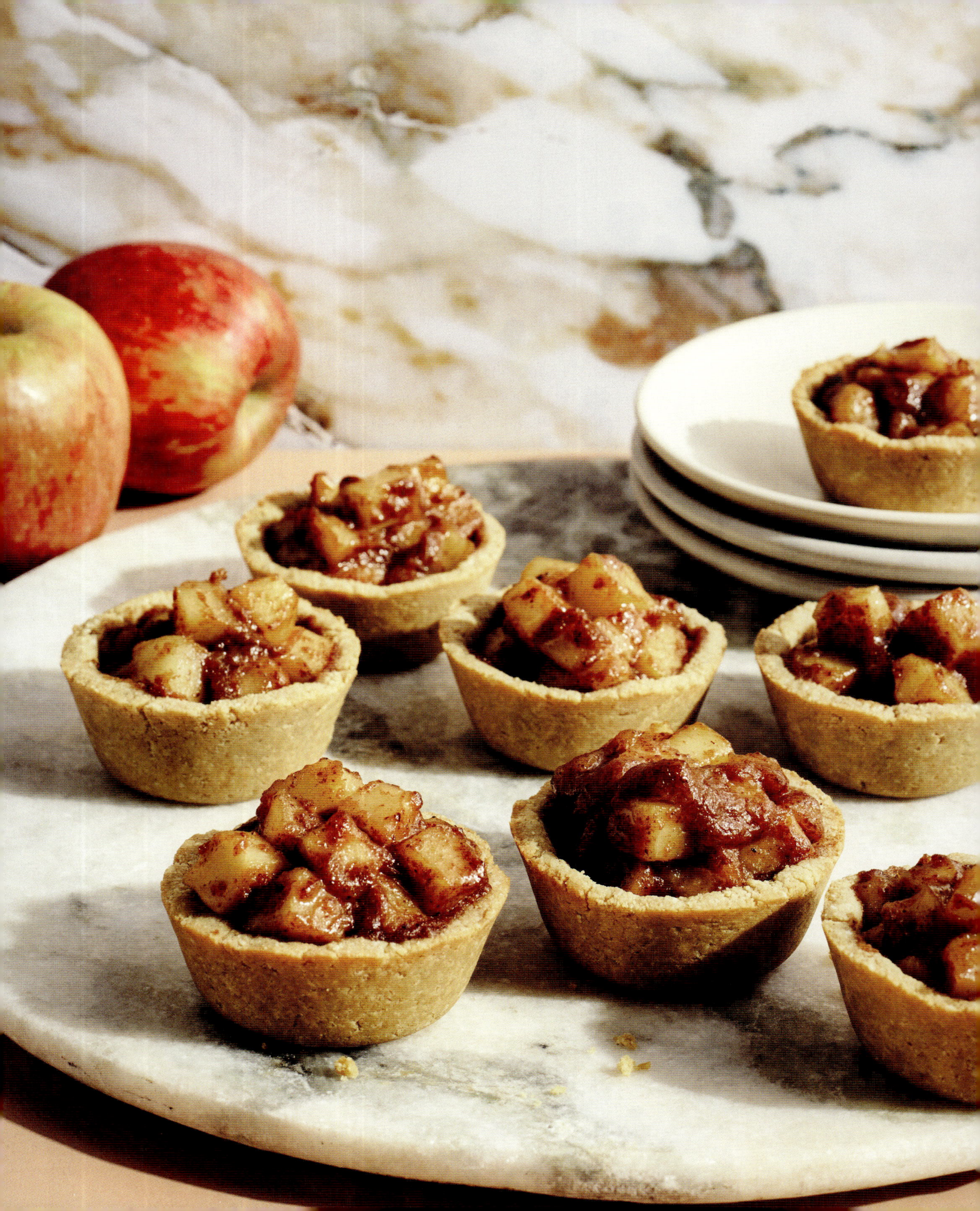

Gluten-Free
Grain-Free
**IF MODIFIED:**
Dairy-Free

# Mini Apple Tarts

**MAKES 8 MINI TARTS • PREP TIME: 10 MINUTES • COOK TIME: 35 MINUTES, PLUS 10 MINUTES COOLING • TOTAL TIME: 55 MINUTES**

**FOR THE FILLING**

- 3 small apples, peeled, cored, and diced (about 3 cups)
- 2 tablespoons maple syrup or coconut sugar
- 2 tablespoons ghee (or vegan butter for dairy-free)
- 2 tablespoons lemon juice
- 2 tablespoons almond butter
- 1 teaspoon vanilla extract
- ½ teaspoon ground cinnamon
- ⅛ teaspoon nutmeg

**FOR THE CRUST**

- 1 cup almond flour
- ¼ cup vanilla protein powder
- 2 tablespoons coconut flour
- Pinch of sea salt
- 2 tablespoons coconut oil, melted
- 1 large egg, beaten
- 1 tablespoon maple syrup
- Optional toppings: 3 tablespoons chopped pecans, 2 tablespoons hemp seeds

These bite-size apple tarts are everything you love about a classic apple pie, just in a perfectly portioned, better-for-you package. With warm spiced apples and a touch of natural sweetness, they make an ideal dessert or mid-afternoon treat. I also love them for holiday gatherings when you might otherwise serve apple pie.

1. Preheat the oven to 350°F. Grease 8 cups of a 12-cup muffin tin or line with silicone liners.
2. **Make the filling:** In a medium saucepan, combine the apples, maple syrup, ghee, lemon juice, almond butter, vanilla, cinnamon, and nutmeg. Cook over medium-low heat, stirring occasionally, for 20 minutes, or until soft but not mushy. Set aside.
3. **Make the crust:** Meanwhile, in a large mixing bowl, whisk together the almond flour, protein powder, coconut flour, and salt to remove any clumps. Add the coconut oil, egg, and maple syrup, stirring until a dough forms.
4. Divide the dough evenly among the 8 muffin cups, using about 1 heaping tablespoon per cup. Firmly press the dough into the bottom and up the side of each cup, ensuring there are no cracks or gaps where the filling could leak. Bake the crusts for 5 minutes, until firm. Remove from the oven.
5. Spoon the apple filling into the parbaked crusts, ensuring the liquid does not rise above the edges. Top with pecans and hemp seeds, if using. Bake for 10 minutes, or until the filling starts to bubble. Let cool for 10 minutes before carefully removing each tart from the tin.

**STORAGE:** Store in an airtight container at room temperature for up to 2 days, or in the fridge for up to 4 days. Reheat in a 350°F toaster oven or oven for 5 to 7 minutes to restore flakiness before serving.

---

**PER SERVING (1 TART)**
Protein: 8g
Carbohydrates: 15g
Fat: 14g

Dairy-Free
Gluten-Free
Grain-Free

# Peppermint Patties

MAKES 16 PATTIES • PREP TIME: 20 MINUTES, PLUS 2 HOURS FREEZING • TOTAL TIME: 2 HOURS 20 MINUTES

FOR THE MINT FILLING

½ cup shredded unsweetened coconut

¼ cup refined coconut oil

¼ cup raw honey

¾ cup almond flour

2 tablespoons unsweetened almond milk or coconut milk

2 tablespoons collagen peptides

1 teaspoon peppermint extract

FOR THE CHOCOLATE COATING

¾ cup dairy-free dark chocolate chips

1 tablespoon refined coconut oil

Flaky salt, for garnish

Forget the peppermint patties you grew up with—these will ruin the store-bought kind for good. With a creamy minty center and rich chocolate shell, they deliver that classic snap and melt combo, minus the junk. Plus, they sneak in some collagen benefits, so you can feel just a little smug while you snack. Keep a stash in the fridge or freezer for when you want something sweet that still feels like a win.

1. **Make the mint filling:** In a high-speed blender or food processor, pulse the coconut for 30 seconds, until it reaches fine shreds.
2. In a medium microwave-safe bowl, microwave the coconut oil for 30 seconds, until liquid. Stir in the honey and whisk until the mixture is totally smooth. Add the shredded coconut and the almond flour, stirring until the mixture becomes a crumbly dough. In a small bowl, whisk together the almond milk, collagen peptides, and peppermint extract until smooth. Pour the mixture into the dough, and stir until well combined.
3. Line a baking sheet with parchment paper. Use a heaping teaspoon to drop the filling into 16 dollops on the baking sheet. Wet your hands and shake off the excess water so they are damp. Roll each dollop into a small ball and press into a thin, flat disk, about 1½ inches in diameter. Transfer to the freezer to set for 1 hour.
4. **Make the chocolate coating**: In a medium, microwave-safe bowl, microwave the chocolate chips and coconut oil in 30-second increments, stirring in between, until the chocolate is smooth and glossy.
5. **Assemble the patties:** Using two forks, dip a peppermint patty into the melted chocolate, coating fully and allowing the excess chocolate to drip off. Place the patty back onto the parchment and sprinkle with flaky salt. Repeat with the remaining patties. Return the patties to the freezer and let set for at least 1 hour before serving.

**STORAGE:** Store in an airtight container in the fridge for up to 1 week or in the freezer for up to 2 months. Enjoy straight from the fridge, or straight from the freezer for a firmer bite—no need to thaw. Let sit at room temperature for a few minutes if you prefer a softer texture.

---

**PER SERVING (1 PATTY)**
Protein: 3g
Carbohydrates: 5g
Fat: 9g

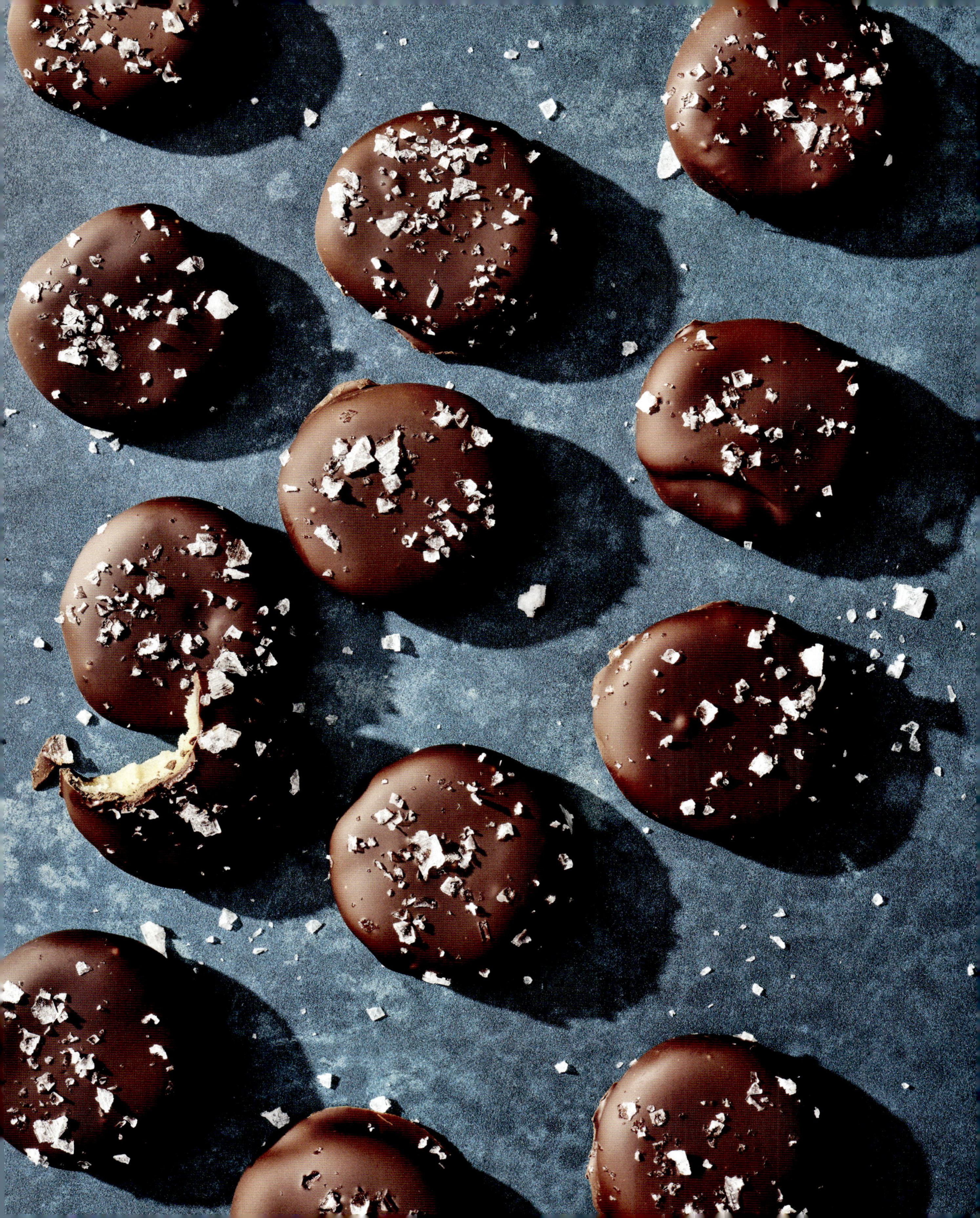

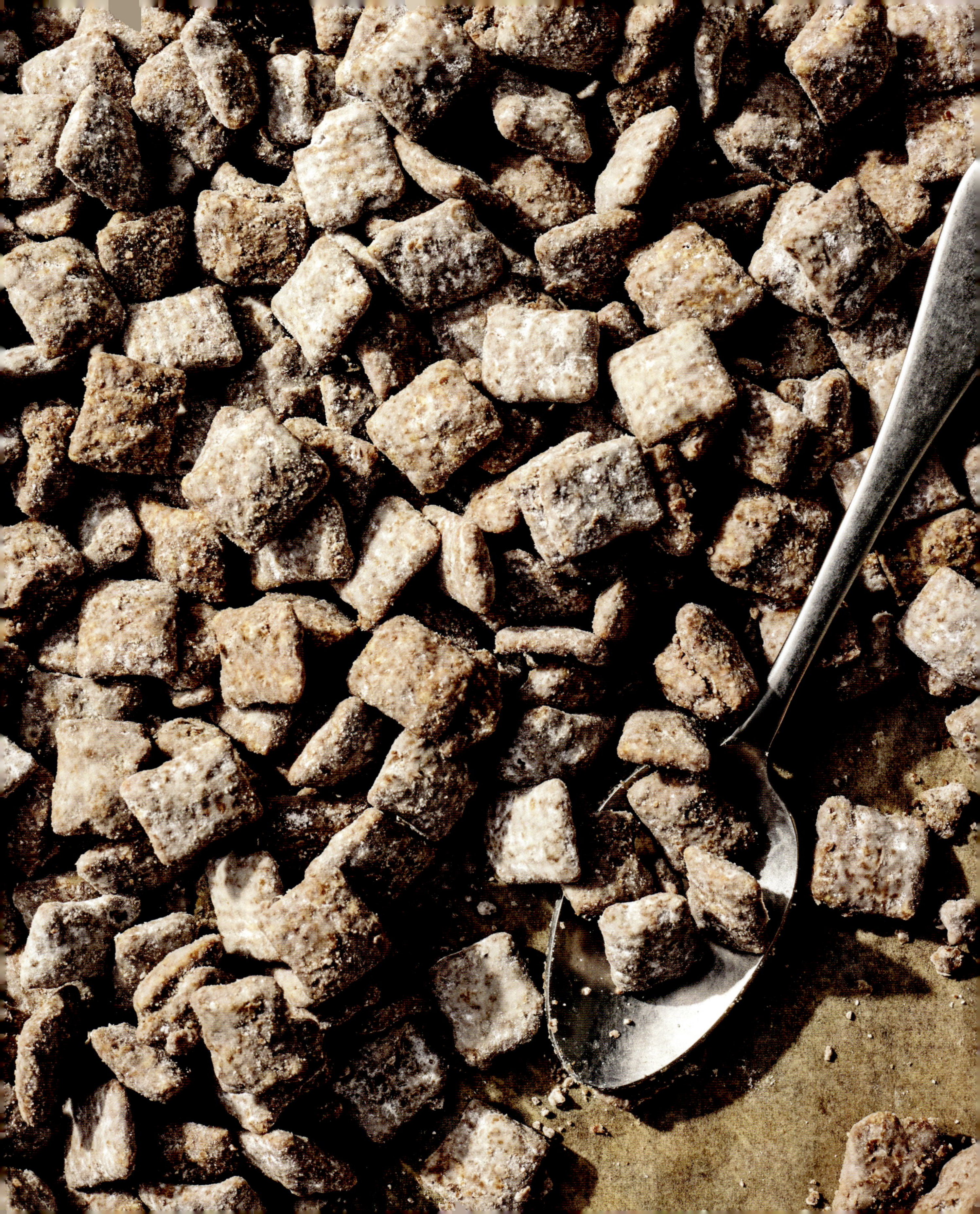

Dairy-Free
Gluten-Free

# Protein Muddy Buddies

**SERVES 8 TO 10 • PREP TIME: 20 MINUTES, PLUS 20 MINUTES COOLING • COOK TIME: 5 MINUTES • TOTAL TIME: 45 MINUTES**

- 1 cup creamy unsweetened peanut butter
- 1½ teaspoons coconut oil
- 1 cup dairy-free dark chocolate chips
- 1 cup unflavored or vanilla protein powder
- ½ cup powdered sugar or powdered monk fruit sweetener
- 8 cups gluten-free rice cereal, such as Chex or sprouted brown rice cereal

When I was in college, our sorority chef Bridget would whip up a massive bowl of muddy buddies and the cereal snack mix would disappear in seconds. This version keeps all the crispy, chocolatey, peanut buttery goodness—but with some protein powder for extra staying power. Snack straight from the bowl, share (if you must), and don't be surprised if it vanishes just as fast. It also makes great holiday gifts, packaged in a pretty bowl or bag and tied with a ribbon.

1. Line a baking sheet with parchment paper. In a small saucepan over low heat, combine the peanut butter, coconut oil, and chocolate chips. Stir continuously for 2 to 3 minutes, until fully melted and smooth. Remove from the heat.
2. In a medium bowl, mix the protein powder and powdered sugar until combined.
3. Place the cereal in a large mixing bowl. Pour the melted peanut butter mixture over the cereal and use a spatula to gently mix until evenly coated.
4. Transfer the coated cereal to a large resealable bag or a container with a lid. Sprinkle the protein powder mixture over the cereal. Seal tightly and shake until all pieces are evenly coated with the powder. Spread the cereal on the baking sheet to cool for 20 to 30 minutes, until set.

**STORAGE:** Store in an airtight container at room temperature for up to 5 days. Let cool completely before sealing to keep the texture crisp.

**PER SERVING (FOR 8 SERVINGS, ABOUT 1¼ CUPS EACH)**
Protein: 15g
Carbohydrates: 42g
Fat: 20g

**TIP:** *Add variety by mixing in nuts, seeds, or unsweetened coconut flakes before coating.*

Gluten-Free
Grain-Free

# Brown Butter–Chocolate Chip Cookies

**MAKES 12 COOKIES • PREP TIME: 15 MINUTES • COOK TIME: 10 MINUTES • TOTAL TIME: 25 MINUTES**

A chocolate chip cookie that feels like a treat but sneaks in a little protein punch? Oh yeah. These are super soft and chewy and loaded with rich almond butter, ghee, and dark chocolate—basically everything you love in a classic cookie, just upgraded with better-for-you ingredients. It may not be your highest-protein bite of the day, but it's one you'll feel good about. I keep the recipe on repeat.

- ¼ cup ghee (or use unsalted butter for browned butter, see Note)
- ¼ cup collagen peptides
- ½ cup unsweetened creamy almond butter
- ¼ cup coconut sugar
- 2 tablespoons maple syrup
- 1 large egg
- 1 teaspoon vanilla extract
- ¼ cup vanilla protein powder
- ⅓ cup almond flour
- ¼ teaspoon baking soda
- ¼ teaspoon sea salt
- ½ cup dark chocolate chips, plus more for topping
- Flaky salt, for garnish

1. Preheat the oven to 350°F. Line a baking sheet with parchment paper.
2. Melt the ghee gently in a saucepan over low heat. Remove from the heat and immediately stir in the collagen peptides until smooth. Let cool for 5 minutes. If using butter, melt it over medium heat, stirring constantly until the milk solids turn golden and smell nutty, 3 to 4 minutes. Remove from the heat, whisk in the collagen peptides until smooth, and let cool for 5 minutes.
3. In a large mixing bowl, whisk together the almond butter, coconut sugar, maple syrup, egg, and vanilla until smooth. Slowly whisk in the ghee-collagen mixture until fully combined. Add the protein powder, almond flour, baking soda, and salt. Stir until a dough forms, then fold in the chocolate chips.
4. Using a cookie scoop or tablespoon, scoop twelve portions of dough and arrange 2 inches apart on the baking sheet. Add a few chocolate chips to the top of each cookie. Bake for 10 to 12 minutes, until the cookie edges are golden but the centers still look soft. Let cool on the baking sheet for 10 minutes and sprinkle with flaky salt.

**NOTE:** *If you're craving that deep, nutty flavor of classic brown butter, swap out the ghee for unsalted butter: Simply brown the butter over medium heat, stirring constantly until the milk solids turn golden and smell nutty, 3 to 4 minutes, then immediately stir in the collagen peptides. This adds an extra layer of flavor to the cookies, though they're still rich and delicious with ghee.*

**STORAGE:** Store in an airtight container at room temperature for up to 4 days, or freeze for up to 2 months. Let frozen cookies sit at room temperature for 10 to 15 minutes before serving, or reheat in a warm oven (about 300°F) for a few minutes for soft, gooey centers.

**PER SERVING (1 COOKIE)**
Protein: 5g
Carbohydrates: 10g
Fat: 8g

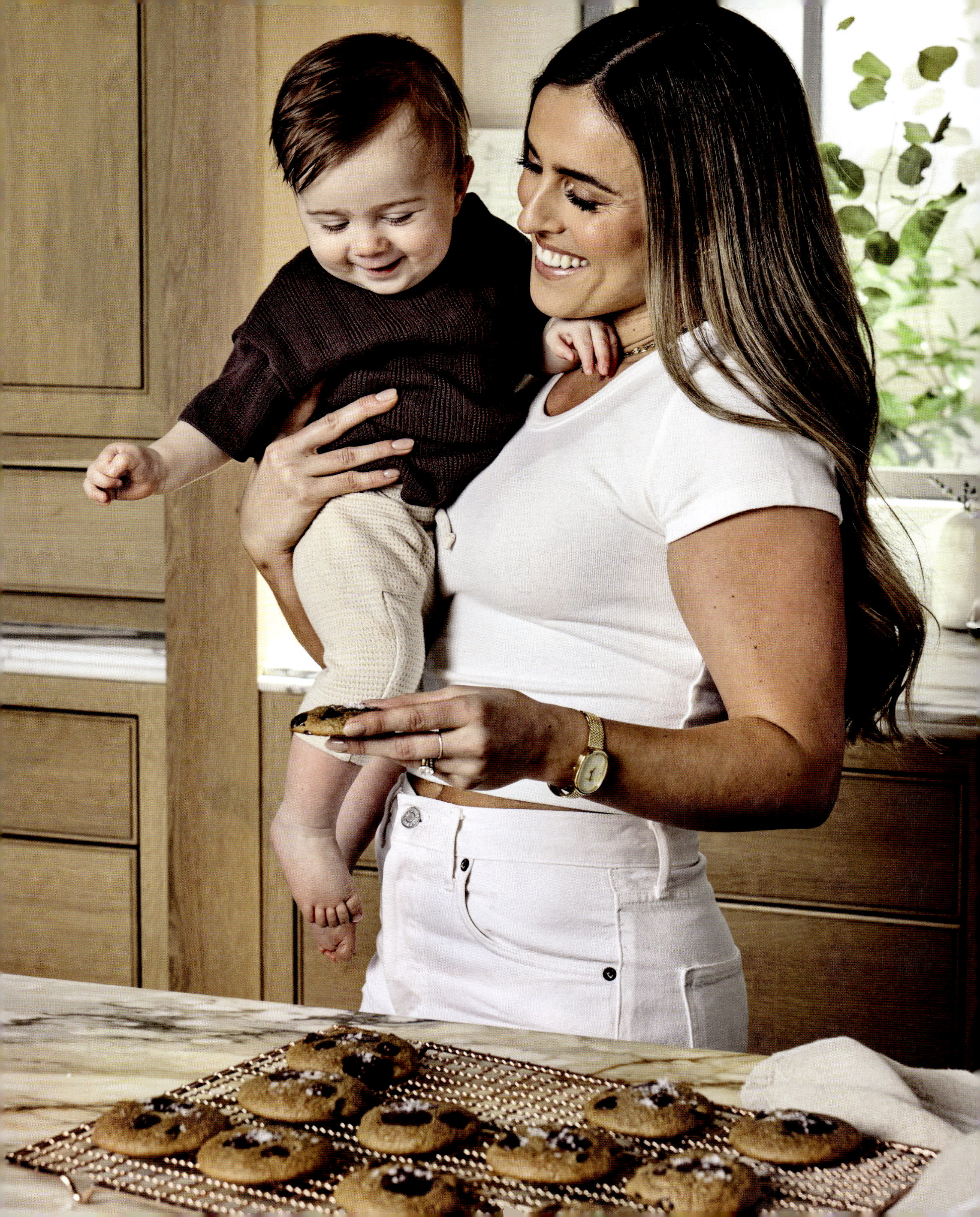

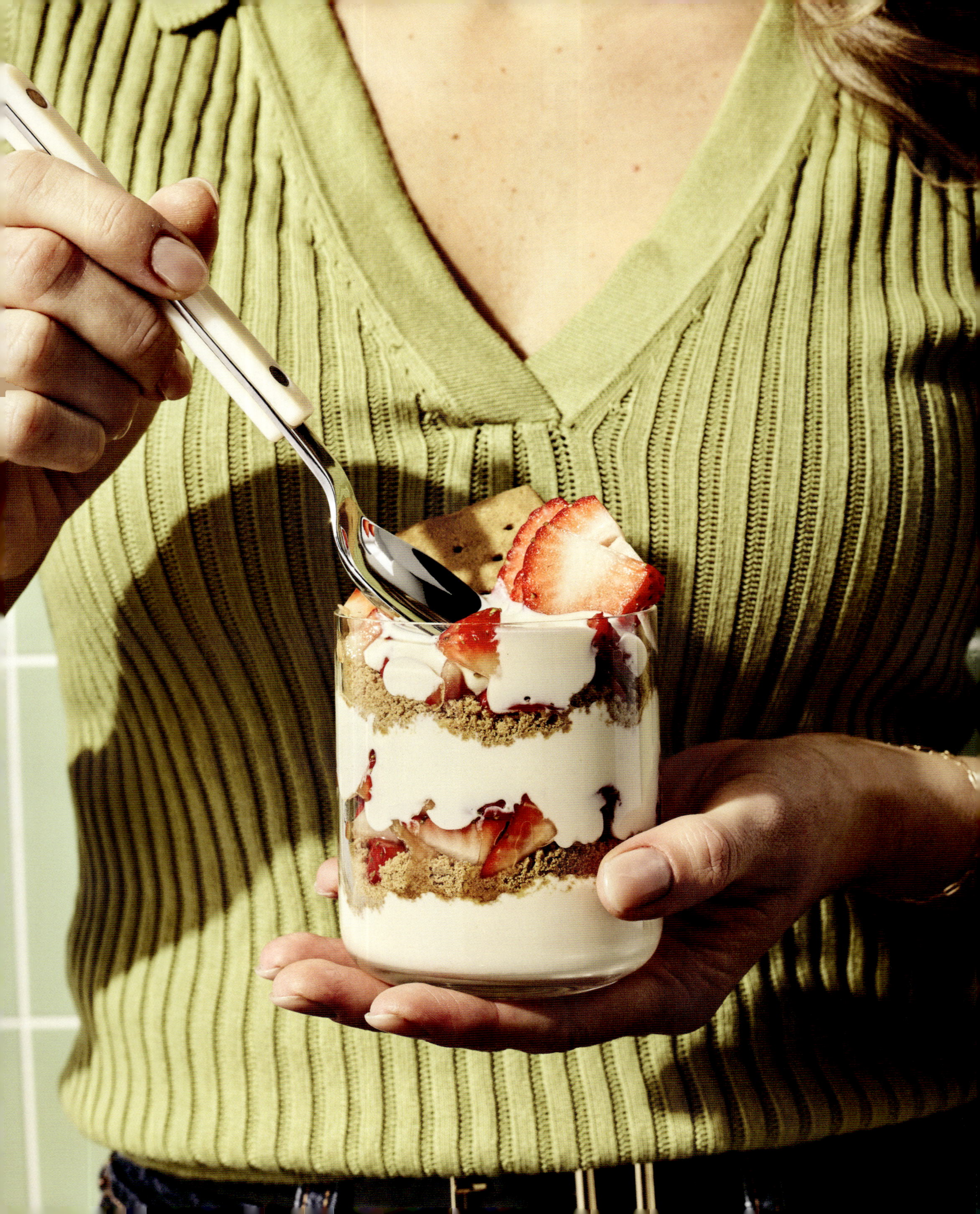

Gluten-Free
**IF MODIFIED:**
Dairy-Free

# Strawberry Cheesecake Pudding

**SERVES 4 • PREP TIME: 10 MINUTES, PLUS 10 MINUTES MACERATING • TOTAL TIME: 20 MINUTES**

- 2 cups diced strawberries (or any seasonal berry or fruit slices), plus more slices for garnish
- 1 tablespoon coconut sugar
- 1 (16-ounce) container full-fat cottage cheese (or coconut yogurt for dairy-free)
- ¼ cup unflavored collagen powder
- 3 tablespoons maple syrup
- 1 teaspoon vanilla extract
- 1 cup crushed gluten-free graham crackers (about 6 graham crackers)

If there's one thing that will make you rethink cottage cheese, it's this pudding. Blended until silky smooth, the cottage cheese is transformed into the dreamiest cheesecake-style pudding—creamy, rich, and full of protein. Macerated strawberries add a juicy, natural sweetness, and gluten-free graham cracker crumbles bring just the right amount of crunch. No baking, no fuss—just layer it up and enjoy. Don't hesitate to swap in your favorite seasonal fruit for the strawberries, then keep the pudding in the fridge for a quick, feel-good dessert anytime!

1. In a medium bowl, combine the strawberries and coconut sugar. Stir until evenly coated, then set aside for 10 minutes, until the sugar dissolves and becomes syrupy.
2. Meanwhile, in a food processor, blend the cottage cheese, collagen powder, maple syrup, and vanilla for 1 minute, or until smooth and creamy.
3. Spoon ¼ cup of the blended cottage cheese into each of four 12- to 16-ounce glasses or mason jars. Add 1½ tablespoons graham crackers and ¼ cup macerated strawberries to each jar.
4. Repeat the layers, starting with the cottage cheese mixture, then the graham crackers, followed by the berries. Finish with a dollop of the whipped cottage cheese mixture and a few strawberry slices for garnish.

**STORAGE:** Store in an airtight container in the fridge for up to 3 days. Serve chilled.

**PER SERVING**
Protein: 21g
Carbohydrates: 35g
Fat: 9g

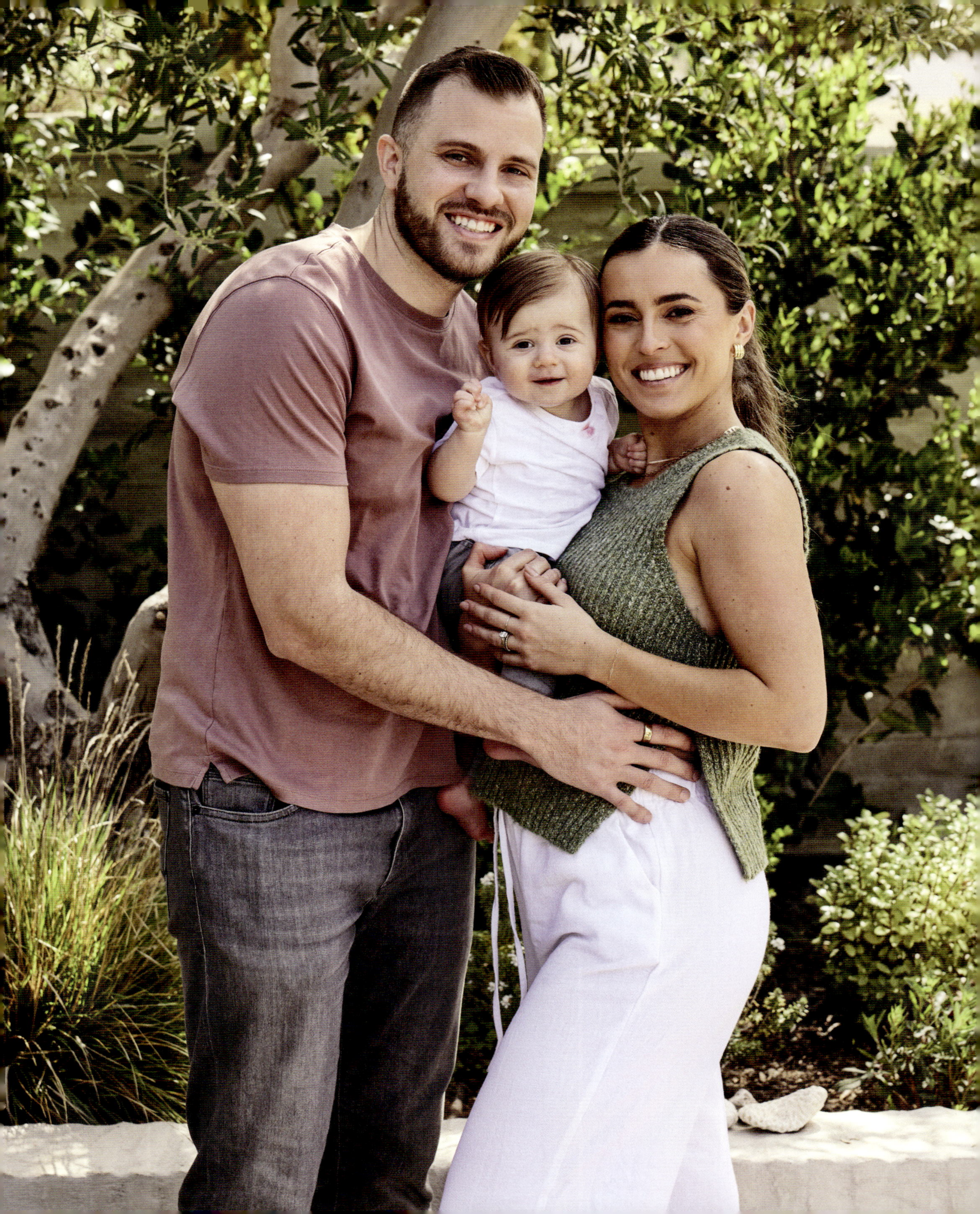

# Acknowledgments

**After writing this cookbook, it's clear it couldn't be done alone. It takes a village—and what a dream village I have!**

To my Good Eats family—you are the heart of all I do. Seeing you cook my recipes in your homes, share them with your people, and tell me how they've made your lives feel a little healthier or happier? That's the part that means the most. You inspire me more than you'll ever know, and I'm forever grateful. Here's to many more meals shared together—thank you for letting me be a small part of your kitchens.

To Bridger, my husband, my calm in the chaos, my ultimate taste tester, and greatest support—thank you for everything. For tasting every bite, encouraging every idea, and giving me all the inspo with your food cravings. And to my littlest sous chef, Hayes, you inspire me in ways I could never put into words. Cooking for you makes every recipe feel even more meaningful. You've given food a whole new purpose in my life, and it's the greatest joy. I love you.

To Maddie, my sister and built-in best friend—you're always the first to say yes to testing a new recipe or inspiring me in the kitchen. Your honest feedback, encouragement, and endless taste-testing make every dish better (and every moment more fun). I'm so lucky to have you by my side, in and out of the kitchen. Getting to cook for our babies is a core memory I'll cherish forever!

To my mom and dad—thank you for cheering me on, for always believing in me, and for telling every stranger you meet about my blog (truly, the best marketing team I could ask for!). Your support never goes unnoticed, and I'll always appreciate the way you show up for me, in big ways and small. Love you both so much.

To Eden—what would I do without you? You dive headfirst into every project, never missing a beat. From our early Good Sweat live workouts to working on this cookbook, I am so beyond happy to have you in my corner.

To my cookbook dream team—Eva Kolenko, you have this effortless way of making every shot look like pure magic. Working with you twice now has been such a privilege. I'm forever grateful for the way you bring my recipes to life in ways I could've only dreamed of. Emily Caneer, you made this whole process feel easy, fun, and endlessly creative. From testing (and retesting) recipes to styling every dish to perfection, you brought so much heart to this book. I feel lucky we got to team up again. Genesis Vallejo, you brought the props and the energy—every day on set felt like a true collaboration, and I'm so glad we got to do this together.

To Melissa—my editing queen. It's your eye for the details that set this apart. You brought so much care and thoughtfulness to making this book feel game-time ready. It wouldn't be the same without you.

To Chelsea Becker—you were there in the editing trenches with me early on, keeping me sane and making this book sharper from the start.

To Alix Frank—you were a huge spark in bringing this book to life. Who else could've motivated me—six months pregnant—to plunge right into such a massive project? Thank you for always being game to test any recipe I send your way—it truly means the most. I'm so grateful to have you by my side as both a friend and manager through this entire journey.

To Nicole Tourtelot, my agent—you've been my biggest advocate, my sounding board, and the one making sure these books actually see the light of day. Your advice, encouragement, and belief in me have been invaluable. I'm lucky to have had you guiding this book into reality.

To Alyssa Johnson and Becca Mader—truly my dream glam team. You both always make me camera-ready and feeling like my best self. Is it too much to have you with me 24/7?!

And to Doris Cooper—thank you for believing in me and in the power of high-protein cooking. You saw the vision for *The High-Protein Plate* and made it a reality. Your belief in this project has been the greatest gift, and it's one I'll never forget. To the entire Simon Element team—thank you for pouring your hearts, brains, and creativity into bringing this book to life. Every thoughtful detail, every brainstorm, every tweak made this project shine, and I so enjoyed working with everyone.

# Index

NOTE: Page references in *italics* refer to photos of recipes.


Air-Fryer Garlic-Butter Salmon Bites, *124,* 125
Alfredo, Homemade, Chicken Milanese with, *94,* 95–96, *97*
amino acids, 14
animal protein, about, 14, 19, 24. *See also* bacon; beef; chicken; dairy; eggs; lamb; pork; seafood; turkey
Apple Tarts, Mini, *264,* 265
Asparagus, Honey-Harissa Salmon with, *116,* 117
avocados
  Avocado Whipped Feta, *244,* 245
  Blackened Shrimp Tacos with Pineapple-Avocado Salsa, 100, *101*
  Chili-Lime Grilled Steak with Zesty Avocado Salsa, 88, *89*
  Chipotle Chicken Avocado Bowls and, *120,* 121

bacon
  Cheesy Bacon and Chive Egg Muffins, 66, *67*
  Savory Herb and Turkey-Bacon Quiche, 46–47, *47*
baking ingredients
  flours, 27
  protein in, 25
Banana Bread Protein Muffins, 246, *247*
BBQ Sauce, Homemade, Super Crispy Chicken Tenders with, 118, *119*
beef
  about, 19
  Beef Bolognese, 108, *109*
  Beef Fried Rice, *162,* 163
  Chili-Lime Grilled Steak with Zesty Avocado Salsa, 88, *89*
  Double Double-Cheeseburger Bowls, *178,* 179
  in Greek-Style Smash Burgers, 92, *93*
  Korean Beef with Glass Noodles, *84,* 86–87
  Mexican Meatballs in Creamy Enchilada Sauce, *136,* 137
  One-Pan Beef and Broccoli, 172, *173*
  Oven-Baked Beefy Burritos, 126–27, *127*
  Philly Cheesesteak–Stuffed Poblanos, *102,* 103
  Savory Beefy Queso Dip, 238, *239*
  Sesame-Ginger Pot Roast, *150,* 151
  Short Ribs with Bone Broth Polenta, 152, *153*
  Sloppy Joe Bowls, 176, *177*
  Slow Cooker Beef Stew, 218, *219*
  in Slow Cooker Picadillo, *154,* 155
  Southwest Steak Salad Bowls, *186,* 188–89
  Steak and Chimichurri Baguette Sandwiches, *98,* 99
Berry Crumble Yogurt Bowls, *60,* 61
Better-than-a-Bagel-Run Bagels, *68,* 69
Birthday Cake Bliss Balls, 234, *235*
Blackened Shrimp Tacos with Pineapple-Avocado Salsa, 100, *101*
bone broth
  about, 28, 32
  Bone Broth Jasmine Rice Three Ways, 198, *199*
  Cheesy Bone Broth Mashed Potatoes, 210, *211*
  Golden Chicken Bone Broth, 226–27, *227*
  Short Ribs with Bone Broth Polenta, 152, *153*
Brats and Potatoes, Sheet-Pan, 164, *165*
breakfast, 42–81
  Berry Crumble Yogurt Bowls, *60,* 61
  Better-than-a-Bagel-Run Bagels, *68,* 69
  Cheesy Bacon and Chive Egg Muffins, 66, *67*
  Chorizo-Style Breakfast Tacos, 58, *59*
  Cinnamon-Apple Protein Pancakes, *48,* 49
  Everything Bagel Egg Wraps, 54, *55*
  Honey-Blackberry Overnight Oats, 50, *51*
  Make-Ahead Coconut-Mango Chia Pudding, *64,* 65
  Maple-Chicken Breakfast Patties, *56,* 57
  Passionberry Smoothie, *78,* 79
  Pick-Me-Up Mocha Smoothie, 72, *73*
  Pumpkin Pie Smoothie, 80, *81*

Ready-When-You-Are Breakfast Sandwiches, 62–63, *63*
Roasty Breakfast Potato Hash, *52*, 52–53
Salted Peanut Butter Cup Smoothie, *70*, 76, *77*
Savory Herb and Turkey-Bacon Quiche, 46–47, *47*
Strawberry Shortcake Smoothie, *74*, 75
Broccoli, One-Pan Beef and, 172, *173*
Broccolini, Garlicky Roasted, 183
Brothy Beans with Zesty Chimichurri, 156–57, *157*
Brown Butter–Chocolate Chip Cookies, 270, *271*
Brownies, Fudge, 258–59, *259*
Buffalo Chicken Baked Tacos, 148, *149*
Burritos, Oven-Baked Beefy, 126–27, *127*

Cake, Mug, Raspberry-Vanilla Protein, *260*, 261
Candy Bark, Sweet and Salty, 262, *263*
Carrots with Hummus, Moroccan-Spiced, *208*, 209
Cheesy Bacon and Chive Egg Muffins, 66, *67*
Cheesy Bone Broth Mashed Potatoes, 210, *211*
chicken
about, 19
Buffalo Chicken Baked Tacos, 148, *149*
Chicken and Peanut Pad Thai Bowls, 130, *131*
Chicken Milanese with Homemade Alfredo, *94*, 95–96, *97*
Chipotle Chicken and Avocado Bowls, *120*, 121
Creamy Tuscan Chicken Soup, *220*, 221
Crispy Lemon-Garlic Chicken Thighs, *10*, *166*, 167
5-Minute Pesto Chicken Salad, *196*, 197
Game-Day Buffalo Chicken Dip, *236*, 237
Golden Chicken Bone Broth, 226–27, *227*
in Grilled Summer Pasta Salad, *200*, 200–201
in Harvest Cobb Salad with Maple-Dijon Dressing, 194–95, *195*
Lemon-Pepper Wings with Dilly Ranch, 232–33
Loaded Chicken Pesto Panini, *140*, 141
Maple-Chicken Breakfast Patties, *56*, 57
Marry Me Chicken, *158*, 160, *161*
in The Rachael Salad, *8*, 206, *207*
in Roasty Breakfast Potato Hash, *52*, 52–53
in Sausage, White Bean, and Kale Soup, 222, *223*
Seasoned Crispy Drumsticks, *90*, 91
Sheet-Pan Greek Chicken and Chickpea Salad, 212, *213*
Sheet-Pan Turmeric Chicken with Romesco, 180, *181*
Shredded Chicken Quesadillas, 138, *139*
Super Crispy Chicken Tenders with Homemade BBQ Sauce, 118, *119*
Szechuan Chicken Lettuce Wraps, *106*, 107
Tomato-Basil Chicken with Spaghetti Squash, 110–11, *111*
20-Minute Shredded Chicken Verde, *132*, 133
chickpeas
Crispy Ranch Air-Fryer Chickpeas, *240*, 241
Hummus, Moroccan-Spiced Carrots with, *208*, 209
Roasted Sweet Potatoes with Spiced Chickpeas and Tahini Drizzle, 202, *203*
Seared Halloumi and Chickpea Bowls with Herby Tahini, 112–13, *113*
Sheet-Pan Greek Chicken and Chickpea Salad, 212, *213*
Chili, Hearty Protein-Packed, *224*, 225
Chili Crisp Tofu and Quinoa Power Bowls, *128*, 129
Chili-Lime Grilled Steak with Zesty Avocado Salsa, 88, *89*
Chimichurri, Zesty, Brothy Beans with, 156–57, *157*
Chimichurri Baguette Sandwiches, Steak and, *98*, 99
Chipotle Chicken and Avocado Bowls, *120*, 121
Chocolate-Coconut Caramel Tart, *256*, 257
choline, 19
Chop Salad, Italian-Style, 190, *191*
Chorizo-Style Breakfast Tacos, 58, *59*
Cinnamon-Apple Protein Pancakes, *48*, 49
Coconut Caramel Tart, Chocolate-, *256*, 257
Coconut-Curry Turkey Meatballs, Saucy, 122, *123*
Coconut-Lime Crema, Roasted Butternut Squash Soup with, 228, *229*
Coconut-Mango Chia Pudding, Make-Ahead, *64*, 65
Cod, Pesto-Crusted Baked, 168, *169*
collagen peptides, 29
Cookies, Brown Butter–Chocolate Chip, 270, *271*
Cottage Cheese Bowls, Savory, 242, *243*
Creamy Tuscan Chicken Soup, *220*, 221
Crispy Lemon-Garlic Chicken Thighs, *10*, *166*, 167
Crispy Ranch Air-Fryer Chickpeas, *240*, 241

dairy
about, 20, 25, 28
Avocado Whipped Feta, *244*, 245
Berry Crumble Yogurt Bowls, *60*, 61
Better-than-a-Bagel-Run Bagels, *68*, 69
Cheesy Bacon and Chive Egg Muffins, 66, *67*
Cheesy Bone Broth Mashed Potatoes, 210, *211*
Magic Shell Yogurt Bowl, 248, *249*

dairy (*cont.*)
Next-Level Mac and Cheese, *192,* 193
Savory Cottage Cheese Bowls, 242, *243*
Seared Halloumi and Chickpea Bowls with Herby Tahini, 112–13, *113*
in Southwest Sauce, *186,* 188–89
Strawberry Cheesecake Pudding, *272,* 273
dairy-free labels, in recipes, 11, 40
dessert, 250–73
Brown Butter–Chocolate Chip Cookies, 270, *271*
Chocolate-Coconut Caramel Tart, *256,* 257
Fudge Brownies, 258–59, *259*
Mini Apple Tarts, *264,* 265
Ninja Creami Ice Cream Two Ways, *252,* 254, 255
Peppermint Patties, 266, *267*
Protein Muddy Buddies, *268,* 269
Raspberry-Vanilla Protein Mug Cake, *260,* 261
Strawberry Cheesecake Pudding, *272,* 273
Sweet and Salty Candy Bark, 262, *263*
DeVaux, Rachael, 33
Dilly Ranch, Lemon-Pepper Wings with, 232–33
dinners, 85–113. *See also* main dishes
Beef Bolognese, 108, *109*
Blackened Shrimp Tacos with Pineapple-Avocado Salsa, 100, *101*
Chicken Milanese with Homemade Alfredo, *94,* 95–96, *97*
Chili-Lime Grilled Steak with Zesty Avocado Salsa, 88, *89*
Greek-Style Smash Burgers, 92, *93*
Korean Beef with Glass Noodles, *84,* 86–87
Philly Cheesesteak–Stuffed Poblanos, *102,* 103
Rosemary-Garlic Lamb Chops with Veggies, 104, *105*
Seared Halloumi and Chickpea Bowls with Herby Tahini, 112–13, *113*
Seasoned Crispy Drumsticks, *90,* 91
Steak and Chimichurri Baguette Sandwiches, *98,* 99
Szechuan Chicken Lettuce Wraps, *106,* 107
Tomato-Basil Chicken with Spaghetti Squash, *109,* 110–11, *111*
Dip, Game-Day Buffalo Chicken, *236,* 237
Dip, Savory Beefy Queso, 238, *239*
Double Chocolate Ice Cream, *252,* 254
Double Double-Cheeseburger Bowls, *178,* 179

Egg Roll in a Bowl, *170,* 171
eggs
about, 19, 25
Cheesy Bacon and Chive Egg Muffins, 66, *67*
Everything Bagel Egg Wraps, 54, *55*
Savory Herb and Turkey-Bacon Quiche, 46–47, *47*
Enchilada Sauce, Creamy, Mexican Meatballs in, *136,* 137
Everything Bagel Egg Wraps, 54, *55*

Farro, 182
fats, about, 20, 28–30
Feta, Avocado Whipped, *244,* 245
5-Minute Pesto Chicken Salad, *196,* 197
freezer staples, 31–32
fridge staples, 30–31
Fried Rice, Beef, *162,* 163
Fudge Brownies, 258–59, *259*

Game-Day Buffalo Chicken Dip, *236,* 237
Garlic-Butter Salmon Bites, Air-Fryer, *124,* 125
Garlicky Roasted Broccolini, 183
ghee, 28
Ginger-Garlic Turkey Skillet, My Weeknight Hero, 142, *143*
Glass Noodles, Korean Beef with, *84,* 86–87
gluten-free labels, in recipes, 11, 40
Golden Chicken Bone Broth, 226–27, *227*
grain-free labels, in recipes, 11, 40
grass-fed and grass-finished organic beef, 19
Greek-Style Smash Burgers, 92, *93*
Greens with Lemon and Olive Oil, Sautéed, 182
Grilled Mahi Mahi with Mango Salsa, 134, *135*
Grilled Summer Pasta Salad, *200,* 200–201

Halloumi, Seared, and Chickpea Bowls with Herby Tahini, 112–13, *113*
Harvest Cobb Salad with Maple-Dijon Dressing, 194–95, *195*
Hash, Roasty Breakfast Potato, *52,* 52–53
Hearty Protein-Packed Chili, *224,* 225
high-protein, defined, 12–14. *See also* protein
Honey-Blackberry Overnight Oats, 50, *51*
Honey-Harissa Salmon with Asparagus, *116,* 117
Hummus, Moroccan-Spiced Carrots with, *208,* 209

Ice Cream Two Ways, Ninja Creami, *252,* 254, 266
ingredients. *See also* protein
baking flours, 27
cooking oils and fats, 28–30
freezer staples, 31–32
fridge staples, 30–31
swapping, 33
Italian-Style Chop Salad, 190, *191*

Jasmine Rice Three Ways, Bone Broth, 198, *199*

Korean Beef with Glass Noodles, *84,* 86–87

lamb
  in Greek-Style Smash Burgers, 92, *93*
  Rosemary-Garlic Lamb Chops with Veggies, 104, *105*
legumes and grains, about protein in, 25. *See also* chickpeas; peanuts and peanut butter; plant-based proteins
Lemon-Dill Sauce, Zucchini Fritters with, *204,* 205
Lemon-Garlic Chicken Thighs, Crispy, *166,* 167
Lemon-Pepper Wings with Dilly Ranch, 232–33
Lettuce Wraps, Szechuan Chicken, *106,* 107
Loaded Chicken Pesto Panini, *140,* 141

Mac and Cheese, Next-Level, *192,* 193
Magic Shell Yogurt Bowl, 248, *249*
main dishes, 82–181
  Air-Fryer Garlic-Butter Salmon Bites, *124,* 125
  Beef Bolognese, 108, *109*
  Beef Fried Rice, *162,* 163
  Blackened Shrimp Tacos with Pineapple-Avocado Salsa, 100, *101*
  Brothy Beans with Zesty Chimichurri, 156–57, *157*
  Buffalo Chicken Baked Tacos, 148, *149*
  Chicken and Peanut Pad Thai Bowls, 130, *131*
  Chicken Milanese with Homemade Alfredo, *94,* 95–96, *97*
  Chili Crisp Tofu and Quinoa Power Bowls, *128,* 129
  Chili-Lime Grilled Steak with Zesty Avocado Salsa, 88, *89*
  Chipotle Chicken and Avocado Bowls, *120,* 121
  Crispy Lemon-Garlic Chicken Thighs, *10, 166,* 167
  Double Double-Cheeseburger Bowls, *178,* 179
  Egg Roll in a Bowl, *170,* 171
  Greek-Style Smash Burgers, 92, *93*
  Grilled Mahi Mahi with Mango Salsa, 134, *135*
  Honey-Harissa Salmon with Asparagus, *116,* 117
  Korean Beef with Glass Noodles, *84,* 86–87
  Loaded Chicken Pesto Panini, *140,* 141
  Marry Me Chicken, *158,* 160, *161*
  Mexican Meatballs in Creamy Enchilada Sauce, *136,* 137
  My Weeknight Hero: Ginger-Garlic Turkey Skillet, 142, *143*
  One-Pan Beef and Broccoli, 172, *173*
  Oven-Baked Beefy Burritos, 126–27, *127*
  Pesto-Crusted Baked Cod, 168, *169*
  Philly Cheesesteak-Stuffed Poblanos, *102,* 103
  Rosemary-Garlic Lamb Chops with Veggies, 104, *105*
  Salsa Verde Shrimp and Rice, *174,* 175
  Saucy Coconut-Curry Turkey Meatballs, 122, *123*
  Seared Halloumi and Chickpea Bowls with Herby Tahini, 112–13, *113*
  Seasoned Crispy Drumsticks, *90,* 91
  Sesame-Ginger Pot Roast, *150,* 151
  Sheet-Pan Brats and Potatoes, 164, *165*
  Sheet-Pan Turmeric Chicken with Romesco, 180, *181*
  Short Ribs with Bone Broth Polenta, 152, *153*
  Shredded Chicken Quesadillas, 138, *139*
  Sloppy Joe Bowls, 176, *177*
  Slow Cooker Picadillo, *154,* 155
  Steak and Chimichurri Baguette Sandwiches, *98,* 99
  Super Crispy Chicken Tenders with Homemade BBQ Sauce, 118, *119*
  Szechuan Chicken Lettuce Wraps, *106,* 107
  Tangy Pulled Pork Sandwiches, *18, 144,* 146–47
  Tomato-Basil Chicken with Spaghetti Squash, 110–11, *111*
  20-Minute Shredded Chicken Verde, *132,* 133
Make-Ahead Coconut-Mango Chia Pudding, *64,* 65
Mango Salsa, Grilled Mahi Mahi with, 134, *135*
Maple-Chicken Breakfast Patties, *56,* 57
Maple-Dijon Dressing, Harvest Cobb Salad with, 194–95, *195*
Marry Me Chicken, *158,* 160, *161*
meal preparation, about, 17, 32, 33, 34–35
Mexican Meatballs in Creamy Enchilada Sauce, *136,* 137
Mini Apple Tarts, *264,* 265
Mocha Smoothie, Pick-Me-Up, 72, *73*
Moroccan-Spiced Carrots with Hummus, *208,* 209
Muffins, Banana Bread Protein, 246, *247*
muscle, protein for, 12, 14–16
My Weeknight Hero: Ginger-Garlic Turkey Skillet, 142, *143*

Next-Level Mac and Cheese, *192,* 193
no-added-sugar labels, in recipes, 11, 40
nuts and seeds, about. *See also* peanuts and peanut butter
  nut butters, 29
  protein in, 23
  seeds, 29
  tahini, 30

Oats, Honey-Blackberry Overnight, 50, *51*
oils and fats, about, 20, 28–30
one-pan meals, 159–80
Beef Fried Rice, *162,* 163
Crispy Lemon-Garlic Chicken Thighs, *10, 166,* 167
Double Double-Cheeseburger Bowls, *178,* 179
Egg Roll in a Bowl, *170,* 171
Marry Me Chicken, *158,* 160, *161*
One-Pan Beef and Broccoli, 172, *173*
Pesto-Crusted Baked Cod, 168, *169*
Salsa Verde Shrimp and Rice, *174,* 175
Sheet-Pan Brats and Potatoes, 164, *165*
Sheet-Pan Turmeric Chicken with Romesco, 180, *181*
Sloppy Joe Bowls, 176, *177*
one-pan sides, 182–83
Farro, 182
Garlicky Roasted Broccolini, 183
Roasted Japanese Sweet Potatoes, 183
Sautéed Greens with Lemon and Olive Oil, 1 82
Oven-Baked Beefy Burritos, 126–27, *127*

Pad Thai Bowls, Chicken and Peanut, 130, *131*
Paleo, labeled in recipes, 11, 40
Pancakes, Cinnamon-Apple Protein, *48,* 49
Panini, Loaded Chicken Pesto, *140,* 141
pantry. *see* ingredients
Passionberry Smoothie, *78,* 79
Pasta Salad, Grilled Summer, *200,* 200–201
peanuts and peanut butter
about peanut butter, 29
Chicken and Peanut Pad Thai Bowls, 130, *131*
in Magic Shell Yogurt Bowl, 248, *249*
Salted Peanut Butter Cup Smoothie, *70,* 76, *77*
in Sweet and Salty Candy Bark, 262, *263*
Peppermint Patties, 266, *267*
Pesto Chicken Salad, 5-Minute, *196,* 197
Pesto-Crusted Baked Cod, 168, *169*
Pesto Panini, Loaded Chicken, *140,* 141
Philly Cheesesteak-Stuffed Poblanos, *102,* 103
Picadillo, Slow Cooker, *154,* 155
Pick-Me-Up Mocha Smoothie, 72, *73*
Pineapple-Avocado Salsa, Blackened Shrimp Tacos with, 100, *101*
plant-based proteins. *See also* chickpeas; peanuts and peanut butter; smoothies
about, 14
about legumes and grains, 25
Brothy Beans with Zesty Chimichurri, 156–57, *157*
Chili Crisp Tofu and Quinoa Power Bowls, *128,* 129
Chocolate-Coconut Caramel Tart, *256,* 257
Fudge Brownies, 258–59, *259*
Moroccan-Spiced Carrots with Hummus, *208,* 209
Ninja Creami Ice Cream Two Ways, *252,* 254, 255
Peppermint Patties, 266, *267*
Protein Muddy Buddies, *268,* 269
in Queso, 238, *239*
in The Rachael Salad, *8,* 206, *207*
in Sausage, White Bean, and Kale Soup, 222, *223*
Sweet and Salty Candy Bark, 262, *263*
Plug-And-Play Meal Prep Guide, 34–35
Poblanos, Philly Cheesesteak-Stuffed, *102,* 103
Polenta, Bone Broth, Short Ribs with, 152, *153*
pork
in Egg Roll in a Bowl, *170,* 171
in Italian-Style Chop Salad, 190, *191*
Sheet-Pan Brats and Potatoes, 164, *165*
Tangy Pulled Pork Sandwiches, *18, 144,* 146–47
Potatoes, Mashed, Cheesy Bone Broth, 210, *211*
Potatoes, Sheet-Pan Brats and, 164, *165*
Potato Hash, Roasty Breakfast, *52,* 52–53
Pot Roast, Sesame-Ginger, *150,* 151
poultry, about, 19. *See also* chicken; turkey
protein. *See also* animal protein, about; plant-based proteins
high-protein, defined, 12–14
importance of, 11–12, 16
meal preparation for, 17, 32, 33, 34–35
for muscles, 12, 14–16
protein guide by food and serving size, 23–25
protein powders, 29
sources of, 14, 19–20
28-Day Protein Reset, 36–40
Protein Muddy Buddies, *268,* 269
Pudding, Make-Ahead Coconut-Mango Chia, *64,* 65
Pudding, Strawberry Cheesecake, *272,* 273
Pumpkin Pie Smoothie, 80, *81*

Quesadillas, Shredded Chicken, 138, *139*
Quiche, Savory Herb and Turkey-Bacon, 46–47, *47*
Quinoa Power Bowls, Chili Crisp Tofu and, *128,* 129

The Rachael Salad, *8,* 206, *207*
Raspberry-Vanilla Protein Mug Cake, *260,* 261
Ready-When-You-Are Breakfast Sandwiches, 62–63, *63*

recipes. *See also individual recipes*
ingredients for, 27–32
labels in (dairy-free, gluten-free, grain-free, no added sugar, Paleo), 11, 40
meal preparation and, 17, 32, 33, 34–35
protein in, 11–17, 19–20, 23–25 (*see also* protein)
reading, 33
for triple challenge of eating, 9
for 28-Day Protein Reset, 36–40
Roasted Butternut Squash Soup with Coconut-Lime Crema, 228, *229*
Roasted Japanese Sweet Potatoes, 183
Roasted Sweet Potatoes with Spiced Chickpeas and Tahini Drizzle, 202, *203*
Roasty Breakfast Potato Hash, *52,* 52–53
Romesco, Sheet-Pan Turmeric Chicken with, 180, *181*
Rosemary-Garlic Lamb Chops with Veggies, 104, *105*

salads. *see* sides and salads
Salsa Verde Shrimp and Rice, *174,* 175
Salted Caramel–Banana Ice Cream, *252,* 255
Salted Peanut Butter Cup Smoothie, *70,* 76, *77*
Sandwiches, Ready-When-You-Are Breakfast, 62–63, *63*
Sandwiches, Steak and Chimichurri Baguette, *98,* 99
Sandwiches, Tangy Pulled Pork, *18, 144,* 146–47
Saucy Coconut-Curry Turkey Meatballs, 122, *123*
Sausage, White Bean, and Kale Soup, 222, *223*
Sautéed Greens with Lemon and Olive Oil, 182
Savory Beefy Queso Dip, 238, *239*
Savory Cottage Cheese Bowls, 242, *243*
Savory Herb and Turkey-Bacon Quiche, 46–47, *47*
seafood
about, 19, 31, 32
Air-Fryer Garlic-Butter Salmon Bites, *124,* 125
Blackened Shrimp Tacos with Pineapple-Avocado Salsa, 100, *101*
Grilled Mahi Mahi with Mango Salsa, 134, *135*
Honey-Harissa Salmon with Asparagus, *116,* 117
Pesto-Crusted Baked Cod, 168, *169*
Salsa Verde Shrimp and Rice, *174,* 175
Spicy Tuna Spring Rolls, *214,* 215
Seared Halloumi and Chickpea Bowls with Herby Tahini, 112–13, *113*
Seasoned Crispy Drumsticks, *90,* 91
Sesame-Ginger Pot Roast, *150,* 151
*7-Day Added Sugar Detox* (DeVaux), 33
Sheet-Pan Brats and Potatoes, 164, *165*
Sheet-Pan Greek Chicken and Chickpea Salad, 212, *213*
Sheet-Pan Turmeric Chicken with Romesco, 180, *181*
Short Ribs with Bone Broth Polenta, 152, *153*
Shredded Chicken Quesadillas, 138, *139*
Shrimp, Blackened, Tacos with Pineapple-Avocado Salsa, 100, *101*
Shrimp and Rice, Salsa Verde, *174,* 175
sides and salads, 187–215
Bone Broth Jasmine Rice Three Ways, 198, *199*
Cheesy Bone Broth Mashed Potatoes, 210, *211*
5-Minute Pesto Chicken Salad, *196,* 197
Grilled Summer Pasta Salad, *200,* 200–201
Harvest Cobb Salad with Maple-Dijon Dressing, 194–95, *195*
Italian-Style Chop Salad, 190, *191*
Moroccan-Spiced Carrots with Hummus, *208,* 209
Next-Level Mac and Cheese, *192,* 193
one-pan sides, 182–83
The Rachael Salad, *8,* 206, *207*
Roasted Sweet Potatoes with Spiced Chickpeas and Tahini Drizzle, 202, *203*
Sheet-Pan Greek Chicken and Chickpea Salad, 212, *213*
Southwest Steak Salad Bowls, *186,* 188–89
Spicy Tuna Spring Rolls, *214,* 215
Zucchini Fritters with Lemon-Dill Sauce, *204,* 205
Sloppy Joe Bowls, 176, *177*
Slow Cooker Beef Stew, 218, *219*
slow cooker main dishes, 145–57
Brothy Beans with Zesty Chimichurri, 156–57, *157*
Buffalo Chicken Baked Tacos, 148, *149*
Sesame-Ginger Pot Roast, *150,* 151
Short Ribs with Bone Broth Polenta, 152, *153*
Slow Cooker Picadillo, *154,* 155
Tangy Pulled Pork Sandwiches, *18, 144,* 146–47
Smash Burgers, Greek-Style, 92, *93*
smoothies, 71–81
Passionberry Smoothie, *78,* 79
Pick-Me-Up Mocha Smoothie, 72, *73*
Pumpkin Pie Smoothie, 80, *81*
Salted Peanut Butter Cup Smoothie, *70,* 76, *77*
Strawberry Shortcake Smoothie, *74,* 75
snacks, 231–49
about quick snacks, 29
Avocado Whipped Feta, *244,* 245

snacks (*cont.*)
Banana Bread Protein Muffins, 246, *247*
Birthday Cake Bliss Balls, 234, *235*
Crispy Ranch Air-Fryer Chickpeas, *240,* 241
Game-Day Buffalo Chicken Dip, *236,* 237
Lemon-Pepper Wings with Dilly Ranch, 232–33
Magic Shell Yogurt Bowl, 248, *249*
Savory Beefy Queso Dip, 238, *239*
Savory Cottage Cheese Bowls, 242, *243*
soups, 217–29
Creamy Tuscan Chicken Soup, *220,* 221
Golden Chicken Bone Broth, 226–27, *227*
Hearty Protein-Packed Chili, *224,* 225
Roasted Butternut Squash Soup with Coconut-Lime Crema, 228, *229*
Sausage, White Bean, and Kale Soup, 222, *223*
Slow Cooker Beef Stew, 218, *219*
Southwest Steak Salad Bowls, *186,* 188–89
Spaghetti Squash, Tomato-Basil Chicken with, 110–11, *111*
Spicy Tuna Spring Rolls, *214,* 215
Spring Rolls, Spicy Tuna, *214,* 215
Steak and Chimichurri Baguette Sandwiches, *98,* 99
Stew, Beef, Slow Cooker, 218, *219*
Strawberry Cheesecake Pudding, *272,* 273
Strawberry Shortcake Smoothie, *74,* 75
sugar, reducing, 11, 14, 17, 20, 33, 40
Super Crispy Chicken Tenders with Homemade BBQ Sauce, 118, *119*
Sweet and Salty Candy Bark, 262, *263*
Sweet Potatoes, Roasted, with Spiced Chickpeas and Tahini Drizzle, 202, *203*
Sweet Potatoes, Roasted Japanese, 183
Szechuan Chicken Lettuce Wraps, *106,* 107

Tacos, Blackened Shrimp, with Pineapple-Avocado Salsa, 100, *101*
Tacos, Buffalo Chicken Baked, 148, *149*
Tacos, Chorizo-Style Breakfast, 58, *59*
Tahini, Herby, Seared Halloumi and Chickpea Bowls with, 112–13, *113*
Tahini Drizzle, Roasted Sweet Potatoes with Spiced Chickpeas and, 202, *203*
Tangy Pulled Pork Sandwiches, *18, 144,* 146–47
Tart, Chocolate-Coconut Caramel, *256,* 257
Tarts, Mini Apple, *264,* 265
30-minutes or less main dishes, 115–43
Air-Fryer Garlic-Butter Salmon Bites, *124,* 125
Chicken and Peanut Pad Thai Bowls, 130, *131*
Chili Crisp Tofu and Quinoa Power Bowls, *128,* 129
Chipotle Chicken and Avocado Bowls, *120,* 121
Grilled Mahi Mahi with Mango Salsa, 134, *135*
Honey-Harissa Salmon with Asparagus, *116,* 117
Loaded Chicken Pesto Panini, *140,* 141
Mexican Meatballs in Creamy Enchilada Sauce, *136,* 137
My Weeknight Hero: Ginger-Garlic Turkey Skillet, 142, *143*
Oven-Baked Beefy Burritos, 126–27, *127*
Saucy Coconut-Curry Turkey Meatballs, 122, *123*
Shredded Chicken Quesadillas, 138, *139*
Super Crispy Chicken Tenders with Homemade BBQ Sauce, 118, *119*
20-Minute Shredded Chicken Verde, *132,* 133
Tofu, Chili Crisp, and Quinoa Power Bowls, *128,* 129
Tomato-Basil Chicken with Spaghetti Squash, 110–11, *111*
turkey
in Chorizo-Style Breakfast Tacos, 58, *59*
in Hearty Protein-Packed Chili, *224,* 225
in Italian-Style Chop Salad, 190, *191*
My Weeknight Hero: Ginger-Garlic Turkey Skillet, 142, *143*
Saucy Coconut-Curry Turkey Meatballs, 122, *123*
Savory Herb and Turkey-Bacon Quiche, 46–47, *47*
Turmeric Chicken with Romesco, Sheet-Pan, 180, *181*
28-Day Protein Reset, 36–40
20-Minute Shredded Chicken Verde, *132,* 133

vegetables, about protein in, 24
Veggies, Rosemary-Garlic Lamb Chops with, 104, *105*

Wraps, Everything Bagel Egg, 54, *55*

Yogurt Bowl, Magic Shell, 248, *249*
Yogurt Bowls, Berry Crumble, *60,* 61

Zucchini Fritters with Lemon-Dill Sauce, *204,* 205

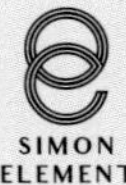

SIMON
ELEMENT

An Imprint of Simon & Schuster, LLC
1230 Avenue of the Americas
New York, NY 10020



First Simon Element hardcover edition March 2026



Photographer: Eva Kolenko
Food Stylist: Emily Caneer
Food Stylist Assistant: Carrie Beyer
Prop Stylist: Genesis Vallejo

Manufactured in Canada

3 5 7 9 10 8 6 4

Library of Congress Control Number is available.

ISBN 978-1-6680-9172-2
ISBN 978-1-6680-9173-9 (ebook)